WHAT OTHERS ARE SAYING ABOUT THIS BOOK:

"... I enjoyed reading the stories of your interaction with patients and the members of the health care team. I appreciated the diversity of acceptance of your role by all the players in the community. I identified with your dilemma regarding the "assembly line" health care. Your decision to stick to your ethics and the tenets of NP practice was admirable.

The book gives an accurate portrayal of the many dimensions of high quality primary care that NP's provide. It informs the public of the many roles NP's play. It gives them valuable information to help them become a better health care consumer and advocate for themselves and their families.

This book will be a wonderful resource for professionals who are considering NP education, consumers looking for answers about NP's and NP's looking for a reminder of why we do what we do.

My best wishes for the success of this book. I'm sure it's a best seller!"

—Marie-Eileen Onieal, MMHS, RN, CPNP
President, *American Academy of Nurse Practitioners*

"... In a lovely way the authors have woven compelling personal stories in amongst helpful facts about common patient complaints. The reader is presented with an excellent education about a variety of human situations (e.g. poverty, poor health choices, mental conditions) along with a deeper understanding about a broad range of disease entities commonly encountered in a primary care practice. Whether the reader is a present/future health care provider or a consumer of healthcare, s/he will finish this book with a greater appreciation of one's own body and mind and the intricacies and devotion required of good health care providers."

—Linda Pearson, RN, MSN, FNP
Editor-in-Chief, *The Nurse Practitioner: The American Journal of Primary Healthcare*

UNFORGETTABLE FACES

THROUGH THE EYES OF A NURSE PRACTITIONER

Elizabeth D. Tate
Michael R. Pranzatelli

ATHENEUM PRESS
Jacksonville, Florida

Cover art by Craig D. Erskine, Creative Director, Imaging Technologies. Portrait photography by Susan Michal. Insert photo by Carlos
Rodriguez, Twenty-First Century Studios. Literary and historical
research, layout, and editing by Michael R. Pranzatelli

First Edition—October 1999

Published by Atheneum Press, Jacksonville, Florida
Place orders at http://www.unforgettablefaces.com

Library of Congress Cataloging 99-095280
ISBN: 0-9673365-0-3

Printed and bound in the United States of America
10 9 8 7 6 5 4 3 2 1

Dedicated

To the Patients

With Special Thanks

To the "regulars" of the North Florida Writers—DeLanie Fant, Doris Cass, Howard Denson, JoAnn Murray, Joyce Davidson, Margaret Gloag, Mary Elliott, Nate Tolar—and other members, for critical listening and keeping the spirit of writing alive;
Kathleen R. Tate, for her avid reading and useful suggestions; Robert H. Johnson, for invaluable advice and encouragement on publishing; and student nurse practitioner mentors Deborah Lipstate and Maryalice Jordan-Marsh

CONTENTS

PREFACE

Health care providers are heterogeneous. Sometimes we choose to focus on important differences in our training, perspectives, roles, and professional genealogy. But in these mercurial times, we must recognize that we all sit in the same camp; we battle a common enemy.

Each of us struggles to maintain high standards of care while working in a less-than-perfect system, in which the clinic can become a human conveyor belt, driven by money-first managed care; bottom-line insurance companies and their lobbyists; non-medical, indifferent administrators; and ever increasing demands for health care.

Based on true stories of more than seventy-five patients, this case-oriented book reveals a unique side of human nature while serving as a teaching guide about the realities and exigencies of the contemporary, health care market place. The book's uplifting and positive human journey through the gamut of emotions makes it a compelling page turner. It will be a must-read for all health care providers.

But the issues addressed in this book apply to health care consumers as well. Knowing more about our own health has never been so important, whether it's information about aging, AIDS, Alzheimer's disease, cancer, depression, diabetes, drug abuse, heart disease, infections, infertility, mental illness, obesity, sexuality, smoking, stress, or stroke. The health care choices and options we all face can sometimes be overwhelming.

For the lay reader and professional alike, the updated medical information that follows each case story keeps pace with rapid changes in medicine and technology. The educational materials are intended to provide clear, succinct, and readily accessible resources. In keeping with the expanding role of the Internet as a health care resource, we have included a list of Websites for medical information, on-line referral centers, and patient support groups. When it comes to health care, the best consumer is an educated consumer.

BEGINNINGS

There is in every human countenance either a history or a prophecy,
which must sadden, or at least soften, every reflecting observer
—SAMUEL TAYLOR COLERIDGE

When I decided to go to graduate school to become a nurse practitioner, I had eight years experience as a registered nurse. Having worked on surgical and medical wards, a burn unit, a surgical intensive care unit, and in a major trauma center's emergency room, I thought I'd seen it all.

I was wrong! All those experiences were just a foundation for my advanced training nursing career. By choosing to be a nurse practitioner, I invited the opportunity to be more actively involved in the decision making process of a patient's care.

Once I left the hallowed halls of UCLA, I was anxious to get a job, roll up my sleeves, and apply my new skills. Although I enjoyed the relaxing southern Californian lifestyle, moving to New York City and adapting to a faster pace seemed like an exciting challenge.

My first job as a nurse practitioner was at an outpatient medical clinic of a large Manhattan hospital. The majority of its clientele were poor, chronically ill, young and middle-aged adults on welfare. The kinds of problems were extreme: HIV on the rise, no preventative care, poor compliance with taking medications. We, as clinic personnel, had to learn Spanish on our own time because of the large Spanish-speaking population.

Among the first of my patients was Consuelo Rojas, a young Hispanic woman who was having symptoms from mitral valve prolapse, a floppy heart valve. She was soft spoken and scarcely looked at me as I elicited a history. As trust was not something that came naturally to her, it took me several visits to establish any rapport. Eventually she allowed me to refer her to a cardiologist.

One day Consuelo came to the clinic unannounced. I found her sitting in the waiting room, bent over, hugging her knees, wearing a black scarf around her head, a stained khaki jacket, and sunglasses. When I called her name, she staggered toward me, holding onto nearby chairs. I reached her just before she fell and managed with help to get her into my office.

Once I removed the scarf and sunglasses, what had happened became obvious: someone used her face and head as a punching bag. After making sure her vital signs were stable, I worked on transporting her to the emergency room. She never disclosed to me why she was assaulted or by whom.

Later, when I asked her why she came to the clinic instead of the emergency room, she said she trusted only me. Her answer surprised me because she had barely made eye contact. Here was the beginning of my real education about the undaunted human spirit. I came to respect the people I met in their daily struggles with life.

After that, I took a job at another hospital clinic. The circumstances were distinctive, but the story was the same. Every day on my way to work, I walked by the many homeless men and women of NYC. The personal and professional journey I'd begun earlier was to continue here. The location didn't matter. There was, however, one very obvious difference: the people were no longer faceless. Some were now my patients. I also worked more with older patients, who had their own set of problems. I wasn't an observer; I was a confidant, a participant. It affected me a lot.

Any nurse will tell you that when nurses get together we usually end up talking about patients who have left their mark on us, happy or sad, good or bad. We don't discuss names; it's what patients have done, said, or endured that moved us. When I saw how much others were affected by hearing about my patients, I realized that I should keep notes on some of the people I saw, how I felt caring for them, and the impact of their lives on mine. I soon found myself dictating in the evenings when I got home from work.

I didn't write much about people with colds, flu, diarrhea, allergies—common things—although maybe one-quarter to one-half of my clientele had minor, non-life-threatening illnesses. They usually weren't the ones who stuck in my mind. Not all of the seriously ill or dying patients were memorable either. There was something unforgettable about certain people.

Before I knew it, fourteen years had elapsed since my first job as a nurse practitioner, and I had accumulated a number of true stories, making changes and composites as necessary to protect confidentiality and improve readability. What started as a personal experience was now something I considered sharing with a wider audience.

To publish or not to publish. I hesitated. Some readers may think the material is too sensitive. Others may find the stories unimportant, saying, people come and go, their problems are found in any big city hospital, what is to be gained by writing about them? Yet, in a way, I had an answer. I came to realize that other nurses in practice and students in training may benefit from my experiences. But it's about more than just sharing this with other nurses.

The stories of patients and their lives matter. The main purpose of such a book is to preserve the memories of these wonderful people so that their courage and suffering have not been in vane, and to present a realistic portrayal of what health care providers face in working in a large inner-city clinic. Too often the essence of taking care of patients is lost in the fast-paced, pressured, and, at times, insensitive medical environment. The truth about the human side of health care also has become distorted in the hyperbole and commercialism of mass media. A glimpse at the lives of real men and women, their trials and tribulations, which they sometimes overcame and other times did not, has some relevance and poignance for everyone. These people are you and I.

Such an endeavor is also timely. Today's health care market utilizes nurse practitioners more than ever, but many people still don't know much about us. Nurse practitioners can set up practice in collaboration with a physician, have our own panel of patients, and, depending on geographical location, write prescriptions and admit patients to the hospital. Unlike physician assistants, we are nurses who have gone for further training. Nurse practitioners have different specialties, such as Adult, Family, Gerontology, Neonatal, or Pediatrics. We all have to pass national boards in our own specialty in order to be certified. Nowadays, nurse practitioners (NP's), sometimes called advanced registered nurse practitioners (ARNP's), also must have a master's degree. We practice in home health services, an outpatient clinic of a hospital, or private practice, rural or urban.

This book is about what it's really like to be a nurse practitioner. It depicts actual practice. Accessing the privileged relation of the nurse practitioner to her patients, the reader follows her through the day as an invisible observer in the drama of a big city clinic. The book explores the bonds between a nurse and her patients, her struggle to be true to herself and her professional role, and the obstacles she encounters.

The role of the nurse practitioner, like other health care providers, has changed in the current health care system under the influence of managed care. With the time of physicians placed more and more at a premium, nurse practitioners are asked to play a greater part in everyday patient care because we are regarded as less expensive commodities than physicians. Unfortunately, the role that nurse practitioners used to play, one of patient advocacy, education, and providing a listening ear, is also under the same intense pressure to change. Administrators, nurses, patients, and physicians are not yet sufficiently aware of the problem and its possible solutions. To provide compassionate and quality care in this cost-minded and downsized health care system remains one of the most important challenges of the next millennium.

1

The Dread Diagnosis

*The more serious the illness, the more important it is for you to fight
back, mobilizing all your resources—spiritual, emotional,
intellectual, physical. Your heaviest artillery will be your will to live.
Keep that big gun going*

—NORMAN COUSINS

*There are no such things as incurable, there are only things for
which man has not found a cure*

—BERNARD MANNES BARUCH

*When I am dead, my dearest,
Sing no sad songs for me;
Plant thou no roses at my head,
Nor shady cypress tree.
Be the green grass above me
With showers and dew drops wet;
And if thou wilt, remember
And if thou wilt, forget*

—CHRISTINA GEORGINA ROSSETTI

"He Told Me Not To Worry"

I remember the day I first saw Anna Monty. Anna came to clinic with three strikes against her: she was congenitally deaf, she had a right radical mastectomy for breast cancer when she was twenty-nine years old, and her mother and aunt both died young from breast cancer. Hispanic and a bit older-looking than her age of thirty-two, Anna kept herself trim and laughed easily. That day she brought her three lovely children, who did hear and were eager to talk.

"I got all A's on my report card," her six-year-old son bragged to me.

"I got mostly A's," her daughter chimed in with a smile. "I'm a good swimmer, too."

"I'm going to go to school soon," added her youngest.

Anna, obviously pleased, signed to them to go to the waiting room so we could talk without interruption. After the usual introductions, I asked what was bothering her. We wrote notes back and forth to each other because it had proven impossible to get a deaf interpreter even with advanced planning. The note exchanges worked, except, when Anna was excited, her handwriting became erratic and illegible. She wrote: *I'm worried about a swelling here.* She pointed to a spot just above her left collarbone.

I asked in writing: *Is it sore?*

Anna wrote: *No.*

Is it getting bigger?

Yes.

Have you gone back to the surgeon who did your mastectomy?

Yes. I told him. He thought it was nothing to get concerned about.

Did he order blood tests or x-rays?

No.

Was a biopsy done?

No.

I was starting to get a very bad feeling, considering the woman's past medical history. I told Anna I'd examine her first, then make some recommendations after discussing her problem with the collaborating physician. Anna indicated she understood. I asked her to disrobe and put on a hospital gown. When she was done, I gestured for her to lie down on the examining table. While palpating her right armpit for swollen lymph nodes, I wondered how things had gone so wrong. Had the surgeon done nothing, or did he recommend tests but Anna was too afraid to get them done or chose to go elsewhere for another opinion? My stomach tightened like a fist.

I palpated her left armpit. Thank God. No enlarged nodes. Then I moved on to the breast examination, the intact left breast first. My fingers made the usual radial movements. Suddenly my worries escalated. I felt two distinct masses, one the size of a walnut and the other almond-sized. The mass protruding near Anna's left collar bone was firm and non-tender. Her physical examination was otherwise normal. After seeing the scarred flesh over Anna's right rib cage and the bony prominences of her ribs, made obvious by lack of breast tissue, I thought she sacrificed a lot in the hope of a cure. But that operation had saved her life—until now. You're in trouble, Anna.

I wrote on the notepad: *Anna, I'll be right back with the physician. I want him to see that mass, okay?*

She signed back to me with her fingers *Okay*.

I was in luck. Dr. Mike Conley was sitting in his office reading a pile of electrocardiograms. As he looked up, he brushed back the swatch of thick, straight hair that fell across his eyes. I reviewed the patient's history and positive physical findings with him.

"Let's go see her." When he stood, he pushed up his slightly oversize wire rimmed glasses, which habitually slid down his nose. "Does she lip-read?" he asked.

"Yes, but we write notes so there's no misunderstanding."

Dr. Conley asked the patient many of the same questions I'd asked earlier. I thought I knew what her answers would be.

"Are you feeling tired or fatigued?"

She shook her head no.

"Have you lost your appetite?"

Again, no.

"Do your clothes feel looser on you lately?"

She paused and looked over at me, then shook her head yes.

Anna's answer stunned me because it wasn't what she told me. It never ceased to amaze me how a patient could give a totally different answer when the same question was posed twice. I felt foolish I hadn't gotten this information, but knew that this was the reality of obtaining a medical history.

"How much do you usually weigh?" he asked.

With her index finger, she traced in mid-air the number *135*. When I said the number out loud, Anna quickly nodded. I jotted down her current weight and showed Dr. Conley: *123 lb.*

"You've lost *twelve* pounds?" he asked her, obviously alarmed. "Since about when?"

She made a gesture with her right hand then wrote: *One month.*

"How long have you felt that lump there?" He pointed to her left shoulder.

It started out small three months ago.

Dr. Conley asked to examine her.

She was uncomfortable lowering her gown this time with a man present in the room.

As a woman, I empathized with her. I mouthed the words for her but did not speak them out loud: *It's important.*

Anna mouthed *Okay.*

When Dr. Conley finished examining Anna, he wrote her a note explaining he wanted to step out and talk with me for a few minutes about her plan of care. We left the room. "I agree with your impression. There are two lesions in her remaining breast, and the mass near her left clavicle suggests possible metastases to the lymph nodes. She needs an urgent biopsy. Refer her to the Breast Clinic ASAP. Tell them to see her urgently. Use my name if it will help and make the call yourself. Get her medical records if possible. It's a shame. I think she waited too long, but we'll see."

Immediately I went about the task of arranging for Anna to be seen urgently. My gut told me it was hopeless, but my mind was holding out for the results of the consultation and biopsy. I did know that if Anna had any chance at all, I had to act rapidly.

Pulling the curtain to give her privacy, I asked Anna to get dressed. When she finished, she sat down in the chair next to my desk. Her face looked grim and she motioned that she wanted to write a note to me.

He thinks the cancer has returned, doesn't he?

Yes. We both felt two masses in your left breast. You need to get that lymph node above your collarbone biopsied.

Anna grimaced. *Will I lose my other breast, too?* Her eyes were searching.

It's possible, Anna, but we're talking about your life here. I need to make you an appointment at the Breast Clinic right away. They handle the treatment themselves. This must seem like déjà vu to you. Tell me what you're feeling.

She scrawled in large, childish, letters: *I'm angry at the surgeon. I saw him when I first noticed the lump. He told me not to worry. I trusted him. I feel betrayed.* She was visibly upset.

I can understand that, but you need to go forward now and get aggressive in taking care of this. You're going to be going through a lot over the next few weeks. You will be making decisions and you will need to make them with your husband. Will he be there for you?

Anna nodded. *He helped me get through it last time.*

Good. Bring your husband with you for moral support. I realized that she had tapped into a deep well of courage and personal strength to make it so far. It seemed almost too much to ask a person to go through this again.

With a sense of urgency, I jotted down a plan of action. I asked her to get a copy of her medical records from the surgeon's office and bring them to the Breast Clinic the next day at two P.M. Then she was to return to see me in two weeks for follow-up and contact me if she had questions in the interim.

Do you understand all this?

Anna looked worried but nodded. *I'll go today and get my records. Thank you for your time. Nobody has ever spent this much time with me.*

I felt the urge to reassure her but was afraid it would only be false reassurance. Instead I touched her arm and told her to take it one day at a time.

After Anna left I looked at my watch. The visit took sixty minutes. However well spent I thought the time was, I would certainly hear about that "excess" expenditure of time from the clinic's financial manager. Nurse practitioners need to spend time listening to their patient's problems, getting the attending physician to come see the patient, then teaching the patient what he or she has to know. It's time spent in consoling and offering words of comfort. The caring, human side of nursing can't be done in a time slot of fifteen minutes.

When I left work that day, I was struck with the lengthening daylight and the lingering warmth of early spring. Yet my heart felt heavy and I could not sustain the uplifting feeling as my thoughts returned to Anna.

Several nights later, I dreamed about Anna. In this dream, my shift had just begun in the ICU. I was making the rounds on my patients. There were five beds with curtains around them. I pulled back every curtain, checked all the respirators and heart monitors with their beeping alarms. I emptied the full urine bags. I inspected the bandages. Some, over chest wounds, were soaked with blood.

Then I noticed another bed, which was isolated from the rest, in a poorly illuminated room. I went inside to see which patient was there. A woman lay on her back, restrained and gagged. A single bright beam of light shone from the center of the ceiling, spotlighting her abdomen. I began to notice men and women in blue gowns wearing masks bent over this woman. They seemed unaware of my presence in the room.

As I stepped closer to see what they were doing, I was stunned. The woman's torso had been filleted open, revealing all of her organs. Blood was everywhere. All the people were up to their elbows working in her body cavity. Their sleeves were dripping with blood when they reached for an instrument from a nearby table. One person was flinging cuttings of bowel over his shoulder towards me. I had to duck to avoid being hit by them. They splattered against the wall behind me and fell to the floor. I suddenly noticed how many pieces of organs were already on the floor.

Somebody yelled, "It's in the nodes, too!"

Then someone else said, "Let's cut out the nodes! We'll get them all!"

The first voice replied solemnly, "No, we're too late. She's a goner. Close her up."

Then the personnel faded away. I was alone with the woman again. I wanted to run from the room, but I forced myself to walk over slowly to look at her face. To my horror, she was awake! She was trying to scream through the gag. I recognized her. Of all people—my dear Anna Monty. I woke up clutching my belly. My heart was pounding and I was sweating.

My subconscious was working overtime on Anna. I realized that the dream was filled with my emotions. It seemed symbolic of my fears and attachment to her. The surgeons were trying to eliminate any trace of cancer, but they couldn't; it was metastatic. They appeared to have lost sight of the patient's best interest in the process. I also seemed to be concerned that Anna was suffering and alone as a result of her cancer. But I was an observer rather than a participant. I wished I could help her, but I couldn't. I felt very strongly about Anna.

When I arrived at the clinic the next day, I found Anna Monty had tried to leave me a message. The note said she couldn't make her appointment with me because she was scheduled for radiation therapy and chemotherapy. I had mixed emotions. I was glad that Anna was being treated aggressively and hoped things would go well, but I was also worried about the lateness of her starting treatment.

A few months later, on my way home from work, I ran across none other than Anna Monty, who was leaving the hospital. Her appearance was shocking. Thin and drawn, Anna looked very tired and seriously ill. I approached and tapped her on the arm. When Anna turned around, I saw she had been crying hard. She started to cry again when she recognized me.

I embraced Anna and we stood there for a moment. When she stopped sobbing, I quickly opened my day runner to write her a note.

Anna put her hand over mine to stop me. She picked up the pen and wrote: *They just told me—the cancer is everywhere!* Anna made a motion with her hand up and down her body.

Those devastating words stabbed into my heart. I looked up immediately into Anna's pained and languid eyes. Then I took the pen. *Are you still being treated?*

They're giving me medication for the pain, and a visiting nurse will be coming to my home when I'm too— She broke off and sighed.

But what about for the cancer? Any more chemotherapy or radiation treatments?

Anna slowly shook her head no.

A sudden chill came over me. So that was it. They had given up. She was told there would be no more treatment; her condition was hopeless; she should prepare herself for the end. I had heard patients told such news before. Even when they expected it and complained about the side effects of chemotherapy and radiation therapy, it always struck home when they were denied further treatment. There was no pleading now; the battle was over.

I could see the hope draining from her. Anna was preparing herself to die. I felt that I was looking at a dead woman, who, though still able to stand and walk, already had one foot in the grave. The news that everyone fears, she had just been told. Angry and distraught, I wondered if there had been some mistake, but I knew from Anna's appearance there could be no error. She had become only a shadow of her former self. The vitality and enthusiasm that were Anna were gone.

My eyes welled up with the tears of many emotions. I was filled with sadness, desperation, and isolation, but most of all anger. I was angry that nothing had helped Anna's cancer. I seethed over Anna's pain and suffering. I raged that Anna slipped beyond her last chance to be saved. The incongruity and irony of it all infuriated me. I had patients who had the opportunity to be treated and saved, but threw away their lives by disregarding the very people who could help them live longer, while Anna Monty, who loved life dearly and wanted to go on living more than anything, had no options and no chance—no chance at all.

People were walking by us, coming in and out of the hospital the whole time. They were strangers, passersby, who did not realize the gravity of what was transpiring between Anna and me. That was the problem with hospitals, I thought: the sublime and the profound mixed with trivial and ordinary interactions between fellow human beings. I wanted to freeze time and just talk to Anna. I wanted to get rid of all the passersby and secure some privacy for Anna. The impersonal coldness of discussing something like death in the hallway seemed intolerable. I started to say, "I'm sorry—"

Anna again interrupted. She put her hand up to my lips for silence. I sensed that Anna stood at a point beyond me, in a stream that was taking her further away by the moment. Anna was past my anger and rage. It was too late for fear or regret. Despite the horrible burden that had been placed on her shoulders, she was already starting to deal with it. Now it was time for her to prepare to leave the earth and everything she held dear.

Anna walked up to me, smiling bravely through her tears, and put her arms around me, giving me as strong a hug as she could. She was so frail. It was a weak and pathetic hug, but perhaps the most dear hug that I have ever received. I knew this would be one of those moments that would later replay in my mind.

With tears streaming down her cheeks, Anna signed *good-bye*. She did it with a sense of finality. It wasn't the good-bye of *See you next week*, or *See you next month*; it was *I'll never see you again*. I will always remember Anna's watery, red-rimmed eyes and the way her lower lip drew up as she tried to suppress the current of tears inside. Those she would try to save for later when she told her family the terrible news, though they would also spill out on the way home—the hot tears of deep sadness and of unplanned departure, of final good-byes.

Anna walked away into the street crowd, alone, carrying the weight of the death sentence she'd just received. As she disappeared into the masses of New York City like a drop of water into the ocean, I felt the sudden impulse to run after her and ask her to come back. I wanted to talk to her, console her, cry with her. But I knew I would never see Anna again. I thought of the husband and three children she would soon leave behind. I thought of Anna drawing them around her and holding them close while she broke the news. I imagined those little children, who had been so proud of their schoolwork, clinging to their mother, trying to make sense of what could make no sense to them. They will all miss her deeply...

And so will I, Anna.

CANCER ALERT

Only one group of people in the world is totally free of cancer: the long-lived Hunza in northwestern Kashmir. For everyone else, cancer is a staggering global problem, accounting for one-tenth of all deaths annually. The World Health Organization (WHO) reports an increase in cancer morbidity and mortality. In the U.S., cancer causes 25% of deaths in adults and comprises more than 150 related diseases. Such diversity makes the problem complex.

Despite the enormous challenge, there is cause for optimism. One-third of cancers is preventable, another third can be cured through early detection, and the pain of the incurable remainder can be ameliorated. Now there are many intriguing approaches to cancer treatment, ranging from herbal remedies, diets, and mind-body techniques for relieving anxiety and pain to the latest scientific advances, such as monoclonal antibodies, designer molecules that selectively target tumor antigens like magic bullets. Cancer vaccines, gene therapy, and drugs that choke the tumor's blood supply, once the stuff of science fiction, are now in clinical trials in the U. S. The use of marijuana to treat the nausea and vomiting associated with cancer chemotherapy and pain continues to stir controversy. These and other strategies will allow scientists and clinicians to close in on cancer.

Although heredity has been shown to play a role in only about 5 to 10% of all cancers, the risk isn't small if you happen to be among that group of people. There are guidelines for who should have genetic testing. Your family history may put you at risk for developing cancer if you have young, close relatives (diagnosed before age 50) with the same type of cancer, or multiple types of primary cancer (breast, colorectal, ovarian, or uterine) run in your family. Count both first-degree (parent, sibling, child) and second-degree relatives (aunt, uncle, niece, nephew, grandparent).

If you are diagnosed with cancer, you should dig for facts about the disease. Look for new treatments. Definitely seek a second or third opinion depending on the severity of your disease and the options you are given. Get a referral from your primary health care provider to a specialist who is able to evaluate the latest therapies. You shouldn't have to face such a problem alone, so seek help and support from family, friends, support groups, and other organizations in your community. With this team of experts and supporters you will have your best chance of defeating cancer.

Breast Cancer

In 1996 the American Cancer Society estimated that more than 184,000 women in the United States, or one woman in nine, would be diagnosed with breast cancer. Other than being female, more than 70% of women with breast cancer don't have known risk factors: excessive alcohol intake, family history of breast cancer, hormone use, poor diet, positive menstrual and reproductive history, and radiation exposure. Aging itself increases the risk, however. Between ages 35 and 55, the risk is 2.5%, but after age 65 it increases considerably.

Inherited genetic mutations cause about 5% of breast cancers. To date five genes affecting the risk of breast cancer have been discovered: *BRCA1*, *BRCA2*, *p53*, *pTEN*, and *HER2/neu*. Commercial testing to determine whether a woman has a gene mutation is available only for *BRCA1* and *BRCA2*. A woman who inherits a mutation in the *BRCA1* or *BRCA2* gene may have a breast cancer risk as high as 85% in her lifetime. Males with the *BRCA2* mutation are also at increased risk for breast and prostate cancer. The *HER2/neu* gene, which promotes tumor growth, is now the target of a new anticancer drug and vaccine.

The American Cancer Society recommends the following screening for breast cancer. *Breast self-examination* should be done monthly, beginning at age 20. The breasts are least tender and easier to examine 5 to 7 days after the onset of menstruation. Post-menopausal women should select any date that will be easy to remember. Women need a *clinical breast examination* every 3 years from age 20 to 40 and every year after age 40. A *mammogram* in women between ages 35 to 40 provides a baseline. At ages 40 to 50, it bears repeating every one or two years; from age 50, yearly.

The health care provider must ask every woman: "Do you examine your breasts and have regular breast cancer screening?" If we strive not to have any more "Anna Monty" endings as our society enters the 21st century, early detection is critical in the war against this killer. Action taken now can control the cancers of tomorrow.

Once an abnormal area in the breast is found, the next step is a biopsy. Depending on whether the health care provider can feel the suspicious area, more than one biopsy technique is available, including fine needle aspiration, stereotactic core biopsy, or open biopsy.

Most women with breast cancer have options. Surgical options may include lumpectomy, mastectomy, removal of the axillary lymph nodes, and breast reconstruction. Depending on the stage of cancer and other prognostic factors, a patient may be a candidate for radiation or adjuvant therapy, such as systemic chemotherapy or hormonal treatment with tamoxifen. She must compare the alternatives, consider the length of treatment, effects over both the short- and long-term, the need for future treatment, and the impact on the quality of life. Chemotherapy given either before or after surgery may shrink a large tumor and control tumor infiltration into the skin at the surgical wound.

Keep these worrisome figures in mind. Although NIH recommends breast-sparing surgery for 75 to 80% of women with breast cancer, the national rate is only 17% and varies regionally. No more than 25% of women with breast cancer require a complete mastectomy. A simple lumpectomy with 6 weeks of radiation therapy is now the gold standard.

For a patient like Anna Monty whose cancer has become metastatic, treatment choices depend on the site of metastasis, how much time has elapsed since the original treatment, and the tumor hormone receptor status. Although metastatic disease is not yet curable, some patients survive for years.

Nurse practitioners and all nurses who work with women are in an excellent position to discuss and teach them about the serious threat of breast cancer. We can make a difference. The first challenge may be determining when a mammographic abnormality is suspicious for cancer. Encourage the patient to bring her husband, significant other, close friend, or relative for the biopsy and include them in discussions about treatment.

Emotional support is just as essential in the healing process. The patient must be made to understand all of her treatment options and be prepared for what to expect after surgery, radiation, or adjuvant therapy. Beyond what you can relate in the clinic, a number of learning materials are available from national organizations or in bookstores and libraries. More than 2 million women in the U.S. are testimony to the fact that breast cancer can be beaten.

RECONCILING GRIEF WITH PROFESSIONALISM

I admit it: I'm a professional and I still cry over some of my patients. I know other professionals who do the same. You don't have to be sorry for having feelings and letting them out. Believing that you need to keep them locked away inside is unhealthy and can lead to problems. C. David Reese, a hospital chaplain, described six techniques to express your personal feelings of loss without compromising your professionalism.

Do what you do best:care. Support the survivors to allow them to grieve. This will help you deal with your sense of helplessness and show them your role as caregiver.

Set a time to grieve. Being professional, health care providers sometimes feel they must be "the strong one" in an emotional situation and delay their own grief. Just be sure to keep that personal appointment with yourself to deal with the grieving.

It's okay to cry. Crying really does ease the pain and at the same time affirms the acceptance of a patient or family member who cries.

A colleague can cover when you need time out to compose yourself.

Call on someone you can count on. What friend would you ask for money? That's probably a person you would trust with your grief. Talking with peers about your grief allows them to reveal emotions that may have been "bottled up" and grants them permission to address their own feelings, too.

Seek institutional support. Talking with a chaplain or staff counselor can help you work through the grieving process. Either may suggest community support groups and other resources.

Say good-bye. Without closure, many health care providers feel unsettled for a long time. Remembrance, personal or organized, offers the opportunity to say good-bye. Take time for a moment of silence. When a patient who's influenced or touched you in some way is dying or has died, it's only human to hurt and to cry. It's okay to grieve.

*   *   *

"I Guess I Make Them Feel Sad"

My stack of clinic phone messages was piling up, so I decided to return a call between seeing patients. I flipped open the chart on Hilda Roak, who had liver cancer with metastases to the lung. "Mrs. Roak? You called the clinic?"

"Yes, dear. I wanted to ask you, is it safe to take prochlorperazine for nausea along with my other medications?" Her sight-reading of the drug name was quite good.

After reviewing her medications, I advised her that they were all compatible.

Mrs. Roak sighed deeply. "Do you have family?"

It was such a quick subject change, I didn't get the drift at first. "Yes, but not nearby."

"I don't have anyone anymore. They're all gone." I didn't know what she looked like, but Mrs. Roak sounded incredibly desperate and unhappy.

"Do you have any friends who could stop by and maybe spend some time?" I asked.

"My friends no longer come around to visit me. You don't understand: I'm dying. I guess I make them feel sad." She was quiet again.

"Yesterday, a neighbor's little girl came to my door selling Girl Scout cookies. I invited her in with her mother to visit. That was the highlight of my month. It took all of five minutes. When they left I realized how alone I am."

Her tone was not one of self-pity. I heard an abandoned child crying for help.

"Does a visiting nurse see you on a regular basis? Do you need a home health aide?"

"A nurse sees me once a week. Twice a week an aide visits, but she speaks and understands little English." Mrs. Roak paused. "I'm marking my time until the end. This is something I never expected. I'd never wish it on anybody." There was a long, pained, melancholy silence.

I was getting that sinking feeling of being overwhelmed by empathy. What did I have to offer her? I just listened. She didn't really call about the compatibility of the antiemetic medication with her other medications; that she already knew. Her real problem was dealing with dying alone. Hilda Roak wanted to talk. Given our schedules, health care providers weren't the best suited to provide such regular social and emotional support. Yet, I knew we were her only support...

Then I got an idea. I told her I'd call her right back. Next I contacted her physician on the telephone. He confirmed that she was terminal and not receiving any further treatment for her cancer.

"Have you considered hospice care for Mrs. Roak?" I asked.

"The last time we talked, she wanted to stay at home until the very end."

"She's lonely, though. The other day a social worker told me about a day-care hospice program. Mrs. Roak could have the best of both worlds."

"That's fine with me if she wants it."

When I contacted Mrs. Roak, she was a little hesitant. "Can you tell me more about it?"

"Sure. After breakfast at home, someone comes to take you to the day-care facility. Activities go on all day there. You can talk with other patients or hospice team members. You can participate in social activities over crafts, games, and music—even set your own schedule to allow time for taking care of yourself, work, rest, and relaxation. Then you go back home."

"And I get to sleep in my own home?"

"Yes."

"And I could stop going if I didn't like it?"

"Definitely."

"Then I think I'd like to try that." When we were done talking, she said, "Thanks for taking the time to listen to me."

THE ART OF LISTENING

When I started working as a nurse practitioner, I focused on the patient's medical complaint—however vague or intangible. Sometimes I couldn't figure out what the problem was. Then I realized they just wanted to talk to anyone about anything. Most were lonely people who had no one else. Theirs weren't the kind of problems to bring them to the social worker or the psychiatry clinic. On the other hand, especially with terminally ill patients, there wasn't enough time in the clinic schedule to deal with the burden of loneliness. I always wished I had more time to listen to people.

The most important thing Elisabeth Kubler-Ross said she learned from terminally ill patients was that they wanted to talk with someone. Dying has become more impersonalized, isolated, and lonely. As a health care provider, it's hard to talk to someone who is dying. Disengaging ourselves from the person dying allows for that comfortable zone of denial. What I always heard in between the words from my dying patients was the unvoiced fear: "Hey! I'm still here, don't give up on me."

I agree with Dr. Kubler-Ross that if we can "stick it out" with them, then we can help terminal patients the most. It's the dying person's wish that we should give them support. What we all hope for is a sense of consolation as we near death. Death is part of life, and when we have accepted death, then maybe we can help our patients, loved ones, and friends learn how, too.

HOSPICE CARE

Nearly 2.5 million Americans—about 1% of the population—die each year: 61% in hospitals, 22% at home, and 17% in nursing homes. For patients living alone with a terminal illness, one of the most important decisions is how and where they will die. Hospice programs in the U.S. serve more than 250,000 patients with terminal illnesses and their families each year, providing counselors, social workers, therapists, and trained nurses. Although hospice care has been most associated with the victims of cancer, more patients with other diseases like Alzheimer's dementia, end-stage organ failure, and intractable pressure sores now partake of the program.

The essence of hospice is simple: to live life fully while dying. The main health care provider and the patient's family have to agree on the concept of terminal care to be considered for a hospice program. A do-not-resuscitate (DNR) status must be obtained or be a part of the patient's living will. Most families understand the DNR status, but acceptance may be influenced by ethnic, racial, and religious background. The patient needs to designate a primary caregiver, such as a spouse, family member, or even a close friend. This designee accepts the responsibility of being the bridge between the hospice team and the patient. Duties include managing the care and, at times, providing hands-on care. If the patient lives alone and has no one to fulfill these functions, one possibility is a hospice daycare.

Cicly Saunders, a hospice pioneer, summarized it best: "You matter to the last moment of your life, and we will do all we can not only to help you die peacefully, but to [help you] live until you die."

*   *   *

"I Head Straight for the Clinic"

I used to dread the clinic visits of Albert Green, a round-faced, stoop-shouldered, black gentleman in his nineties. His prostate cancer had metastasized to bone, making it stage four. The cancerous lesions were erupting from his forehead. To touch certain bones hurt him. Chemotherapy was tried but to no avail. He came to the clinic almost daily to see any available nurse practitioner or physician. The conversation always began the same way.

"What can I do for you, Mr. Green?" I asked.

"I don't feel well."

"Tell me what's bothering you."

"My aches and pains are worse." He sighed.

I didn't have to review his chart to recall that he already took potent pain medications like hydromorphone, methadone, and codeine just to get him through the day. "Where does it hurt?"

He paused. "I don't know. All over I guess." He removed his black-framed eyeglasses, which were firmly anchored on his large ears, and rubbed his eyes. But the look of chronic fatigue persisted.

As much as I talked to him about his disease, he tended to develop vague physical complaints. I always tried to reassure him and give him some comfort by providing a listening ear. What else could I tell him? He came in so repeatedly that I finally had a talk with him one day.

"Mr. Green, why do you come to the hospital so often? You were here yesterday for the same problem. When you visit that frequently, I don't know what we can do differently than the day before. Isn't it hard on you to come here so often?"

He showed no hesitation in answering. "If it's a good day and I don't hurts too much once I wake up, I'll go to the senior citizens center and get a hot meal. I takes my medication, then goes home and sits and watches television. But if it's a bad day 'cause I didn't sleep good all night, I heads straight for the clinic."

I was frustrated I couldn't make a difference. Then I noticed that Mr. Green kept rubbing his legs. "Do you have bone pain there?"

"No, they're swollen."

When I examined him, he did have pronounced leg edema. After speaking with his physician, I prescribed a diuretic. "Mr. Green, try this 'water pill.' It's for your legs."

"Do you think it will help?"

"It certainly won't do any harm and it might work. It's worth a try." Given his terminal condition I couldn't convince myself it would make a huge difference.

Four days later, he returned. "Thank you."

"What do you mean?"

"For really helping me. The swelling—it's gone down in my legs. My pain ain't as bad. I can walk easier."

I was amazed. A simple diuretic made a difference. It wasn't a cure, but it did improve the quality of his remaining days. I had assumed that nothing could be done for him. When you have constant, severe pain, getting rid of a little helps a lot.

PROSTATE CANCER

Prostate cancer exacts a high toll. More than 40,000 men died of it in 1996, making it the second leading cause of cancer death (after lung cancer) and the sixth leading cause of death overall among American men. It's cause is unknown. Digital rectal examination, prostate-specific antigen (PSA) testing, and transrectal ultrasound (TRUS) have greatly improved detection rates.

The PSA blood test can lead to the diagnosis of cancerous prostate five or more years before symptoms arise. Prior to PSA testing, the majority of prostate cancers had already spread beyond the prostate before producing any symptoms. Once prostate cancer reaches an advanced stage, there is no effective therapy. PSA detects cancer early, when it is most likely to respond to treatment. Because of this, both the American Cancer Society and the American Urological Association currently recommend that healthy men older than 50 have both the rectal examination and PSA testing annually. Men at high risk for prostate cancer, including African-Americans and those with a family history of this cancer, should begin testing at age 40.

What options does a man with prostate cancer have? The decision of how best to treat the cancer must be tempered by several factors. Most prostate cancers are small and are neither aggressive nor prone to metastasize. In men older than 70, they are unlikely to produce clinical disease during the remaining life expectancy.

Once the cancer spreads beyond the prostate, it is incurable despite hormonal therapy or removal of the testes. As two-thirds of detected prostate cancers are confined to the prostate and can be eliminated by radiation or surgery, early screening programs are essential. All it takes is a phone call for an appointment.

Prostate cancer is different than benign prostatic hypertrophy (BPH), a common, non-malignant neoplasm usually of men 55 and older. By the age of 60, about 35% of men have symptoms of urinary hesitancy, intermittency, straining, weak urine stream, or the need to use a catheter. When symptoms affect the quality of life, therapy is needed. The options include medications (α1-adrenergic receptor blockers, hormones, 5α-reductase inhibitors) and surgical treatments (transurethral incision [TURP] or prostate resection, intra-prostatic stent placement, prostate ablation).

TACKLING CHRONIC PAIN

The results of a national telephone survey of 1,000 Americans concerning pain medications were startling. More than 80% worried about becoming addicted, especially when they heard the word *narcotic*. Only about 40% believed that the pain could be controlled.

Patients with cancer have voiced similar reluctance to report pain and use strong analgesics because of worries about addiction, adverse drug reactions, injections, not being viewed as a "good" patient, becoming tolerant to the medication, and a certain fatalism about the inevitability of pain. Those with access to a patient-controlled analgesia (PCA) pump, flustered by the IV apparatus and bedside technology, may not press the button for fear of making a mistake. All this worsens matters, and pain is undertreated.

Setting aside the negative connotations, effective treatments for pain are available. Pain lasting more than three months is by definition chronic. Bone pain, body (somatic) pain, and nerve (neuropathic) pain are the major types. Long-standing pain creates an emotional burden, giving rise to negative emotions such as anger, depression, guilt, and loss of self-esteem. The goal is to return the patient to normal activity as soon as possible. The payoff is huge.

The type of pain determines the choice of analgesic. Bone pain, which is caused by too much of the inflammatory chemical prostaglandin, responds to anti-inflammatory agents (NSAID's). For somatic pain, acetaminophen or NSAID's may suffice. Long-acting opiates are more potent for severe pain but do have addictive potential. Extended-release morphine helps prevent "breakthrough pain." Neuropathic pain is better treated with a low dose of tricyclic antidepressant, which, taken at bedtime, also aides sleep. A combination of drugs helps treat pain due to muscle spasm, nerve damage, and inflammation. Dose adjustments need to be made for older patients.

Non-drug therapies, like biofeedback, cognitive-behavioral techniques, hypnosis, and relaxation techniques, give added benefit. For pain that eludes standard treatments, invasive therapies may prove necessary. Acupuncture, which releases endorphins, provides short-term relief to specific areas. Trigger-point injection of corticosteroids with an anesthetic also offers temporary relief. Nerve block or ablation and morphine pumps have a place in the treatment of chronic, refractory, cancer pain.

2

Confessions of a Smoker

The wretcheder one is, the more one smokes;
and the more one smokes, the wretcheder one gets—a vicious circle
—GEORGE LOUIS DU MAURIER

It is now proved beyond doubt that smoking is one of the leading
causes of statistics
—FLETCHER KNEBEL

For thy sake, tobacco, I
Would do anything but die
—CHARLES LAMB

A life-renouncing meal of smoke
—MONA VAN DUYN

To the average cigarette smoker the world is his ashtray
—ALEXANDER CHASE

"Give Me a Damn Cigarette"

"You've got to see this patient," Dr. David Morrell insisted as he stopped by my office in the clinic one morning. The excuse was the usual one. "I have a full schedule today. He walked in without an appointment, demanding to be seen. You know him as well as I do. Just see him, check him over, reassure him, and send him on his way." He tossed the chart on my desk before I had a chance to open my mouth.

Seeing how stressed and irritable the physician was, I took the chart, walked to the waiting room, and called out the patient's name. Although I didn't complain, I had my own full schedule of patients, too, and felt stretched.

Frank Svelton, a man in his seventies, had the same complaint he always had: trouble breathing. As he perched on the edge of his chair, leaning forward, clutching onto the sides of the seat to help himself breathe, his neck muscles strained to support each breath. Habitually disheveled, Mr. Svelton wore the same old khaki workman's pants, soiled and baggy, with a short sleeve shirt and dirty suspenders. He usually kept a pack of cigarettes in his left upper pocket. Today he didn't have any on him.

"Goddammit, give me a cigarette," Mr. Svelton said in a low, grainy voice. He was always demanding cigarettes. Then he wiped his moist brow with his forearm. Now that it was getting warmer outside, most people with emphysema were finding it more difficult to breathe.

"Mr. Svelton, you can't smoke. It's killing you."

"Do you know that millions of Americans smoke and they do quite well?" he argued.

"You tell me that, but that doesn't help you breathe, does it?"

"Look, girlie, I've smoked three packs a day for fifty years. *I'm* still here aren't I? I've lived a long time, too. *You'll* be lucky to live this long."

I looked him over as he spoke. A man who always breathed like he just finished a marathon was bragging about smoking and living to tell about it. What kind of life did he lead? Didn't he think he paid too high a price? As I watched him, it dawned on me for the first time that the patients with severe emphysema look more like each other than like their own family members. They all have that same exhausted look.

"Damned doctors," he muttered as he wiped his nose and coughed into a dirty-white handkerchief. His teeth were stained yellow-brown from tobacco and his nail-beds were also brown. The fingers of his thick, flat, stubby hands were calloused from years of working with machines.

"Why didn't you call ahead to see if you could see your own doctor?"

"I didn't pay my phone bill, so they disconnected my phone. Damned phone company." His bulbous nose, with its pitted skin and vessels at the end near his nostrils, looked especially red in the clinic lights.

Still annoyed that his own doctor "turfed" him to me, I was short with him. "If you don't stop smoking, why do you bother to come back to the clinic?"

"I don't feel good. I can't breathe."

"You have emphysema, a lung disease that makes it difficult to breathe. Smoking is making it worse. It's destroying you!" I was exasperated. Why did I have to care for people who were on a suicide mission? If he wanted to eliminate himself, that was his business, I supposed. But my efforts would be better spent with patients who wanted to get well.

"I just don't feel right," he insisted.

While talking to him, I automatically started to take his history. I'd been through the drill so many times before.

Then he said the words that jarred me out of my complacency: "I've been coughing up blood."

"Is that new?"

"Yes," Mr. Svelton confessed.

"How much?"

"A little."

"Specks of blood?"

"More than that." He pulled out his handkerchief again and unfolded it.

I was aghast. There, at the center of the unwashed, yellowed, sputum-ridden handkerchief, was a quarter-size area of old, dried blood. On further questioning, he admitted to weight loss and poor appetite with intermittent bouts of fever.

I wanted to kick myself for not listening to him. I hadn't given him the benefit of the doubt. Maybe it was because he cried wolf so often, but that was no excuse for my attitude toward him.

When I listened to his chest, I heard no breath sounds in the lower lobes of his lungs and his respiratory rate was elevated. He was slightly sweaty and faintly bluish around the lips—the way he usually looked. This time his temperature was 100.6° F, which was a little high, but not terribly abnormal. Taken together, these were the signs and symptoms of pneumonia, but they were so difficult to interpret given his emphysema.

"After I draw your blood, I'm sending you down for a chest x-ray."

Mr. Svelton shook his head that he understood. He was a veteran of the x-ray machine.

I knew I could send him down to the clinical laboratory to have the blood drawn, but there was frequently a waiting line. I didn't think he could afford to wait, so I spent the extra time to draw the blood. When I filled out the stat x-ray requisition, I took the patient to the secretary to arrange for a wheelchair transport. I handed over the tubes of blood and paperwork to be sent off to the lab stat. Then I went to see another patient. After I finished with the next patient and was writing my note, the radiologist phoned.

"Hey, this guy Svelton is sick."

"I know. That's why I ordered the chest film," I replied, somewhat irritably.

"I sent him to the ER. They're going to admit him."

"Why?" I didn't anticipate an admission.

"The chest x-ray showed a white-out. He's developed more difficulty breathing. Looking at this x-ray, I'm surprised he was able to walk to the hospital."

I sat up straight in my chair. Massive pneumonia, I groaned inwardly. "I see. Thank you for calling me."

I went over to the lab computer terminal and sat down to get a look at Mr. Svelton's blood work. After I typed in the clearance code and the patient's name, it seemed like forever until the lab results came up on the screen. There they were. Abnormalities flashed before me like neon. He had an elevated white blood cell count with a predominance of cells that suggested a bacterial infection.

I continued to see my regularly scheduled patients the rest of the day, but was preoccupied. Full of remorse I wanted to visit Frank Svelton in the hospital. I realized that he was caught up in a miserable life, which he wouldn't have wished for himself when he was young. Now that I found it within me to sympathize with the human being trapped in his ravaged body, I planned to apologize to him for my harsh words and to see how he was doing. Hopefully, antibiotics would eradicate the pneumonia and he might feel a bit better. Even though his lungs were in such bad condition from smoking, perhaps the pneumonia accounted for some of his shortness of breath.

When I went upstairs to the third floor, I found out that Mr. Svelton was in room 345 on the south wing. Around the corner and down a long hall, I came to a partially open door. I knocked, but no one answered. When I entered, I saw that he occupied the bed closest to the door. The curtain was pulled; I couldn't tell if his roommate was in or not. At first I noticed the IV in Mr. Svelton's left arm and the oxygen nasal prongs in his nose. In the dim and sallow lighting of the room, I could not appreciate his cyanosis. He looked a shade of gray, as he always did. I said hello and was about to ask him how he was when I got a whiff of a strange smell. It was a familiar smell, but one out of context. Cigarette smoke? In a hospital room? From a man who was on oxygen?

"Mr. Svelton," I said with horror, "Have you been smoking?"

"No." His guilty look gave him away.

"You're on oxygen, for heaven's sake!"

"Oh, mind your own goddamned business. It's no damned concern of yours what I do." A severe bout of coughing interrupted his words. He turned bluer as he coughed. I walked over to assist him, but he waved me away. Finally he managed to catch his breath.

"Yes, it *is* my business. You could blow yourself up and take everyone with you. Even if you don't care about yourself, your roommate and the people on this end of the hallway don't deserve that. What's wrong with you?"

"Oh, go to hell! Get the hell out of my room. Who asked you to come up here anyway with your preachin' and your high-minded ideas? Just let me alone. I'm goin' to die and I just want to be left alone. *Now, get the hell out!*" Glaring, he pointed toward the door.

The argument ended abruptly when the trash can in the corner of the room ignited, a few feet away from the head of the bed. Flames leapt about a foot. Mr. Svelton had tossed the lit cigarette in the can. I must have startled him when I came into the room. He was beside himself. His little secret was exposed. Now he'd started a fire.

My initial reaction of fear swiftly gave way to action. I sprinted to the head of Mr. Svelton's bed where the oxygen meter was and instinctively turned the dial to off. No one else was in the room. I tried to get him out of bed, but he froze. Where was the fire extinguisher? Every hall in the hospital was required to have one. I ran outside the room and spotted the fire box on the wall. Propelled by the jolt of my own adrenaline, I opened the door and yanked out the extinguisher. I dashed back into the room.

The fire had grown taller and more intense. Brilliant yellow and orange flames lit that corner of the room. It was hard to believe a trash can could pack such heat. I pulled the pin and the extinguisher's white, wet vapors sprayed out of the conical dispenser with a blast. Within seconds, smoke poured from the trash can where flames had blazed. I blasted it again and again, unaware of the overkill. Shaken, I set the extinguisher on the floor.

Mr. Svelton, normally tough and incorrigible, looked like he was facing judgment day. He sat cowering at the head of the bed, wide-eyed, his feet drawn up near him as far away as possible from me as if the nurse-avenger herself stood before him.

I was incensed and beyond reasoning. "If I *ever* catch you with a cigarette," I yelled, "if I *ever* even so much as *see* you with a cigarette in your mouth, you won't have to worry about dying, you won't have to worry about *anything* anymore."

As I turned to leave the room, I caught a glimpse of Mr. Svelton's stunned face. My hands were trembling and my head felt like it was going to explode. What had I done? What words did I hear myself saying? Who was this person inside me? I couldn't believe what had just transpired. I'd *never* spoken to a patient that way before.

When I stopped at the nurses' station on the way out, I felt like saying *BOOK HIM!* Instead, I admonished them about the fire. "You'd better keep an eye on Mr. Svelton in 345," I warned, "if you don't want to be blown to bits tonight. He has an open oxygen line and he loves to smoke! I had to turn it off, so you better go check on him."

Unaware that there had been a fire they looked at me as if I were crazy.

"And, by the way, find out why that smoke alarm didn't work!" I stomped off the ward knowing some nursing supervisor would remind me to first dial the fire code.

On the way home that night, as I stared mindlessly at a smoking ad in the subway station, my thoughts instantly reverted to Mr. Svelton. Why didn't they place *his* picture in their ad? After all, wasn't *he* their best customer? He was willing to use his last feeble breath to inhale one of their cigarettes. They could display pictures of him as a teen-ager puffing on his first cigarette. Then they could depict him in the future, a sickly, ashen shade, removing his oxygen line to beg for a cigarette. Through special filters, they could block out the stains on his teeth and fingernails. The desperate look of air-hunger in his eyes—*that* would be harder to disguise. They would have to work on it. Maybe through trick photography and manipulation of information, it would be possible to convince the public that cigarettes aren't really harmful.

That night I slept restlessly. I dreamed I somehow ended up in a room with cookie jars. They were very colorful crockery jars. I went to the bright yellow one and removed the lid. Inside were the most wonderful oatmeal-raisin cookies. They were large and thin and chewy. I ate one. It was *so* delicious.

My curiosity drew me to a different jar. It was bright red. I put my hand inside and pulled out another cookie—black, thicker and crunchier. Under the assumption it was chocolate, I chewed and chewed. At first it tasted good, but gradually I became aware of a strange, unpleasant aftertaste. The more I chewed, the grittier the cookie became. My mouth began to burn. Suddenly, my nose was stinging with the odor of formaldehyde. I looked at the jar's white label. Horror seized me when I read the name: FRANK SVELTON.

I spit out the so-called cookie onto the tabletop. It was pieces of his cigarette-blackened lung. I kept on trying to spit out all the particles in my mouth. My saliva was carbon black. My mouth was filled with soot. I leaned over and vomited a bucket of pure black soot. Then I woke up in a panic.

The next day didn't go much better for me. In the cafeteria, I encountered Susan Crawley, another of our clinic nurse practitioners, and sank down beside her near a window overlooking the courtyard. Outside, preparations were underway for medical and nursing school graduation. Seeing the activities made me think about being a new graduate. How idealistic I was—so anxious to get a job and start helping people.

"Do you remember feeling that way, Susan—all fired up and eager for new experiences?"

"Sure. We were young and naive then." She laughed as she opened her brown bag lunch. Her hair was short and sandy, and she wore little make-up—just mascara and some blush.

"I don't know anymore. When I spend time teaching patients about their diseases, they don't listen. It seems like a no-win situation."

It didn't take Susan long to figure out something was bothering me. "Do you have a problem with a patient?"

"I have this patient who is killing himself by smoking, and I can't get him to stop. He wants my help, but he won't do the only thing that could really make a difference."

She nodded. "You can't stop everyone trying to self-destruct. If you or I knew how to do that, we'd never have to work again. In the case of smoking, you are really dealing with two patients."

"How so?"

"One is a person with a lethal lung disease and the other is someone with a drug addiction. They can't help each other; the needs of the one aren't the needs of the other. You're not going to rehabilitate drug addicts with lecturing, right? You'll be as blue in the face as your patient probably is, and he'll still crave his nicotine. Failure to make him change his ways can't be interpreted as your personal failure. It's endemic."

I hadn't looked at it that way.

I had the opportunity to see Mr. Svelton again. Recently released from the hospital, he came in for a follow-up visit. I was quite surprised he returned to the clinic to see me.

"I thought you weren't coming back after what I told you," I said.

He looked at me. "Well, I shouldn't have," he said curtly, followed by a little cough. Then he took a couple of extra-heavy breaths.

"So why did you?"

"I thought I could get back at you more," he said, pausing to breath, "if I returned and you got stuck taking care of me." He studied my face carefully with a twinkle in his eye, while his chest heaved as forcefully as the gills of a fish out of water to capture some air.

Secretly I thought he was right. With the same inimitable outspoken irreverence, he'd laid out the plan for his ultimate revenge. What if every clinic day began with finding Mr. Svelton sitting in my office waiting to be seen? The misery of those thoughts.

"You know I'm only going to tell you to quit smoking those damned cancer sticks," I said.

"So now they're cancer sticks, are they?"

"You heard right." I went over and listened to his lungs. He was returning to his own baseline before the pneumonia, but had clearly lost ground.

Mr. Svelton made an indistinct sound of discontent. Then, unexpectedly, he said, "I smoke because I'm already a dead man." He gasped for air. "What's the use. I just want to hurry it along and be done with all of this mess." He licked his lips and swallowed. "This is no life. The Frank Svelton I once was died long ago."

As he struggled to gather his air, Mr. Svelton had the forlorn look of a human trying to stay alive on another planet that lacked sufficient oxygen. Paradoxically, he was now an alien on earth unable to live off the atmospheric mix of life-giving gases.

"But that trash can," he said, "that fire was so close to my oxygen line. When I realized it might blow up," he gasped, "I didn't want to die. I was afraid to die." He searched my eyes.

I knew that Frank Svelton wasn't the kind of man who poured out his heart to anyone. This was as close as he would come to an expression of insight to a near stranger. But he and I had been through something together that day in the hospital and he knew it, too. *He* was the man who stood on top of the bridge tower with the wind in his face, looking down at the water far below and seeing in it a merciful oblivion that would swallow him up and take him to a restful place where he did not have to struggle to breathe. And *I* was the woman who stood nearby, extending her arm and telling him of the cold, hard, merciless death that awaited him below, seeing a river that was ready to steal his last precious breath of life. That day, we both knew where we stood and the irreconcilability of our perspectives, but we each had a better appreciation of the other person's point of view and pain.

He coughed. "You know, I have nightmares about it."

"So do I, Mr. Svelton." I returned to my desk.

Then he buttoned his shirt and tucked it into his trousers. "Now give me a damn cigarette."

I peered up from writing my note. He was grinning.

"I'm glad you're feeling better. Just remember to finish all your antibiotics and I'll see you back in a week. Deal?"

"Yeah, yeah, deal."

THE NICOTINE SCANDAL

Smoking and the American dream. Ever since Christopher Columbus introduced tobacco to Europe in 1493, the practice of smoking tobacco spread like wildfire. In the U.S., mass marketing and assembly-line production of cigarettes boosted cigarette smoking to the level of a national pastime. Billboards, TV, and the movies, with their sensuous allure, have wooed generations of youths to light up, embarking on the most dangerous undertaking of their lives.

Now 46 million Americans smoke a billion cigarettes daily. Each day more than 6,000 teenagers puff on their first cigarette and half go on to smoke chronically. If they smoke 1 pack a day for 35 years, they can expect to pay $225,000 to support their habit, at least twice the average cost of raising a child. More than 3 decades after the U.S. Surgeon General declared that "Cigarette smoking may be hazardous to your health," one quarter of the adult population still smokes.

All the more incongruous that a practice so common could be so devastating. In 1577 tobacco was proposed as a cure for many ailments ranging from arthritis to bad breath. Now we know better.

What's so terrible about smoking? Tobacco smoke contains carbon monoxide and 43 carcinogens. Smoking causes almost 90% of all lung cancer, which has the highest fatality rate of any cancer in the U.S. Cigarette smoking also keeps company with cancers of the bladder, esophagus, kidney, larynx, mouth, pancreas, pharynx, and uterine cervix. Maybe this is what Henry David Thoreau meant: "Some circumstantial evidence is very strong, as when you find a trout in the milk."

Who would chronically engage in a behavior that increases their chance of dying of cancer by 10 to 20 times? It's irrational. Although the lungs take the brunt of it, smoking catapults the risk of cardiovascular disease (heart disease, stroke), complications from oral contraceptives (stroke) and pregnancy (low birth weight or premature infants, maternal hemorrhage, and spontaneous abortion), gastrointestinal disorders (ulcers, reflux), and osteoporosis. Parents who smoke threaten the health of their children, who breathe secondhand smoke and have higher risk of asthma, sudden infant death syndrome (SIDS), and respiratory infections. Why don't smokers just quit?

Nicotine, the active ingredient in cigarettes, is an addictive drug.

How addictive? Ahmed Zogu—commemorated on an Albanian stamp as the world's greatest smoker—reputedly smoked an average of 240 cigarettes or 12 packs a day? In a 16 hour day, that's 15 cigarettes an hour—a human smokestack.

Only 10 seconds after inhalation, nicotine reaches the brain and causes a "nicotine rush." By binding to receptors in the brain, nicotine triggers a cascade of chemical events that alters the release of neurotransmitters, such as dopamine and noradrenalin, the chemical messengers between cells. Nicotine effects, which are dose-related, include arousal, muscle relaxation, stimulation, and a number of autonomic effects (increased blood pressure, cardiac output, heart rate, and oxygen consumption due to catecholamine release and peripheral vasoconstriction).

Chronic smoking leads to physical and psychological dependence and tolerance. Those who have to smoke a cigarette within 30 minutes of waking and who smoke brands with a nicotine level of 1.3 mg or more are highly addicted. When long-term smokers quit abruptly, they experience intense withdrawal symptoms: anxiety, depression, difficulty concentrating, frustration, gastrointestinal disturbances, headache, impatience, insomnia, irritability, restlessness, tobacco cravings, and weight gain. The symptoms last days to months.

Breaking the habit. To reduce nicotine withdrawal symptoms, the Food and Drug Administration (FDA) approved several nicotine replacement therapies: chewing gum, nasal spray, and transdermal patches. Despite the risk that patients may transfer their dependence to nicotine alternative delivery choices, they won't be exposed to the carcinogens and other toxic components of cigarette smoke. Both the gum and patch may double smoking cessation rates.

The only drug approved for smoking cessation that is not based on nicotine is buproprion, an antidepressant. Thought to interrupt addiction by acting on the brain neurotransmitters affected by nicotine receptors, buproprion can be used alone or in combination with nicotine replacement and is available as a sustained-release tablet.

Pharmacological supportive treatments work best when used adjunctively with psychosocial interventions, such as individual counseling and smoking cessation programs with a behavioral group session, a hypnosis audiotape, self-help printed materials, and even a cigarette replacement device that looks and feels like a real cigarette. Because the average smoker gains about 8 pounds after quitting smoking, offering a plan for weight reduction allays fears.

MAKING A DIFFERENCE

Do we tell smokers not to smoke? Apparently not. Only about one-third of patients who smoke report receiving advice about smoking from their health care provider. As many as 70% of heavy smokers say they might consider quitting if so advised. What if health professionals intervened with every patient to achieve even a 10% smoking quit rate? There would be several million fewer smokers in the U.S. each year. The challenge is to reduce the 400,000 tobacco-related deaths that occur annually.

But the task is arduous. About 34% of adult smokers try to quit each year, but only 2.5% succeed on their own. The success rate of smoking cessation programs is only about 20 to 30%. Motivation is essential. The National Cancer Institute (NCI) recommends the *4 A's*: *ask* about a patient's smoking history, *advise* smokers to quit, *assist* with information and treatment options, and *arrange* a follow-up visit.

How can nurses make a difference in getting patients to stop smoking? The waiting room can set the example. The office should be smoke-free. Display no-smoking signs, remove ashtrays and tobacco advertising, and make smoking cessation materials available. Counsel the smoker. Motivate and educate, listen and support.

In one outpatient setting, nurse-assisted smoking cessation counseling nearly doubled smoking quit rates compared to physician advice alone. The nurses provided specific suggestions and techniques on quitting with follow-up phone calls to patients. Short-term smoking abstinence in patients with cancer was 75% in those who received a nurse-delivered intervention compared to the usual-care quit rate of 43%. The Nursing Center for Tobacco Intervention is dedicated to reducing tobacco use.

The rewards of quitting smoking are tangible and immediate. Even 8 hours later, carbon dioxide and oxygen levels in the blood normalize. In a few days, the sense of smell and taste improves and mucus in the airways starts to break up. By 3 months, walking becomes easier. In 1 year, coughing, fatigue, and shortness of breath decrease substantially. The risk of smoking-induced cancers drops by 50% at 5 years and becomes similar to that of non-smokers at 10 years. By 15 years the risk of heart disease is no greater than for non-smokers. So there *is* a pot of gold at the end of the rainbow.

DON'T LOSE IT, USE IT

Let's face it: working with some patients can make health care providers lose their usual equanimity at times. Patients like "Mr. Svelton" tend to anger us with their expert manipulation. The resentment and frustration can be consuming. Suppressing anger or expressing it in a hostile way won't achieve the therapeutic goals necessary to help the patient. Many nurses and nurse practitioners turn their anger inward through self-disparaging comments. They devalue their work by referring to it as "scut work" and "being dumped on." Negative staff feelings often lead to rejection of the patient, the patient's needs are not met, and the manipulative behavior escalates.

Self-understanding is key to identifying manipulative behavior. Anger is an alarm going off in our heads. It's saying: "Something just happened here and on a gut level I feel violated." If we acknowledge our anger, then we can identify solutions. Anger can liberate when channeled into productive action or problem-solving that helps us be more effective with our patients and colleagues.

What's the solution? To be therapeutic, the health care provider must search for the meaning of the patient's behavior. While being noncritical in tone and content, the practitioner can access the antecedents and explore the consequences of manipulative behavior with the patient. Issues of self-esteem and control are at the core. Limits must be set without being punitive, and new appropriate behaviors, such as assertiveness, improved problem-solving skills, and development of a more positive outlook, must be taught. Though difficult and time consuming, the efforts are well worthwhile.

*   *   *

"Something Bad Is Going to Happen to Me"

Over the Christmas holidays, I saw Mary Sedgewick as a *walk-in*, an unscheduled patient who literally walks in off the street and wants to be evaluated. Such patients have to register so a chart can be made up on them, but that's all. If it weren't for a clinic like ours, they would go directly to the ER, which is supposed to be reserved for true emergencies.

Mary was an old, short, incredibly thin woman whose partially shaded bifocal lens were as thick as the bottom of a cola-bottle. She had severe, chronic obstructive lung disease.

"I've been coughing and not eating," she said. "I'm feeling worse."

"How long has this been going on?"

"A couple of weeks."

"Do you smoke?"

"Oh, yeah. I used to smoke two packs a day for the past forty years, but I got it down to one pack." The way she said it, the feat was nothing short of a miracle. I supposed it was, too. The lines at the side of her nose and mouth were deeply etched as if cut in clay. Her lips were slightly dusky and her nail beds were cyanotic. She looked older than her sixty-four years. Through the dehumanizing mask of her chronic disease, Mary appeared distraught. She seemed afraid to answer my questions.

"I'm tired of it all and tired of being alone," she complained. "Something bad is going to happen to me and I don't want to be alone when it happens."

It was hard to imagine how it must feel to breathe three times faster than normal all the time—perhaps like running a ten-kilometer race or doing the one-hundred-yard dash continuously. "Let me examine you and arrange for a few tests. We'll see if we can't get you feeling some better."

She had a low grade fever. Her breathing was rapid and labored and her pulse was fast. With each exhaled breath she pursed her lips. When I listened to Mary's chest, I noticed she was hardly moving any air. I kept checking to be sure, and she started wondering what I was doing for so long. She was having trouble breathing and talking at the same time.

After I discussed her with my attending physician, he came back into the room with me. "We think you should go to the emergency room to have blood gases done," he said.

"I can't go today because I can't get a ride home. I'll ask my neighbor's son to take me in tomorrow morning."

The attending sighed. Here was another of the endless compromises and negotiations of clinical medicine. He knew it could probably wait if we treated her in the meantime. "All right, but I'm going to hold you to your promise."

Mary's chest x-ray did not show any signs of pneumonia, so we thought she had a bronchial infection, which was making her lungs decompensate. I put her on an oral antibiotic, an inhaler, and the oral steroid prednisone. It was a big gun, but she had little margin for error.

The next day I took a call from the laboratory. Mary kept her promise to have the blood test done, but the results were worse than we expected. Her arterial oxygen level or pAO2 was a low forty-eight. The carbon dioxide level was nearly twice normal. With these values, she was at risk for respiratory failure. I called in home oxygen for her and made a referral to a pulmonologist for the following day. I also had a home health nurse assigned to her for several weeks.

On Christmas Day, Mary Sedgewick felt especially anxious and thought she was going to die. She called 911 and was rushed to the ER, where she waited for eight hours to be seen. "I didn't mind the wait," she later divulged, "because I got to talk to other people in the waiting room. I just didn't want to be alone. I wanted to be around other people. "

When I saw her in the clinic a few days afterward she looked better. There was no more fever and she was able to muster a laugh. "What kept you from coming in sooner for your chest infection?"

"I was afraid."

"Of what?"

She hesitated.

"Afraid you were going to die?"

"Not exactly. I was afraid you were going to tell me I had lung cancer. That's the way my husband died. It was terrible to watch him waste away. His suffering was the worst part of his dying."

We talked about her lung disease and how important it would be to stop smoking. I offered to see her weekly for awhile.

On the next visit Mary proudly announced she'd cut back to eight or nine cigarettes a day. She still required oxygen and couldn't walk from her house to the mailbox without becoming breathless. However, her convalescence was off to a good start.

By her next appointment she had started to dress up and wear make-up. It was wonderful to see red lipstick over the once bluish lips. She'd been to the salon and had her hair dyed.

Three months later, still on oxygen, Mary was cracking jokes and didn't seem to be the same person. I referred her to the hospital's pulmonary classes to learn more about her disease. It was a good deal for her because the hospital van picked up patients for free. She claimed to have almost stopped smoking.

But when I was listening to her lungs I smelled a familiar odor. "Your hair still smells of smoke."

"It's hard to give them up completely," she confessed. "They've been so much a part of my life. They're like—"

"Family?" I interjected.

"Or like old friends. We've been through a lot together. They were there for me when nobody else was: when my children left home; when my husband died."

"With friends like cigarettes, you don't need enemies."

"I know it's pathetic to say so. Smoking's one of the few things in this life I enjoy."

As I reflected on her words, she gathered her belongings, and wheeled her squeaky, green, portable oxygen cylinder to the door.

"Keep trying," I said. "You're doing well."

She smiled. With a nod Mary Sedgewick was gone.

You can't take away everything all at once from somebody.

CHRONIC LUNG DISEASE AND SMOKING

In healthy adults, the lungs—paired organs only 10 to 12 inches long—draw in about 3 to 5 liters of air in a single breath. They filter out incoming organisms and dangerous particles and exchange life-supporting oxygen for carbon dioxide (alveolar respiration). Although their resilience in the face of pollution is remarkable, it is not limitless.

As the fifth leading cause of death in the United States and a source of serious morbidity, chronic obstructive pulmonary disease (COPD) is a major health concern. It has increased more than 40% since 1982, suffocating 85,000 people every year and costing society about $12 billion annually. Cigarette smoking, now causally linked to COPD, accounts for more than 80% of the cases. An estimated 10% to 15% of smokers develop extensive lung damage and clinical symptoms of disease. Even breathing secondhand smoke is risky: it kills 53,000 people a year.

Patients with COPD *do* clinically start to look alike. They tend to cough, be thin, grow short of breath on exertion, purse-lip breathe, and wheeze. Breathing becomes progressively difficult and tiring.

COPD runs an insidious course, and after prolonged respiratory disability, death occurs. The emphysematous lung retains air because the wall between the air sacs ruptures and traps the air. Air retention expands the rib cage and flattens the diaphragm. Muscles in the rib cage and abdomen take over the work of breathing when the diaphragm is no longer effective. As the disease progresses, the shortage of large air sacs to exchange oxygen and carbon dioxide prolongs expiration.

Although Frederich Ruysch first diagnosed COPD in 1691, it wasn't until about 300 years later that scientific clues to COPD emerged. Previously believed to be a purely mechanical lung injury from excessive coughing, the lung damage in COPD is now thought to result from a chemical imbalance. A deficiency of lung α1-antiprotease (α1-antitrypsin) allows protease enzymes released from inflammatory cells in the lung to destroy elastin, the flexible substance that gives the lungs their elastic recoil.

The chronic respiratory infections of patients with emphysema only add insult to injury. *Haemophilus*, the most common offending organism, accounts for more than one-third of the cases. Due to constant inflammation of the smaller branches of the airways (bronchioles), excess mucus leads to chronic cough. Patients with emphysema and chronic bronchitis are prone to respiratory infections such as pneumonia. They may even develop asthma.

The first goal is to get the patient with emphysema to stop smoking. Set a specific quit date. By stopping, the patient will experience less coughing spasms and copious expectoration. Other goals in treatment are to help the patient breathe easier and prevent respiratory infections. Physical exercise, such as walking, improves physical stamina by allowing the lungs to use the available oxygen more efficiently, so a patient can do minor chores without being so winded. Breathing exercises improve the use of the diaphragm. Pulmonary rehabilitation is essential.

Don't forget the simple things we can do. It's important to immunize patients with COPD against pneumococcus and influenza to decrease their risk of life-threatening lung infections. Use antibiotics early in an upper respiratory infection and provide supplemental oxygen for severe emphysema. Many bronchodilator drugs, such as anticholinergics and beta agonists, may be delivered by inhalers. Steroid inhalers reduce lung inflammation, but if used for too long, cause high blood pressure and diabetes. Oral medications include the bronchodilator theophylline and intermittent use of anti-inflamma-tory steroids.

A new procedure, volume reduction surgery or "lung shaving," is now being performed at many medical centers. Removing damaged air sacs reduces the size of the lungs, which helps the diaphragm work more efficiently. Lasers are also being applied, but have not proven as effective as surgery. Within the last decade, lung trans-plant has become a final option when other approaches have failed, but donors are limited.

THE ILLUSORY NATURE OF DYSPNEA

We all breathe hard at times, whether it's from carrying groceries, running to get the phone, climbing stairs, jogging, swimming, or working out. *Dyspnea* is something more. When breathing is uncom-fortable or inappropriately difficult for the situation, it may meet the definition of dyspnea. The search for the cause takes the examiner from superficial inspection of the nose, throat, and chest to listening intently for abnormal sounds emanating from deep within the thorax.

When it comes to breathing, we think first of the airway and lungs. Obstructive and restrictive lung disorders are the principal pulmonary causes of dyspnea. In chronic lung disorders, the diameter of the chest increases and accessory breathing muscles work over-time. Abnormal breath sounds, such as rales, rhonchi, or expiratory wheezes, prevail. While lung diseases are a major reason for dysp-nea, problems with the heart or other systems are also important eti-ologies.

The heart is a superb pump, but when it fails, blood backs up in the lungs and body veins. This pulmonary and systemic congestion labors breathing. Once called "dropsy," congestive heart failure (CHF) affects about 5 million people in the U.S. and carries a mor-tality rate of 65 to 80%. To sleep at night, patients with CHF may have to prop several pillows under their heads as fluid drains into their lungs.

Reversible causes of CHF include anemia, aortic stenosis, ar-rhythmias, and thyroid disease. Coronary artery disease, enlarged heart (asymmetric septal hypertrophy, left ventricular hypertrophy), heart attack (myocardial infarction), heart valve dysfunction (aortic stenosis, mitral insufficiency), and inflammation of the heart's outer lining (pericarditis) are other sources of cardiac dyspnea and CHF. Cardiovascular examination reveals abnormal heart rate or rhythm, extra heart sounds, heart murmurs, neck bruits, or poor peripheral perfusion and edema. In addition to treatment of the underlying cause, the management of systolic CHF entails exercise, sodium restriction in the diet, and use of angiotensin-converting enzyme inhibitors (ACE) inhibitors combined with the usual "heart medications" (digoxin, diuretics, and vasodilators).

Sometimes two must share the blame. Both the heart and lungs contribute to dyspnea in patients with chronic pulmonary emboli, COPD with pulmonary hypertension and right heart failure (cor pulmonale), deconditioning, and trauma.

Neither the heart nor lungs is directly responsible for other causes of dyspnea. Psychiatric conditions such as anxiety, hyperventilation, and panic disorders can leave a person breathless, sweating, and tremulous. Airway stricture (supraglottic or subglottic), enlarged tonsils, and nasal obstruction by polyps or septal deviation are otorhinolaryngeal explanations for dyspnea. Neuromuscular diseases, such as muscular dystrophy or spinal cord disorders, weaken mechanical breathing mechanisms. Even bad posture from the spine deformities of kyphosis, osteoporosis, or scoliosis restricts the lungs.

The chest x-ray and electrocardiogram (ECG) need no introduction as tools for evaluating dyspnea. Arterial blood gas measurement identifies retention of carbon dioxide (hypercapnia), abnormal pH (respiratory acidosis), and low blood oxygen (hypoxemia). If the patient can give a maximum effort, spirometry helps differentiate obstructive and restrictive lung diseases, but complete pulmonary function testing is preferable. Pulse oximetry measures hemoglobin oxygen saturation by infrared light. A search for structural (echocardiography) and functional heart problems (treadmill exercise testing) or the overall function of both heart and lungs (cardiopulmonary exercise testing) completes the list of available tools. On the horizon are new blood tests for difficult diagnoses, such as measuring natriuretic peptides for diagnosing CHF.

3

Mortal Pain

We cannot truly face life until we have learned to face the fact that it will be taken away from us
—BILLY GRAHAM

After great pain, a formal feeling comes—
The nerves sit ceremonious, like tombs
—-EMILY DICKINSON

An hour of pain is as long as a day of pleasure
— ENGLISH PROVERB

Pleasure is oft a visitant; but pain
Clings cruelly to us.
—JOHN KEATS

The sorrow which has no vent in tears may make other organs weep
—HENRY MAUDSLEY

"I Deserve This"

At the end of the day I walked into the clinic waiting room. Although it was Friday after five o'clock—the clinic usually looked like a ghost town—checking to make sure there were no more patients was a force of habit.

My mind already was wandering to plans for the weekend when, to my surprise, I saw a tall man sitting in the corner. He leaned forward clutching his chest. Ashen and with a pained expression, he had the unmistakable look of a heart attack victim. I knew I had an emergency on my hands.

I whisked him into my room and gave him nitroglycerin and oxygen. How could they have left a sick patient in the clinic, I wondered.

Suddenly, he grabbed my arm. "Am I going to die?" His hand was cool and clammy. His eyes looked plaintive and fatigued. I noticed the streaks of gray through his mostly brown hair.

"Not if we can help it." I was more startled than I should have been at the question.

He shook his head at me, but I wasn't sure if he was trying to say something. Clean but not fastidious, he didn't seem well enough to talk more.

"Don't try to speak," I said. "Just take it easy."

After a short time he was doing better and I was able to get some information from him. I ran a brief electrocardiogram, which showed no acute ischemic changes. Satisfied that he was stable for the moment, I contemplated getting him to the ER. "I'll be back in a minute."

I rushed out of the room to look for the clinic physician.

"Hey, nurse practitioner-extraordinaire!" a voice called out behind me from the other end of the hallway. "Where are you off to in such a hurry? Wait up!"

Even without turning around, I knew it had to be Dr. Carlos Santini, wanting to regale me with a story about one of his patients. Always upbeat and positive, Dr. Santini loved cracking jokes with all the nurse practitioners and was our most sympathetic ear. He was a handsome Hispanic with a type-A personality—fast-laughing and fast-talking—always enjoying being the center of attention. Sometimes it was hard to get a word in edgewise. I thought he missed his calling and should have been an actor, but I respected him as a physician.

"I've got to tell you this joke I heard," he said with a crescendo of animation.

"Where's Dr. Morrell?" I interrupted. "He's supposed to be my clinic attending today."

"Bad news. He left over an hour ago to pick up his wife or something."

"Carlos, come over here. I've got a late walk-in patient. Can you eyeball him for me?"

"Do I look like a glutton for punishment?" Dr. Santini retorted playfully.

"I need you in here *now*," I insisted.

"Did we have a little too much coffee, my friend?" he bantered. "Perhaps you should add some water to the grounds."

"He's got chest pain," I said, ignoring his remarks. "An attending needs to see him; he looks acute. I can't leave him for too long. There are no medical records here and everyone seems to have left the office, including the secretary."

Dr. Santini's smile evaporated. "Let's go."

We stood just outside my room. The door was ajar, so I could keep my eye on the patient.

"Okay, what do you know about him so far?" Dr. Santini asked.

"Mr. Boone is a fifty-three-year-old, white male with recent onset of shortness of breath, left anterior chest pain with intermittent left hand numbness, slow pulse, and diaphoresis. The brief history I could get is that he was climbing the stairs out of the subway and felt as if a ton of bricks landed on his chest. The pain was squeezing and radiated down his left arm. He claims he's never had this kind of pain before, he hasn't been seen at our clinic, and he is on no medications. He's roughly fifty pounds overweight, smokes two packs of cigarettes a day over thirty years, and he puts away a six-pack or two of beer on the weekends."

"And what have you done for him so far?"

"I've hooked him up to oxygen by nasal cannula at two liters per minute, but his lips remain cyanotic. I gave him a sublingual nitroglycerin tablet and obtained the electrocardiogram. I wanted to get this guy to the ER stat, but felt he was too unstable to transport by wheelchair."

"Let's see him."

Gary Boone looked transformed as he sat on the examining table. Only a little short of breath, he was much pinker and more relaxed.

"Doc," he said to me, "I feel better since you put this thing in my nose and that pill under my tongue, but wow—what a headache, just like you said." Then he got off the table and started dressing.

"Where are you going?" I asked in bewilderment.

"I've got to leave."

"You're not ready to leave," I cautioned.

"Oh, I don't want to bother you people, so if you just get me unhooked, I'll be on my way. Thanks a lot."

Dr. Santini flashed me a puzzled look as he introduced himself to the patient. "Mr. Boone, do you have a plane to catch?" he quipped, trying to inject some levity. "Seriously, though, I must ask you a few questions. I am responsible for your care today."

Mr. Boone sat down again. "Okay, but please hurry."

Dr. Santini questioned him about previous episodes of chest pain. Mr. Boone's answers were vague. Santini keep hammering at the point. Mr. Boone now looked down at the floor sheepishly and then over at me. My intuition told me he was about to diverge from his previous story and confess to something troublesome.

Mr. Boone returned Dr. Santini's gaze. His explanation stumbled out. "Ah—well, sure, I had chest pains before, just not this bad."

"Why didn't you mention this?" Dr. Santini asked.

"I don't know. Look, I have to be honest with you. I don't want to waste any more of your time. It comes down to this: it's not easy for me to say so, but I'm not a great husband to my wife. I've beaten her when I was drunk and only knew it by the bruises on her face the next day. I know the ticker is giving out, but I hope to redeem myself in my wife's eyes with the seven-hundred-fifty-thousand dollar life insurance policy I have.

So I don't want anymore help or any emergency rooms or anything like that. I deserve this pain. Lord knows I've caused her years of heartache. Now it's my turn. I just came by to pick up my wife from her appointment and got a little lost. I stumbled into this clinic, thinking no one was here and I would finally die and everything would be over. This nice lady saw I was hurting and helped me out. But that's as far as it goes."

He proceeded to strip off the nasal cannula that was supplying him with oxygen, stood up, and buttoned his shirt. "I'd better get going. My wife will wonder what happened to me. Can you tell me how to get to the kidney clinic? She has bad kidneys, you see."

I stared at Dr. Santini with consternation and was about to say something to Mr. Boone when Dr. Santini cut me off. His face was uncharacteristically stern. "Mr. Boone, I strongly advise you to be fully evaluated. It goes against medical advice to let you go, knowing you're bound to have a massive heart attack soon based on today's symptoms. I really think you're doing the wrong thing by not going to the emergency room immediately."

"I don't want to stay and you can't make me stay." He was emphatic.

"No, that's true, I can't." A look of resignation came over Dr. Santini's bright face like a shadow. He turned to me. "Do you have any paperwork on Mr. Boone?

"No, I don't."

"Why not?"

"It turns out he never got registered. He looked so ill and in such pain, I just assumed he was a walk-in. Otherwise, I would have transported him straight to the ER." I felt rather foolish.

"Well, let's stamp up some papers on him, write down his information and what was done for him."

Addressing the patient, Dr. Santini remarked officiously, "I'm going to ask you to sign your name to acknowledge that we advised you to stay and to have a full cardiac work-up. You can take a copy of this with you. Is that agreeable?"

Mr. Boone nodded.

"Then I'll have the nurse practitioner take your vital signs again and write you a prescription for nitroglycerin tablets. Put one under your tongue when you get that chest pain, and if the pain doesn't subside in ten minutes, take another one. If the pain is still bad, call 911. The nurse practitioner will write those instructions on your discharge copy. Do you have any questions?"

"No. I thank you kindly."

Dr. Santini turned on his heels and left the room.

As I handed the patient the prescription and papers, I asked him seriously to reconsider. Torn over how much more I should presume to say, I decided to take the plunge.

"Mr. Boone, look, you obviously have regrets about your drinking and the way you treat your wife. Have you thought of other options? You could get counseling, join Alcoholics Anonymous, or go through an alcohol rehabilitation program. It doesn't have to be this way."

He gazed at me blankly.

"Surely your wife would prefer you alive and well rather than dead."

Mr. Boone seemed to consider what I said. Then that recondite look. He smiled slowly and replied, "I'll think it over. Give me your card and I'll call you about it later."

I escorted Mr. Boone to the main hallway of the medical building and told him where to find the nephrology clinic. I advised him to use the elevators and avoid stairwells at all cost. He thanked me again and we parted. I reassured myself that he heeded my words by taking his prescription.

When I returned, Carlos Santini was back in my office. In a serious tone, he said, "Now, if you think that patient is going to count as a number on the clinic revenue ledger, you're sadly mistaken. Remember, register the patient first, then see the patient."

"When I saw Mr. Boone in the waiting room, I recognized the symptoms of an acute MI and went to work. Registering him was not on my mind."

Dr. Santini burst out laughing and held up his hands defensively, leaning against the door jam. "I'm joking, I'm joking. All kidding aside, you did the right thing. Good job. But a piece of advice: lighten up. You look so serious and sad. You can't save the world. You really have got to stop trying to save patients who don't want to be saved. Help those who ask for your help and then let it go."

"Is that why you didn't fight harder to make him stay?"

"You mean rant and rave and make a big scene?"

I nodded.

"If I thought it helped, I would have. He's an adult; I'm not a parent. Besides, he's made up his mind. I've met many Mr. Boone's before. You can't change them."

I had no reply. Inwardly, I disagreed. I felt we'd made a difference.

"Well, enough fun for now. Got to go. My patients await me in the hospital wards."

"Thanks for your assistance."

"I can't turn down a nurse practitioner in need." He saluted me in mock military style as he walked out of the office, whistling the song, *I Did It My Way*.

I gathered my purse and jacket and arranged my desk for Monday morning's clinic. Feeling I might need it later, I tucked a copy of Mr. Boone's clinic record in my top drawer.

Enrico, the housekeeper, peeked in the room to see if he could empty the trash. He was an affable, small-framed man with a broad face and thinning hair. From his downcast eyes and tendency to nod too agreeably, I thought he was self-effacing. I motioned him in and indicated I was leaving for the night. Although he wore headphones, he nodded that he understood.

My thoughts returned to the surreal encounter with Mr. Boone. Now with the stress of the medical emergency ebbing, I was left with the incongruities, the harsh realities, and the cruel irony. Strangely I did not feel all that bad about him. Was it a value judgment about a self-admitted wife abuser and alcoholic? As pathetic as the situation was, it seemed to follow the ethics of some B-grade Hollywood movie: a man atones for his wicked ways by making the ultimate sacrifice. The idea of giving up his life was not something I understood or could identify with, but he seemed to be at peace with himself, believing he was doing the right thing. He'd been informed about his situation. The choice was his to make.

Did the wife have a right to know? What were my ethical obligations? In a tangential flow of thoughts, I found myself wondering what his wife was like and what she would do with the seven-hundred-fifty-thousand dollars.

By coincidence, as I walked through the hospital lobby on my way out of the building, I caught sight of Gary Boone and a woman I presumed to be his wife. They were walking a little ahead of me. Although I didn't get a look at her face because she was in front of him, she seemed like an average, middle-aged woman. The thought occurred to me that she might not be his wife. Maybe he was having an affair, felt guilty about it, and wanted to leave his wife the money. That seemed awfully involved. My suspicions broadened. Had he taken something to induce a heart attack? My imagination was running away with me.

Should I try to meet the woman? Should I run up and urge Mr. Boone to fill his prescription? I couldn't believe he was prepared to go through with his plan. If he didn't fill it, the die was cast. I thought of him collapsing somewhere from a massive heart attack. *I give you maybe two months, Mr. Boone...less if you use the stairs or run for a bus.* Maybe Benjamin Franklin was right: nine men in ten *are* suicides...

Mr. Boone stopped near the exit. I watched as he pulled out my business card and prescription. He lingered a moment—*come on, come on, make the right choice*—then nonchalantly tore them up and pitched them in the trash can. Catching up with the woman outside the door, he disappeared down the street. She never looked behind.

HEART ATTACK

It rests but never stops. It beats 2.5 billion times over a lifetime, beginning in the fourth week of fetal life. It pumps 4,000 gallons of blood daily, over 50 to 100 million gallons in a lifetime. The size of a fist and shaped like a cone, it weighs only 10 to 12 ounces and has walls 3.5 inches thick. From the Greek "myo" for muscle and "kardia" for heart, the heart muscle (myocardium) is an engineering feat. Man's heroic attempts at building an artificial heart, aided by modern engineering and space-age technology, are primitive by comparison. But the heart is not invincible.

The cold, hard facts. Sixty-six million Americans have heart disease. An estimated 1.5 million Americans each year suffer a heart attack or myocardial infarction (MI). One quarter of all MI's are silent, without chest pain. The peak time is the morning hours between 4 and 10 A.M. when blood adrenaline levels are high. The location of pain in an MI may be misleading, seeming to arise in the arm, back, jaw, or stomach. A little less than half of all patients with an MI die, often abruptly due to cardiac arrhythmias, which occur in 95% of them.

By initiating cardiopulmonary resuscitation (CPR) within five minutes, a bystander can breathe for the victim and externally apply chest compressions to pump blood from the heart. CPR buys time until the paramedics arrive with medications and a defibrillator. About 90% to 95% of heart attack victims who arrive at the hospital survive, but the first 6 hours are crucial, and no one is completely out of the woods for 10 to 14 days.

What happens? A heart attack strikes when cardiac muscle does not receive oxygen from the heart's blood supply. Most occur on the left side of the heart. They are classified as anterior, posterior, inferior, or lateral, depending on their location. If the coronary artery is blocked by a cholesterol plaque or blood clot (coronary thrombosis), the blood-starved heart muscle starts to die (infarction), causing chest pain and electrical disorganization of the heart beat. Erratic electrical transmission in the heart can lead to the deadly arrhythmia ventricular fibrillation. Once the heart is in this rhythm, its ineffectual quivering cannot deliver oxygenated blood to the brain, and permanent brain damage and death occur within five minutes.

How can you ascertain whether someone has had an MI? Beside the traditional measures, new, rapid, bedside blood tests are available. One recent study suggests that patients who have acute chest pain may be discharged from the ER safely if they have negative results on troponin T and troponin I tests when first drawn and six hours after the onset of chest pain.

In spite of its grim nature, heart disease *can* be treated. Percutaneous transluminal coronary angioplasty (PTCA) involves threading a small, plastic balloon catheter to the blocked artery site and inflating it to decrease the clot or plaque. PCTA reopens up to 95% of arteries, usually within one hour. Over 300,000 angioplasties are performed each year at hospitals with a cardiac catheterization lab.

Clot-dissolving medications (thrombolytic agents) like TPA (tissue plasminogen activator), if given early (prior to 6 hours after the onset of chest pain), have an 80% success rate of opening clogged arteries within 90 minutes. Antiplatelet drugs and anticoagulants prevent recurrent artery closure by their anti-clotting effect. Nitroglycerin, placed under the tongue, dilates the coronary blood vessels and liberates blood flow to the area of ischemia. Angiotensin converting enzyme (ACE) inhibitors, taken orally after a heart attack, reduce stress and promote healing.

If patients fail PTCA and medications, a coronary artery bypass graft (CABG) may be indicated to open the coronary arteries surgically and replace them with vein grafts. About 350,000 coronary bypass surgeries are done in this country yearly.

Other methods? New blood-thinning medications, such as bivalirudin, are being tested. Research with direct laser energy and ultrasound to break up blood clots and plaques is underway.

PREVENTING HEART DISEASE

What's your cholesterol? The blood cholesterol concentration has gained the status of a vital statistic in everyday conversations. It's not surprising because more than 96 million Americans have a level above 200 mg/dL. For 38 million others, it's above 240 mg/dL. While the media have heralded the dangers of high cholesterol throughout the U.S., cholesterol, only one of a number of "red flags," does not tell the whole story.

Major risk factors for coronary heart disease are abnormal blood lipid panel, advanced age, current cigarette smoking, diabetes, family history of premature coronary heart disease, and high blood pressure. Men over the age of 45 and women older than 55 or having premature menopause without estrogen replacement therapy may be in jeopardy.

The fasting blood lipid panel includes total cholesterol, "bad cholesterol" (low-density lipoprotein cholesterol, LDL-C), "good cholesterol" (high-density lipoprotein cholesterol, HDL-C), and triglycerides. Risk factors are low HDL-C (<35 mg/dL) and elevated LDL-C (>100 mg/dL), triglycerides (>200 mg/dL), and total cholesterol (>200 mg/dL). The likelihood of heart disease also climbs with high blood levels of homocysteine (>13 μmol/mL), a product of folate metabolism; fibrinogen, a clotting factor; and insulin.

All risk factors must be considered. The more risk factors a person has, the greater the chances of a heart attack, and the more vigorous the efforts at prevention should be. There are, of course, no quick answers. How patients at risk should be managed is controversial and subject to change. Case in point. Most experts agree that there are different levels of risk, such as borderline abnormal, mild, moderate, or severe abnormalities, but they disagree on how those levels are defined.

The first step toward risk reduction is usually lifestyle intervention: dietary modification, physical activity, stress reduction, and elimination or treatment of any possible major risk factors such as diabetes, hypertension, or smoking. Walking, one of the best forms of cardiovascular exercise, burns about 300 calories an hour and can reduce stress. Telling patients to "Take a hike" may be sound advice. Don't think walking is for sissies: the walking record is 142 miles in 24 hours! Comparatively, a mere 30 to 60 minutes a day sounds very doable.

How hard should the heart be pushed by exercise? For healthy individuals, subtract your age from 220; then take 75% of that number. The result is the optimal exercise heart rate—your "training zone." For patients with medical problems, the figure should be reduced on an individual basis.

Failure of these approaches after 3 to 6 months in the presence of more than two major risk factors and moderate or severe blood lipid abnormalities usually requires drug treatment. In post-menopausal women, estrogen replacement therapy may suffice to correct blood lipid abnormalities. Otherwise a cholesterol-lowering drug should be prescribed. Some of the newer ones, which are competitive inhibitors of cholesterol biosynthesis (HMG-CoA reductase), have been demonstrated to reduce the risk of first heart attack. Older drugs include cholestyramine, clofibrate, colestipol, and niacin. Many have potentially serious side effects and require monitoring. A daily folic acid supplement of 400 micrograms remedies high homocysteine.

*   *   *

"I Ran Out of My Medicines"

"Hector Rodriguez," I shouted.

There was no answer from the forty or fifty bored patients who languished in the clinic waiting for their turn to be seen.

"Mr. Rodriguez," I repeated louder over the buzz of conversation and the hospital intercom.

Those engaged in idle chat or reading a paperback looked up and glanced around the room. A woman knitting a baby blanket nudged a sleeping man. He sat up straight.

"Rodriguez?" I asked.

He shook his head yes.

"Are you two together?"

"No."

The short, older man with dyed black hair, a black shirt, and black pants roused himself and stood up slowly, picked up his broad-rimmed, white hat, and ambled over to me. "Sorry, I haven't been sleeping too well. It must be some kind of indigestion I'm having."

I motioned that he precede me. As we walked down the hall to my examining room, I thought about how many of my patients attributed all sorts of medical problems to indigestion. My job was to pick out the patient whose indigestion was actually heart pain or an ulcer brewing.

While I sat and searched through his chart, I inquired, "Why are you here?"

His records showed a history of chest pain and irregular heart rhythms and one small heart attack in the past. He was placed on digoxin and nitroglycerin.

"I ran out of my medicines."

Of all the things to worry a health care provider, that was one of the most effective. So many of my patients let themselves run out of critical medications. They didn't appreciate the dangerous game they were playing with their own lives.

"When did you run out?"

"It's been awhile." He glanced away. I knew that look, too.

"You know, these are important medicines, Mr. Rodriguez. You don't want to run out. They help your heart get more oxygen when it needs it."

The patient nodded.

"Have you been taking a lot of these lately?"

He shrugged. "The usual. I don't like taking them. They give me a headache."

"That's a common side effect of nitroglycerin."

Mr. Rodriguez looked at me blankly. I never knew how much of such looks were due to a language problem or apathy.

"You mentioned indigestion."

"Yes."

"Describe the pain."

"It feels heavy, like a weight, almost like it's squeezing. It builds up in my chest and I get short of breath. My heart feels like it's going very fast. I put one of those small pills under my tongue and that helps it right away."

"Are you having chest pain now?" I searched his face carefully.

"No."

"How often are you getting these pains?"

"About once a week. I had a bad pain yesterday, but I didn't have any pills. I got sweaty and felt sick to my stomach. But then it passed. That's why I'm here today—to get more pills."

"Does it happen when you are relaxing or doing something physical?"

"Anytime, mostly when I'm doing something."

I didn't like the sound of that. The problem with chest pain was it could be caused by anxiety and any number of minor conditions. Even medical professionals had difficulty describing it accurately. The big worry was an impending heart attack.

"Please take off your shirt and lie down on the table. I want to examine you and then run an electrocardiogram."

He gave me a puzzled look.

"You know, that heart test with all the wires put on your chest."

"Ah, *si*," he said, and began to undress.

After finishing his examination, I brought the ECG machine into my office, attached the leads to his chest and limbs, told him to lie still, and hit the start button. The machine did the rest. The signs of the old heart attack were apparent on the paper tracing. The patient had mild atrial fibrillation, a common and usually chronic irregularity in heart rhythm, which was unchanged from his previous tracing. Things looked stable. There were no new changes.

With tracing in hand I stepped out of the room and flagged the physician covering for me that morning. "Janet, got a minute?"

"Well, make it quick. I still have five more patients to go."

Dr. Janet Ressor was a tall, lean woman who recently joined the group practice. She dressed plainly but neatly, not one to lavish much time on personal appearance. Usually thoughtful and pleasant to work with, she was starting to show the strain of meeting the patient quotas.

"I'm seeing a patient with angina."

"Is he having acute chest pain now?"

"He denies it."

"Do I need to see him?"

That question could be a double-edged sword. The physicians, who were dealing with their own scheduling pressures, relied on me to know when to say *You need to drop what you're doing and see my patient.* Most cases weren't at issue; it was the gray-zone patients I worried about. If you asked a physician to spot check a patient right away and he or she didn't think it's was an acute problem, you often got a look like, *That was no big deal and you should have known it.*

"Yes, you do," I answered.

After I reviewed the pertinent information, Dr. Ressor registered her concern. "Do you have an ECG yet?"

"Yes."

"How does it look?"

"Here, see for yourself. I don't see anything acute."

Dr. Ressor poured over the tracing. She agreed. "He has some atrial fibrillation. I don't see any digoxin effect, so it may have been awhile since he ran out," she said with a frown. "Let's go see him together."

When we walked back into my room, Mr. Rodriguez was lying quietly on the examining table. After introducing herself, Dr. Ressor asked, "Are you having chest pain now?"

"No."

"Are you *sure*? *No* chest pains."

"Yes," he insisted.

"Are your chest pains getting worse every day?"

Mr. Rodriguez paused. "No."

"Can I have a listen?"

He nodded.

Dr. Ressor took the stethoscope from around her neck, where internists were in the habit of carrying it, and listened to his chest methodically.

I knew what she was doing. Here in the middle of a busy clinic, she was making a judgment call that she would have to stand by. It was her call. That's why she was the attending physician.

Dr. Ressor raised her head slowly and put the stethoscope back around her neck as easily as laying a phone receiver in its cradle. "Well, Mr. Rodriguez," she said thoughtfully, "things sound okay. Your heart rate is a little irregular, but I think you'll be all right once you get back on your medications. That's very important. Start them today and don't run out of them. We want you to return to this clinic in one week and have some heart tests done in the meantime. If you have any more problems, call or come back sooner. Okay?"

"Will you give me a refill on my prescriptions?"

"Yes. The nurse practitioner will write them for you."

"Okay, Doctor. *Gracias*."

Dr. Ressor cued me to follow her out of the room. Her blond ponytail swung around as she turned. "Call him in a day or two and see how he's doing. If you get the feeling that he's no better, bring him in. Let's also order a thallium scan with exercise testing."

When I returned to my room, I wrote out each prescription. Having prescriptive rights was an aspect of my job I liked because it was a privilege and made me feel independent. As I handed the patient instructions on what to do in case of an emergency, I emphasized, "Please go and get these prescriptions filled right away. Don't wait. Promise?"

Hector Rodriguez looked up at me. His eyes were dark and inscrutable. I was uncertain of his compliance, but he'd given me no reason to doubt him. "I'll go to the local druggist in my neighborhood," he said. "I have an account with him. He knows me."

"Okay. But *don't* put it off until tomorrow. You mustn't forget," I warned.

"I won't." His smile didn't falter.

I reached into my desk drawer and pulled out a few free samples of nitroglycerin from the drug rep. "Here are some samples to get you started. Put one under your tongue if you have chest pain."

"*Mucho gracias*," he said appreciatively.

When he left, the thought that he might not comply crossed my mind, but I tried to dismiss it. After all, he had allowed himself to run out of medications, yet he came to the clinic because he knew he needed them. I had no rapport with Mr. Rodriguez, not having taken care of him before. Attaching a sample of the ECG to his chart, I completed my note.

It was an especially busy day. I caught a quick bite in my office, glad to have brown-bagged it, and went on to see three more patients.

Later, Thelma Townsend, the unit secretary to the outpatient clinic, stuck her head in my doorway. Her gold, dangling earrings, accentuated by her short hair, tinkled with her movement. She was an aristocratic-looking African-American.

"Do you know a Hector Rodriguez?" she asked with a hint of a West Indies accent. "Nobody else seems to know him."

"Yes."

"Well, there's a family member on the phone who is *very* upset. She wants to speak to someone *right now*."

"Put the call through to me."

"Do you want the chart?"

"No, I still have it on my desk." The phone rang in my room. With trepidation, I picked up the receiver.

"Are you the person who saw my father this morning?" the caller asked in a voice brimming with emotion.

"Yes." My concern was mounting.

"I don't know what you people are doing over there, *but you killed him!*" she yelled.

"*What?*" Cold sweat. The woman's words, my worst nightmare, were the last thing that I expected to hear. But even they had less impact on me than the desperation in her voice did. My insides were trembling.

"My father was on his way home from his visit with you for his heart problems and died from a heart attack. Someone called 911, but he didn't make it."

I fell silent for a few moments, processing this unexpected and tragic news. Harsh reality soon took hold. I sat back in my chair and closed my eyes.

"I don't know what to say. This is terrible." Reproach and devastation.

"Are you a doctor?" the caller asked.

"No, I'm a nurse practitioner."

"Maybe if a *doctor* had seen my father he would still be alive."

Shocked silence, then the sting of those words. The angry way in which she spoke them attacked my vulnerability and insecurities as a nurse practitioner. Doctors could do no wrong; it was always the nurse practitioner's fault.

"Both the doctor *and* I saw your father together," I asserted. My voice was so calm it didn't seem to be mine. "We renewed his prescriptions. Did you know he let himself run out of medicine for his angina and irregular heart beat?" I asked. "That didn't help his heart."

The daughter paused. "I didn't know."

"We were trying to help your father," I added. "He told us he wasn't having heart pain today. Otherwise we would have admitted him to the hospital."

"He shouldn't have died," the daughter pleaded. "It wasn't his time yet." She cried.

The crying made matters all the worse. As much as I was hurt by the woman's anger, it would have been preferable to hearing a stranger in pain crying over the phone and feeling responsible.

"I know this is as much a shock to you as it is to us," I said. "He had a bad heart condition, but we wouldn't have sent him home if we thought this was going to happen."

There was no response on the other end of the line, just sobbing.

"Do you have someone at home with you?"

"Yes," the woman answered between sobs.

"Good. Let me discuss this with the doctor and have her call you back."

"Okay, but promise to call me back today." The sound of the voice changed from angry to pathetic.

"I promise."

When I replaced the receiver, I grabbed Mr. Rodriguez's chart and searched frantically for Janet Ressor. The French roast coffee I just drank from my thermos now felt like sulfuric acid churning in the pit of my stomach and bubbling up to my throat. Dr. Ressor was talking with a colleague, but I signaled her frantically. She came over. "What's the matter?"

"I just got a call. Mr. Rodriguez is *dead*."

Her face paled. She looked stunned. "What happened?" When I told her, she managed to ask, "Did he get his nitroglycerin?"

"I gave him a handful of free samples besides the prescription."

"Good. Let me see the chart. I want to look at his ECG again." Her voice sounded urgent and nervousness. She riffled through the chart. Her eyes were glued to the tracing. "No, no, he *was* stable," she mumbled to herself. "This ECG is not acute." She looked relieved to know that she hadn't missed blatant evidence of an acute myocardial infarction.

"I'm feeling real bad about this," I confessed. "Maybe we should have admitted him." The wave of peculiar dizziness I felt was one I recognized as guilt.

"No. It was a judgment call and I made it. You did everything right. I stand by the decision. It seemed correct at the time."

"I still feel bad." Tears welled in my eyes. "I talked to the daughter who is very upset. Would you speak with her, too?"

"Yes. I'll call her." The doctor put her arm around me. "I'm sorry this happened and I feel very badly, too. It's not your mistake. He had a serious heart condition for years. This is the down side of medicine. We can't predict the future. We can't admit every person with angina to the hospital. Had we known this would happen, we would have admitted him. You never know. They told us in medical school, about half of such patients can go home and have a heart attack even after seeing their doctor that same day."

"Dr. Ressor," the unit secretary called out. "Your three-o'clock patient has arrived. So did your late two-thirty."

Janet Ressor shook her head. She looked like she wanted to say more. "I've got to go." She rushed down the hall and disappeared into her office.

I returned to my room and sat at my desk, reflecting on Hector Rodriguez. He seemed to have no idea he was about to die. Was he being stoic? Was he having chest pain? Was he trying to avoid being admitted to the hospital? I agonized. I had been involved in a life-

and-death decision over a man who walked in off the street. His survival depended on my ability to discern stoicism or cultural macho behavior from denial. It was all too imprecise. We made an educated decision and the patient died. We sent many other people out who have not died. How could such important decisions be made on so little information and such limited tools? I stared at the open chart on my desk, trying to find a clue. But I realized the answer was not to be found there.

Although I saw three more patients, my mind drifted back to Mr. Rodriguez. The self-critical voices of doubt, uncertainty, and reproach were clamoring in my head, undermining what remained of my confidence. I wondered if there were some way we could have foreseen his heart attack. That was a question I would ask myself every day in the weeks that followed.

Now the unsettling day was drawing to a close. One minute I'm raging...*Life isn't fair...Nothing makes sense...* the next I'm in tears. I shook my head. *No more tears...I have work to do.* I finished my chart notes with difficulty, still rattled by what had happened. It was one of the worst days in my life. I didn't know then I'd hardly feel alive for days at a time until the hurt became less raw.

When I left, Enrico from housekeeping was trying to resuscitate the old green linoleum floor of the clinic. Worn and dirty, scraped and scuffed by the shoes of countless thousands in the community, the floor had succumbed long ago. Now it matched the beat-up, dark brown, wooden chairs with their soiled, paper-thin seat cushions; the small, defunct ceiling fan that hung in the corner; and the ugly, framed, yellowing prints, hanging crooked on the walls. The fatigued hands of the wall clock fell incrementally further and further behind the time of the rest of the world, like a runner who continues to run, but knows he has lost the race.

"Don't work too hard, Enrico."

"No, no. Good night, señora."

ORIGINS OF CHEST PAIN

This worst case scenario lays the risks on the line. Nothing replaces the role of patient education and a long-standing relation of trust between a patient and health care provider.

Angina must be the first thought. Patients who complain of a heavy sensation or squeezing behind their sternum or breast bone, pain radiating to the neck, shoulder, or down the left arm—especially with exercise, and relieved by sublingual nitroglycerin—are probably having angina. An anginal episode usually lasts less than 5 minutes. When the pain is severe and persists 30 minutes, with nausea, vomiting, shortness of breath, but no relief from nitroglycerin, a myocardial infarction may be in progress. Angina may be stable or unstable. People with unstable angina are difficult to diagnose and manage because of the wide range of their symptoms and risks for an MI.

Although the possibility of heart disease as a cause of chest pain is the immediate concern, there are many other causes, too. A detailed history is crucial to determine the duration, intensity, location, pattern of radiation, and quality of the pain. Many conditions mimic heart pain, some of which are benign and self-limited, while others are serious and sometimes fatal.

Medical tips. When anxiety and hyperventilation cause chest pain, the clue is the patient's emotional state. Esophageal pain is relieved by antacids. Musculoskeletal chest pain, from arthritis or strained chest muscles and ligaments, is reproducible by palpation of the chest and is triggered by movement of the shoulders or neck. Pleuritic chest pain or pleural catch is the sharp localized stab unmistakably linked to deep inspiration or coughing.

Make no mistake: chest pain may warn of more serious disorders. Blood clots in the lung (pulmonary embolism) bring on bloody sputum (hemoptysis), sudden shortness of breath, and substernal pain. Lacerating pain radiating to the back signals aortic tearing (dissection) in hypertensive patients. The pain of pericarditis, an inflammation of the pericardial lining, lasts longer and shadows a viral upper respiratory infection. Lessening when the patients sits, it is left-sided and unaffected by exertion.

MEDICATION NONCOMPLIANCE

It's a mini-epidemic: the unwillingness of patients to take their medication correctly is a serious problem. Up to one-half of patients fail to achieve full compliance and a third never take their medication at all. Noncompliance is sometimes revealed only by measuring drug levels. Patients tend to comply better with short-term, self-administered therapies than with long-term therapies.

Why don't patients comply? In the geriatric population, the problem may be difficulty reading labels and inserts. By one estimate, as many as 90 million adults are unable to understand the instructions. Socioeconomic factors, such as illiteracy and the high costs of medications, also contribute to the problem. Compliance decreases when the medical prognosis is poor, as in diabetes, heart disease, or uncontrolled hypertension. Denial is a root cause.

True, there is no one solution to the problem, but the health care provider can take steps to help prevent noncompliance. Writing instructions in plain language, especially in the patient's first language, is important. Relations between caregivers and patients should be strong, trusting, and collaborative. Patients must participate in decisions about their own treatment regimen. By asking them how they plan to take medications after hearing the instructions, simple misunderstandings can be prevented.

CIRCUMSTANCES OF DEATH

How often are health care providers caught unaware when a patient is about to die? In about 25% of the cases, a patient's death in a primary care practice is unexpected and abrupt, according to the North American Primary Care Research Group. The rest of the time death was anticipated, but sudden in about half. Only slightly more than 50% of the patients had an advance directive in place to tell how they wished final matters to be handled. The commonest causes of death in the U.S. in 1995? From the most to the least common they were heart disease, cancer, stroke, COPD, accidents, pneumonia and influenza, diabetes, HIV, suicide, and chronic liver disease.

4

Keeping the Peace in the Family

Happy families are all alike; every unhappy family is unhappy in its own way
—LEO TOLSTOY

Problems are not stop signs, they are guidelines
—ROBERT SCHULLER

Stress is an unavoidable consequence of life
—PAUL ROSCH

The reason that husbands and wives do not understand each other is because they belong to different sexes
—DOROTHY DIX

"I Won"

"Shut up, mother!"

Lynn Friedman, a fourteen-year-old, sat on the edge of the examining table. Her blue-gray eyes and milky fair skin belied the contempt in her voice.

"I'm trying to get a woman doctor to examine you so it will make it easier for you," her mother said calmly. The short, middle-aged woman was a little overweight, but not obese, well-dressed and nicely made up. "You've never had this—"

"I don't need it. I didn't do anything wrong. I don't want your help and I don't need you." She tugged on her miniskirt.

I watched the exchange in disbelief, a reluctant witness to this embarrassing moment. The mother looked reprimanded. *If a daughter can talk to her mother like that in front of a total stranger, what kind of arguments got on at home? The control this girl wields over her mother is clear.*

"Hold on, now," I interjected. "One person talking at a time. I don't want any fighting in here. I need to find out what happened."

Lynn glared at me as if to ask: "Who the hell are you?" Now I was an authority figure, no longer a neutral party. I would not be forgiven for this transgression.

I noticed that the mother withdrew and looked abashed. She hung her head and said nothing. Strands of hair over her ears came unclasped. I asked her to step out so I could speak with the teenager alone.

When the mother left, I told Lynn this was our confidential time. "Why are you here, Lynn?"

"I'm clueless. I don't want to be here." She made no eye contact. The silence was punctuated only by her sighs of exasperation.

"I understand you ran away with some friends."

"Who told you that?" She studied me for a moment before her eyes darted away.

"Well, I already talked with your mom, but I want to hear *your* side of the story."

Lynn looked down without responding. As she swung her feet back and forth, her platform shoes tapped against the metal side of the examining table. Finally she nodded.

"So how did you get home? Did you come back on your own or

were you picked up by the police?"

"The cops found us." Her voice was almost inaudible.

"Why did you run away?"

"Because they're my best friends and I hang out with them. We do things together and they were going to run away from home. I wasn't happy at home so I went with them."

"Are things that tough?"

Lynn stared out the window without answering. She fingered the silvery beads of her short necklace.

"I understand there was some trouble with your girlfriends. They got raped."

Lynn became very emotional. "They just went out to get something to eat. Then they met these two guys who offered them food, so they went in the car with them. When they came back, my friends told me they got raped several times. But they protected me."

"Did you go along, too?"

"No. I stayed with another girlfriend at a friend's house."

"Did they know these men?"

"No."

"Were you doing any drugs?"

"Yes," she answered reluctantly. "We smoked some joints and drank some alcohol. I smoked cigarettes, but that was about it."

"I can't figure out why you want to pal around with these girls?"

"We've been best buddies since we were in fourth grade. No one can separate us, not even my mom." Her tone grew more defiant.

"How can you call them good friends if they take you into a situation that's so violent and dangerous?'

"They didn't mean it to happen. It just happened. I told you, they were *protecting* me. Why do I have to be here?" she scowled. "I don't understand."

"It's important, Lynn. I used to work in the emergency room. I remember seeing young runaways beaten up. That might have happened to you, too."

She rung her hands as I spoke. Raising her fist in front of her eyes, she shook her head like a two-year-old, as if to blot out what I was saying. Her light brown hair became disheveled.

"Friends don't do this to friends."

"They were *protecting* me," she repeated.

"You keep saying that. What does it mean?"

"They warned me to keep back because there might be trouble."

"They weren't protecting you, Lynn, they were endangering you."

I could see that in her mind, her friends somehow were helping her. Tempted as I was to feel like the parent, which was not my role, there were other pressing matters.

"Are you sexually active?"

She shot up her head. "What do you mean?"

"Have you had intercourse?"

"I haven't gone all the way."

"Has sex ever been forced on you?"

"No."

After taking a gynecological history from her, I did a physical examination. There were no bruises or scratches or other signs of physical violence. Then came the difficult part.

"I need to do a pelvic exam on you, Lynn."

"No. I'm not going to let you. There's no reason to. Nobody did anything to me." Her eyes were now impudent.

"Because of the circumstances you were in, I need to."

"You don't believe me," she complained.

"It's not whether I believe you. You've lost some credibility with your family because of your running away and lying to them."

"I never lied to anybody."

When I realized that Lynn was not going to allow me do a pelvic examination, I made a decision. "I'm going to bring your mother back in. Go ahead and get dressed."

I found the mother standing in the hallway in utter anguish. "Tell me what's going on with your daughter?" I asked.

"I don't know. Somehow she got caught up with these wild girlfriends and her whole life changed. They were a bad influence. She started cutting classes, getting herself in trouble at school, not talking to us anymore. She didn't used to be this way. We had this beautiful little girl who played flute in grade school and junior high. She was good. She was going to go to music school. Somewhere along the line we lost our daughter."

Tears welled in her eyes, her lower lip trembled and her voice cracked. When she could no longer fight it, she broke down and cried. "It's a terrible feeling," she managed to utter between sobs, "when your daughter doesn't come home one night and you have to call the police. We didn't know what happened to her for five whole days. When the detective called, you can't imagine what runs through a person's mind. We felt relieved they found her alive. Then you realize she hates you when they bring her back."

"Are you okay?"

"Yeah, I'm okay." On regaining her composure, she continued, "The worst of it is, I found out about the rapes not from my daughter, but from the mother of one of her girlfriends. My *own* daughter wouldn't even tell me."

"Have you tried counseling?"

"We've been in counseling for months. It hasn't helped."

"She's refused a pelvic exam. Legally, I can't force her."

The mother shook her head. "If she's been raped and gets pregnant over this, I'm not going to be able take it."

"Come on back in the room with me," I said. "I want to talk to both of you."

When I returned, Lynn looked away.

"Lynn, I have your mother's permission to draw some blood for a drug screen and HIV testing."

"You won't find anything," she said flippantly. "I didn't do anything wrong."

"Well, that may be, but we have to be sure. Because you won't let me do a pelvic exam here, I have no choice but to send you to the rape crisis center."

Her eyes flashed rage at me. "I won't let *them* do it either," she insisted. "They're not going to touch me."

"That will be up to you and them." When I gave the mother the address to the rape crisis center, they both left.

The last image I have is the broken mother walking solemnly down the clinic hallway followed by her defiant daughter who cast a backward glance at me. Her eyes and the lift of her chin proclaimed loudly *I won, bitch.*

Several days later, I called Mrs. Friedman. She was relieved to hear that the blood tests were negative. The rape crisis center honored her daughter's refusal to have a pelvic exam, but did make arrangements to have a pregnancy test done later.

"How is Lynn?"

"She's already gone to Oklahoma."

"Oklahoma?"

"The whole purpose was to separate her from her girlfriends. We've got family there who live near an adolescent center for troubled young girls. Hopefully, we'll see her at the holidays. When

Lynn comes back, we'll put her in a private school. We may even have to move to keep them apart." The mother's voice was sad but surprisingly resolute and hopeful.

I felt sorry for both of them. No one won. The girl had no idea of the long-term consequences of her actions. The odds were against her. She had found her mother's vulnerable spots and eventually dominated their relationship, but what good did it do? The mother, trying to put her world back in its previous order against relentless change, seemed unaware of how arduous a task lay ahead to reclaim her daughter.

THE ADOLESCENT IN CRISIS

Trapped between childhood and adulthood, teen-agers have special needs. When they seek the help of a health care professional, it's usually for an acute, often sexually-related problem. More than one million girls become pregnant each year. Conservative estimates have it that about 80% of boys and 70% of girls have intercourse by age 19. Many young adults who die with AIDS were infected as adolescents. Teen-agers have the highest rates of sexually transmitted diseases and hospitalizations for pelvic inflammatory disease (PID). These and other behavioral problems contribute to the three leading causes of teen death: accidents, homicides, and suicide.

Success in caring for minors demands effective communication skills and careful assessment. Confidentiality is a legal mandate unless it's a life-or-death situation. The practices of talking to the teenager and parents separately as well as together, adopting a non-judgmental demeanor, and being direct and honest encourage trust. Beginning with the least personal and threatening questions about afterschool activities, home, and school, the health care provider can gradually broach more sensitive issues such as depression, eating disorders, sexual activity, and substance abuse. Making teens feel comfortable and providing them with explanations and positive reinforcement may allow them to talk freely.

Knowledge is power. Educating teen-agers is crucial because they often do not consider the consequences of their behavior or how to counter peer-pressure. Teen-agers may be relieved to talk to an interested health care provider about matters they do not feel comfortable discussing with their parents. The adolescent's orientation to the present rather than to the future, the need to gratify immediate needs and to be like everyone else, and feelings of invulnerability act as barriers to changing attitudes about risky behaviors and mask underlying fear.

Although some patients can be quite difficult to work with, the effort is worthwhile. Don't underestimate yourself. Health care providers can influence their young patients for a lifetime.

SEXUAL ASSAULT

Sexual assault is on the increase. According to the American College of Obstetricians and Gynecologists, the annual incidence in 1994 was 200 per 100,000 persons in the U.S. These figures are undoubtedly low because many victims do not report sexual assault due to embarrassment, fear of retribution, feelings of guilt, or lack of knowledge about their rights. Sexual assault affects people of all ages, genders, races, and socioeconomic groups.

The health care provider assumes both a medical and a legal role. The medical priorities are to assess and treat physical injuries, obtain cultures and provide treatment or prophylaxis for sexually transmitted diseases (*C. trachomatis*, hepatitis B virus, HIV, *N. gonorrhoeae*, syphilis), offer therapy to prevent unwanted conception, provide counseling, and arrange for follow-up care. Pelvic examination allows the status of reproductive organs to be determined.

Victims of sexual assault must give informed consent before they can be examined and specimens can be collected. A third party should be present during the entire process to reassure and support the victim. It's important to talk to the victim about the injuries and likelihood of infections or pregnancy as well as possible emotional and physical consequences of the assault.

The legal role of the care provider is to accurately record events, collect samples (blood-stained clothing, fingernail scrapings, pubic hair, saliva, vaginal secretions), document injuries, and provide the "chain of evidence" to authorities. The injured areas need to be documented by drawings or photographs.

*   *   *

"I'm Pregnant"

"How long has it been since you had your baby?" I asked Marie Acevedez, a young Hispanic woman, who was back for a routine follow-
up visit.

"Seven months," she answered softly with a pretty smile, her
hands folded in her lap. Her long, wavy, dark brown hair hung down
to the middle of her back. Born in the Bronx, second generation from
Puerto Rico, Mrs. Acevedez had the sadness of an inner-city kid. Her
heart-shaped face had tiny features. She was such a pixie and looked
so childlike, it was hard to believe she was the mother of four.

"A baby girl, is that correct?"

"Yes."

"How is she doing?"

"She's okay. I'm starting to wean her. With the other children and
all, breast-feeding takes up too much time."

"How are *you* doing?" I searched her eyes. Mrs. Acevedez had a
history of panic disorders and anxiety.

"Not so good."

"What's wrong?"

She looked embarrassed. "My husband and I were having sex
about two weeks ago, but I had no suppository in me."

"Why not?"

"I forgot," she said self-consciously.

I remembered the last time I saw Marie Acevedez. She was emphatic about not having another child. "But you just had a baby. You
said you didn't want to get pregnant again."

"I know." She hung her head.

"What did you do then? Did you douche or use a spermicide?"

"I laid in bed and didn't do anything about it. I just worried."

I sat looking at her. The critical seventy-two hour window for
postcoital contraception had slammed closed.

"I don't want another baby. The new baby is very difficult for me
and I already have three other children at home. I feel very nervous.
Sometimes I feel like my children are an octopus around me. That's
why I wanted to have my tubes tied, but the doctor didn't want to do
it because I am only twenty-two-years old."

"What does your husband think?"

"My husband doesn't want a vasectomy because he had a friend who had one done and lost the use of it completely! He told me that if he gets a vasectomy, I'd have thousands of babies, but not by him."

I looked puzzled. "What did he mean?"

"He thought I would wander because he couldn't use his thing anymore." I was accustomed to the use of *thing* or *it* to indicate *penis*. It wasn't something I read in the journals.

"Marie, it seems to me, based on what you are saying, that you need to use some kind of birth control."

"I know. My mother tells me it's wrong to use anything, but I can't take care of another baby. What should I do?"

I talked to her about the available choices such as birth control pills, an IUD, a diaphragm or a condom with spermicide. Marie declined pills, didn't want to put any devices inside her, but had no problem with her husband wearing a condom. She said she would try that for a while.

"How is it going at home for you?" I inquired.

"A little better. For the time being, my sister-in-law's helping me out at the house for two hours a day, three days a week. It frees me to come out and visit my friends or come here without my children."

"That's good. I'm glad to hear that."

"By the way, what's an echocardiogram for?" Mrs. Acevedez asked nonchalantly.

"Echocardiogram? Why do you want to know about that?"

"I saw a doctor near where I live."

"Why?"

I noticed Marie Acevedez's dark brown eyes as she said, "My heart was going so fast, I thought something was wrong with it. I thought I was going to die." She described palpitations. "My doctor ordered a heart test on me. I had the test done, but I never went back for the results because I was afraid. Can you get them for me?"

"Sure. Tell me who to call."

"I have his number here." She teased a crumpled slip of paper from her choked purse.

"Have you had any more panic attacks?"

"Yes, at night. I worry constantly that I have cancer of the skin or lungs or I have heart problems." I noticed her lack of eye contact and fidgeting hands on her lap. She grew anxious just by talking about it.

"Remember now, your anxiety disorder is what's behind your worries. It will help to keep that in mind. You have worried about cancer and heart problems in the past. You don't have cancer or heart problems for real. When you feel anxious, you worry about everything. When people get anxious, their heartbeats can seem stronger and they may be aware of their heart beating in their chest. It's a common reaction to anxiety. Some people think their heart isn't working right when that happens. But that's natural. I will call about the echocardiogram, but I don't want you to be worried about it. Okay?"

"Thanks." She looked calmer.

"If you need to go back on your medicines for anxiety, we will do that. But we want to wait until you are no longer breast feeding the baby."

"I understand."

When I called about her echocardiogram, I found out it was normal. I gave her an appointment in one month and said good-bye. If the appointments were too far apart, her anxiety galloped out of control. She needed small doses of reassurance on a regular basis.

Later my office phone rang loudly. *Who could be trying to get me now instead of leaving a message with the secretary?* I picked up the receiver. "Hello."

"Oh, thank God, it's you. *Thank God.*" The caller was nearly hysterical.

"Calm down, please. Who is this?"

"Marie."

"Marie Acevedez?"

"Yes."

"What's the matter?"

"I'm *pregnant!*"

I had all I could to refrain from saying *Tell me it's not true.* Instead I said simply, "Are you absolutely sure?"

"Yes. My doctor did the test this morning."

"I'm sorry, Marie. I know you didn't want to get pregnant. I was afraid this might happen."

"I can't be pregnant," she exclaimed. "This *can't* be happening to me again."

I heard the abhorrent recrudescence of the demon Panic. "Okay, go easy. Take a few deep breaths." Over the phone it sounded like a Lamaze class. "What are you going to do?" I asked calmly.

"I don't know. That's why I called you."

"Have you told your husband?"

"No, he's at work. I told him anyway that I didn't want to get pregnant, but he didn't listen to me. Now look what happened."

"What do you think he'll want to do?"

"He doesn't care. He doesn't understand why I don't want another baby," she said with exasperation. "*He's* not the one who has to take care of all the children. *I* do."

"Have you thought about your options?"

"I don't want to have the baby. My friends think I should have an abortion."

How the whole world's gone topsy-turvy. Now that she was pregnant, I couldn't restart the very medications for anxiety that Marie needed so desperately. I felt hand-tied.

"You have choices. There's also adoption."

"I could never give up a baby."

I reviewed the various options with her. "I'm not going to push one option over the next, Marie. That's up to you and your husband. You have to talk to him. Don't put it off. I would also suggest talking to your gynecologist face to face, not over the phone. In the meantime, start taking a folic acid prenatal vitamin. It prevents birth defects. You need to take it no matter what your plans for the pregnancy turn out to be."

As I recalled her childlike manner, I felt that Marie Acevedez wanted the decision to be made for her. Given the woman's emotional state, it seemed that life was asking too much of her with this unwanted pregnancy. Medically speaking, it was probably unwise for her to have another child. Her anxiety disorder wasn't helping matters. She was already maximally stressed. I made a referral to a therapist to explore family issues and other factors. Secretly I did not feel optimistic about the outcome and wished Mrs. Acevedez had heeded the advise about birth control.

"MORNING AFTER" CONTRACEPTION

What can you do *after* the fact? Practicing a regular, reliable method of birth control is more effective than "morning after" methods, also called emergency or postcoital contraception. However, women have unprotected sex for many reasons, and postcoital contraception could prevent more than 2 million unintended and unwanted pregnancies in the United States each year.

A need for intervention: health care providers must educate women about issues related to both fertility and contraception. Women are potentially fertile up to six to eight days in the cycle and the symptoms of ovulation are easily recognizable. Oral contraceptives (OC's), the most commonly used postcoital contraceptive, must be taken within three days of unprotected sex or up to day 21 of the menstrual cycle. Their rate of preventing pregnancy when used in this manner is about 98%.

The chief types of OC's are combination OC's (ethinyl estradiol plus norgestrel or levonorgestrel) or progestin-only OC's (minipills). To use combination OC's as postcoital contraceptives, patients must take two to four pills, depending on strength, as soon as possible after unprotected sex and two more 12 hours later. Patients who cannot tolerate estrogen take progestin-only OC's: 20 pills within 48 hours of unprotected sex and 12 hours later.

Before prescribing the pills, obtain menstrual information and consider contraindications such as history of breast or liver cancer, heart disease, or stroke. Several procedures, such as breast, pelvic, and cervical mucus examinations, a PAP smear, tests for sexually transmitted diseases, and a urine pregnancy test, may be indicated. Rape victims should be referred to a rape crisis center.

In selected women, an intrauterine device, such as a copper-bearing IUD, is an effective alternative. It's not recommended for women who have not given birth, have a history of ectopic pregnancy, or are at risk for PID.

Follow-up examination should take place in three to five weeks. Postcoital contraception fails when the pregnancy is already established, the patient has multiple sexual encounters, or the dosage of medication taken or prescribed is inadequate. Rest assured. If implantation has already occurred, the pills will not cause abortion or harm the fetus.

PANIC DISORDER

What affliction did Charlotte Brontë, Robert Burns, Emily Dickinson, Sigmund Freud, Barbara Gordon, Abraham Lincoln, Edvard Munch, Sir Isaac Newton, Alfred Lord Tennyson, and Nikola Tesla—economists, painters, politicians, scientists, and writers—have in common? Panic attacks.

The admonition "Don't panic!" may not be so easy to heed. Panic, the sudden overwhelming sense of fright or terror, springs up recurrently and unexpectedly in patients with panic disorder. Unlike ordinary nervousness or anxiety, panic disorder is an intense and often debilitating condition associated with numerous physical symptoms and the sense of loss of control or dying. First appearing between late adolescence and the mid-30's, panic attacks grip about 1 to 3% of the population, have a strong familial pattern, and are diagnosed twice as frequently in women as they are in men. Repeat visits to the primary care provider or ER are characteristic.

Break the cycle; otherwise, panic evolves into a full blown syndrome. Panic attacks usually first appear during routine tasks. With education, reassurance, and support, they may not progress. Stage 2 involves fear and avoidance of events or activities associated with panic attacks and preoccupation with bodily symptoms. The final stage is agoraphobia, the fear of places or situations for which help or escape may be unavailable. Avoidance behavior leads to isolation, becoming homebound, and loss of normal functioning and relationships.

Eyes open: physical disorders that mimic panic attacks include hypoglycemia, hyperthyroidism, mitral valve prolapse, and temporal lobe epilepsy. Screening for these disorders is a priority, but failure to recognize panic disorder may lead to invasive and unnecessary diagnostic procedures.

Many conditions exacerbate, interact with, or precipitate panic disorder. Although some patients with panic disorder self-medicate with alcohol and antianxiety agents, both substances worsen the situation. Caffeinism and street drug use may precipitate panic attacks.

Patients with panic disorder are prone to major depression and suicide. Early patient education and psychiatric intervention help prevent long-term disability. For severe cases, medications are necessary. Although imipramine and alprazolam have been the standard drug treatment for panic disorder, selective serotonin re-uptake inhibitors are being used more frequently. There's room for optimism.

*   *   *

"I Hate the Person I've Become"

Just when I was trying hard to keep the morning on schedule, the worst possible thing happened: Mrs. Leslie Steiner walked in. Well-known to the group practice, she came in often to complain about *everything* in her life. Each of us groaned inwardly when we glimpsed her in the hallway if we were on walk-in duty. Mrs. Steiner's primary physician, Dr. Stan Macky, saw her weekly for fifteen minutes to reassure her. Her atrial fibrillation, degenerative joint disease, and mild hypertension were well controlled. One visit was not enough for Leslie, who stopped by three times a week with vague complaints.

"Hi, Mrs. Steiner," I said. "I just saw you with your doctor two days ago. What brings you back in so soon?"

"Oh honey, I don't know what to do with all this pain I have. It hurts to walk, sit, or stand. I feel better in my bed with my heating pad on; it's my best friend. I hope you never have to get old." She sighed from the bottom of her lungs.

Repetitive sighing was Mrs. Steiner's trademark. As she aged, she gave up on her appearance. Now she had a haggard "woe is me" look, was on the short side, and forty pounds overweight. Her arms were flabby and wiggled when she gestured. Her round visage displayed deep lines and her complexion was chalky. I was amused by the woman's unkempt hair, which gave her the appearance of Bozo the Clown.

"Well, the *bad* news is I will get old, but the *good* news is that it will be gradual," I said with a smile.

Mrs. Steiner continued to pout. "Easy for you to joke, you're younger. Just wait till you're in your seventies like me, then you'll suffer."

"Mrs. Steiner, I can't seem to locate your funny bone."

She didn't reply. I sensed an inner sadness. Mrs. Steiner was hurting.

"You seem so unhappy," I said. "Tell me why."

Mrs. Steiner looked at me then down at her hands. She turned her wedding band around and around on her finger. In a small voice she answered, "You don't need to look at my joints; they're no different than two days ago. I just want to talk to somebody who will listen to me."

"Okay."

"I am lonely and unhappy. I hate the person I've become. My son, who is fifty years old this year, calls me just twice a year—Mother's Day and on my birthday. He makes excuses why he can't travel to visit with me. I haven't seen my grandchildren in five years."

"Why is that?"

"He hates me. We had a big fight a long time ago over something trivial. Then it was a big deal; now I even forget the details. Anyway, tempers were running hot on both sides and I felt he had to bow to my will. He never did, and I didn't budge an inch toward his. That stubbornness was our undoing. I wouldn't call him and he wouldn't call me. At first his wife called to check on me and put my grandkids on to talk, but that soon stopped, too. This went on for a few years. Eventually I swallowed my pride and called one night to apologize. I'm getting older and more frail, and I'm afraid I'll never see my son and his kids again before I die."

"Did that solve the problem?"

"No. He's cool and standoffish towards me. I beg him to visit me with the kids. I complain to him about my health so that he gets the hint that I'm not doing well. I can hear the whining in my own voice. I think that pushes him away even more."

"Are you trying to make him feel guilty?"

"Yes, I suppose I am. When I was your age, I never dreamed for a minute that I would be a bitter, manipulative, old women. You wouldn't have known it, but I was something to look at back in the old days." Mrs. Steiner smiled as she reflected.

"What was the young Leslie Steiner like? I haven't a clue."

"First of all, my maiden name was Leslie Goshen. I was a pretty girl. I had shiny, naturally curly, black hair and didn't need to wear make-up. I wore a size six. I use to have a choice of which boy would walk me home after class and had lots of girlfriends at school and in my neighborhood. At the age of eighteen, I wanted to get a job in the garment district.

My father was a tailor and I had an eye for designing clothes for women. I hoped to set the world on fire, but my father was—I guess you could call him—the fireman in my life. He was set on marrying me to a nice Jewish boy with a future in business. He told me the purpose of my life was to have babies, be a loyal wife and a good mother. I had no skills, no training, and no job. I lived with my parents and I didn't have options like women do today. I loved my parents and never would have disobeyed them. Sure I was disappointed, but I did what my parents told me to do."

"So what happened next?"

"My father introduced me to my husband of forty-five years. I was a mere nineteen-years old. My husband passed away from a heart attack when I was sixty-four-years old. God bless him. He was a good man and a good husband. We had a son and I miscarried three times after that and was told I shouldn't keep trying to have babies. The doctors thought something was wrong with my womb. We had Joseph and considered ourselves blessed to have him. I was the happiest in my life being a mother. My only regret was that Joseph grew up too fast; I wished I had more children.

When Joe went away to college, I had the 'empty nest' problem real bad. I looked at my husband one day over our morning coffee and realized I didn't have a thing in common with this man. I loved him, but didn't know what made him tick. My husband was a jeweler by trade and did a nice business in the diamond district—you should have seen my engagement ring—but all in all, not a terribly interesting man. I think that was when I started complaining. I wanted some attention from my husband. Joe use to shower me with it, but not a drop from my husband."

I reflexively looked at my watch. I knew other patients were not far behind.

"I'm so sorry for taking up all your valuable time talking about my past," she said. "I guess my point was that I wasn't always like this and Joe knows it. I miss my husband these days, too. I didn't realize how lucky I was when he was with me. I would do things differently now. If you do find a nice young man and settle down, make sure you never forget the person you fell in love with and why. By the way, are you Jewish?"

"No, why?"

"Too bad, I know this nice Jewish boy about your age in my apartment building. All he needs is the right Jewish girl and his life would be complete."

I took the woman's hand in mine and said, "You need to call your son and tell him what you just told me today. Don't complain about your symptoms, he already knows them. Don't cry; he's heard you do that, too. Tell him from your heart what you're really afraid of and that you're aware of how you must sound to him. Tell him you love him and need his love. For now, work on re-establishing a link with him. Give him some time to think about what you've told him. Maybe it will seem like a breath of fresh air to him and he will be more willing to talk with you. And Mrs. Steiner, call tonight."

Mrs. Steiner looked at me with red-rimmed, watery eyes about to overflow. "Thank you, I will. I'd better be going. You've got sicker people than me to care for." She gave my hand a big squeeze. "You're a good listener."

I offered her a tissue, which she took on her way out. Expecting to find another chart, I looked outside my office. To my relief, there was none. Thinking back on Mrs. Steiner, I realized that patients who were physically ill often took less time than people who just came to talk did.

About a month later, I remembered Leslie Steiner and realized I hadn't seen her in a long time. I asked the other clinic staff about her over lunch, but no one else had seen her either. Dr. Macky said that Mrs. Steiner had canceled two weeks of appointments. He was totally surprised. I decided to call and make sure that she was okay.

The voice of the person who answered the phone was unfamiliar to me, and for a moment, I thought I might have misdialed the number.

"Hello, I'm looking for Leslie Steiner. Is she in?"

"No, my mother is out with my wife and kids at the Brooklyn aquarium. Can I take a message for her?"

I smiled. "No, that's all right, thank you."

Good for you Leslie Goshen Steiner. Good for you.

STRESS

We are living in stressful times. As many as 30 to 50% of marriages end in divorce. One in three Americans is a member of a step-family and 60% of such families disintegrate. Nearly one-third of all people in the U.S. who are 45 years of age and older are unmarried and living alone, according to the 1994 census. In an era of workaholism, habitual planning, and future orientation, Ralph Waldo Emerson's words are as true today as they were in 1834: "We are always getting ready to live but never living."

But history is full of examples of consequential family stress. Take England's early 16th century ruler Henry VIII. His efforts to annul his marriage and divorce Catherine of Aragon brought about a break with the Roman Catholic Church and started the Church of England!

Stress slices across family life. It occurs when an individual is having trouble adapting to life events and becomes overwhelmed. The significance of the events is individually defined. Objectively they may seem insignificant, even positive, such as a promotion or transfer requiring new responsibilities or relocation. Whether it's the estrangement of a elderly mother from her son or a young mother from her husband over the issue of how many children she can raise without losing her mind, the common denominator is stress.

Family stress motivates many visits to the medical clinic. "Life events" can be disruptive and stressful. It's not "all in your head." Moving, changing jobs, and marital problems are among the most stressful of the "stressors."

At different ages, the causes of stress differ considerably. Young adults face concerns over employment, careers, financial stability, marriage, and parent-child relationships. Middle-aged people are apt to be worried about changing family or spousal relationships and problems with aging parents. In old age, personal losses, physical deterioration, retirement, and thoughts of death predominate. Women, who are often caregivers of the elderly and infirm and of grandchildren, are subject to burnout as caregivers and depression. Some frenetic people overfill their lives and create extra stress.

So far not surprising. Yet it may not be as obvious that stress is every bit as deleterious as a major medical disease. Stress influences our physical as well as mental health through many mechanisms, which are now only coming to light. It compromises our immunity through interactions between the brain and immune system. Interacting with hormones, stress may tamper with fertility.

The body's stress reaction—rapid heart rate, increased blood pressure, heightened alertness—evolved to allow ancestral humans to cope and survive in a world with constant physical threats from animals and the elements. As a temporary measure, it poses little problem. Sustained stress is a different matter.

Is there "good" stress and "bad" stress? A little stress is not necessarily bad. It prevents apathy, boredom, and dullness. Exactly when stress becomes too much is an individual matter.

People react to stress in different ways. Small wonder; the possibilities are almost limitless. We become anxious, depressed, develop physical symptoms, drink alcohol, run away, or have an extramarital affair. We experience a gamut of emotions such as fear, guilt, rage, or shame, have intrusive thoughts, and manifest fatigue, hyper-alertness, impulsivity, inability to concentrate, irritability, night-mares, restlessness, sleeplessness, and tension.

Maladaptive behavior to stress becomes an adjustment or situa-tional disorder. When there is a re-experiencing of a traumatic event, the syndrome may be a post-traumatic stress disorder. Patients fre-quently self-treat with alcohol or drugs.

UNWINDING THE TENSION

The goal of treatment for stress is a quick return to satisfactory func-tion. A behavioral approach identifies the precipitators, responses, and alleviators of stress, keeping a daily log if necessary. Stress reduction techniques remove oneself from the source of stress or lim-it the reaction to stress by exercise and relaxation.

As many as one-fifth of Americans are "down shifting," delib-erately seeking less stressful employment even if it means reduced pay and less opportunity for advancement. Marriage counseling and supportive psychotherapy have a role. Limited and judicious use of sedatives as an adjunct to these other measures may allow the patient to keep functioning through the worst phase.

For those who practice yoga, the key to relaxation is the control of breathing. It becomes slower and more regular as we relax. Taking a deep breath stops the sympathetic nervous system from producing the physiologic overdrive triggered by stress. It helps normalize the heart rate and slows the release of glucose into the blood. If you're a skeptical sort, give it a try. Such a little step can provide a panoply of benefits. Get control of your life. Take one thing at a time. Put prob-lems in perspective. Concentrate on the positives.

Women may be right: having a good cry can reduce stress. Although boys and girls cry through adolescence, men are less likely to cry than women are. When surveyed, both admitted that crying was a release, but 45% of men say they don't cry, whereas only 6% of women could say the same. Researchers claim that women's pro-lactin levels, which are 50 to 60% higher than men's levels, may be involved.

Laughter is the cheapest medicine. It is a "form of internal jogging ..., an igniter of great expectations," says Norman Cousins. Laughter, part of the vocabulary of socialization from very ancient times, conveys a reassuring message of non-dominance. Besides it feels so good.

By the way, when was the last time you had a belly laugh?

PEOPLE WHO CHRONICALLY COMPLAIN

The ancient Greek physician Hippocrates, *Father of Medicine*, knew the answer to a question frequently asked by modern health care providers: "Why does this patient keep complaining?" At one time or another, especially in managing geriatric patients, the problem of the chronic complainer is enigmatic and vexing. The solution is to determine what the complaining really signifies. All complaining means something, but the meaning may be hidden.

Many patients judge health care providers more on listening skills than on medical competency. Does the patient feel rushed through the visit? Perhaps he or she did not have enough time to explain the full problem or felt that no one listened. Repeating the complaint may be an attempt to be sure the health care provider understood the problem. Listening carefully the first time actually may save the health care provider time. With geriatric patients especially, an initial comprehensive assessment is more effective at getting at the patient's needs compared to troubleshooting problems as they arise.

Is the complaint a sign of psychological or social distress? Older people go to a lot of funerals. They talk about death and see their friends die. The grief can be so upsetting they appear to be developing dementia. They may require only a dose of grief counseling rather than tests and medications.

Is the patient lonely? Perhaps the complaint is merely an excuse to visit someone who is a nice person, a companion of sorts, someone who will listen. A support or therapy group may do wonders for a lonely patient.

Does the patient remember previous conversations about the same complaint? If not, are there other indications of memory loss?

Did the treatment fail? Was the diagnosis correct? About 86% of geriatric patients have chronic illnesses, an average of four unrelated diseases, some of which are serious. Their care is difficult and time consuming because of atypical symptomatology, a higher incidence of adverse drug effects, and multi-systemic diseases. Women are more likely than men are to utilize outpatient care because they tend to suffer from chronic disease. Geriatric medicine often must deal more with managing symptoms and slowing disease progression than with curing the disease. It's not for all health care providers. We must know when to refer.

Healthcare providers should ask ourselves the following questions, advises Dr. Lu Nahemow. Do I know who my patient is? Do I understand what my patient wants from me? Am I helping my patients take charge of their care? Do I encourage patients to comply? Do I pay enough attention to the families? Do I like taking care of geriatric patients? Have I come to terms with my own feelings about aging and death? Do my patients feel comfortable talking to me about their problems? The answers may be revealing.

*　　*　　*

"I'm Not Crazy, Am I?"

"I think I might need some medication or something. I practically assaulted my husband the other night over a stupid accident. My emotions are way out of control."

Annette Long, a pretty woman in her thirties, fluffed her curly, dark hair, and fidgeted in her seat. She wore a pale, pink-and-gray jogging outfit with walking shoes.

"Did you actually hit him? Tell me what happened."

"Well, I'm a cat lover and my husband's a cat tolerator. I had a terrible pounding headache all day at work last week and it was my turn to fix dinner that night. The kids were quiet and working on their homework, thank God, but my husband kept bugging me to hurry up with dinner. I was feeling tired, stressed-out, and ready to jump out of my skin. I remember telling him to get off my case and that I could get the damn food ready if he stayed out of the kitchen."

"All right, and what's this have to do with cats?" I asked, waiting for the other shoe to drop.

"This is the inane part. I'm *so* embarrassed. Jay, my husband, stormed out of the kitchen pissed-off. Just then, Moxie—my feline companion—crossed his path and got tangled between his legs, causing my husband to take a swan dive to the carpet. Jay has quite a short temper and, while cursing, he picked up the cat and flung it practically into the stratosphere. Well, it was obviously an accident, but when I saw my husband wasn't hurt and had taken his temper out on the cat—which by the way landed fine—I just lost it."

"What did you do to him?"

"I starting throwing my prized homemade ceramic plates at him in rapid-fire sequence. Plates were flying, he was dodging, the kids started yelling, the cat was yowling, and I was crying. I think I would have finished off the eight-piece plate setting, but the sound of them breaking snapped me out of it. All of a sudden it seemed very quiet and I remember looking at all the broken plates on the red tile floor thinking why didn't they land on the carpet. Isn't that strange?"

"Was anyone hurt?"

"No, to his credit, Jay's quick on his feet. I looked up warily and found everyone's eyes on me, including the damn cat's. It's like they were thinking, 'What's wrong with you?' At that moment, I realized I needed some space and made a quick dart for my keys and purse and ran out of the house. When I came home later, of course, I apologized to my family and told them I hadn't a clue what happened earlier. Jay told me in bed later that night that I seem to act kind of crazy for a week or so every month, then I'm normal again. Do you think I need to see a shrink or is this about my hormones?"

"Do you have these feelings before, during, or after your menstrual period?"

"It seems like I'd feel bad four or five days beforehand. But over the past six months, it's longer—like seven or ten days. Half the month is living with headaches, tension, irritability at the slightest provocation, crying while watching a funeral advertisement on television, and not being able to stop for ten minutes. Would you believe that my husband is so conditioned that when we watch television, he'll gauge when my periods are due based on how quickly I start crying over a sappy commercial? The thing is, he's usually right."

"How are you with the kids? What are their ages again?"

"Oh, they're so sweet. Kim is ten years old and Jason is eight. They tend to keep a low profile and have instinctively learned to stay clear when I have my invisible war paint on. I don't like feeling this way and treating my family, friends, and coworkers like they're always wrong and I'm right. You know, maybe I inherited this emotional roller coaster. I remember my mother being bitchy at times and my siblings and I would avoid her like the plague. I can't believe it. I'm turning into my mother. ARHHG!"

"Mrs. Long, do you have any food cravings during these times you're upset?"

"Are you kidding? God, yes. I go out of my way to get chocolate snacks and anything salty. I should have known something was wrong with me when I ordered a take-out pizza loaded with anchovies for our Friday family night at home. Needless to say, I was very unpopular with my family, who let me know about it as they picked out all the anchovies. I ate all the unloved fishies and had the swollen fingers to show for it the next morning. That's another thing: I gain about three to four pounds right before my periods. Is that normal?"

"Some women get bloating due to fluid retention. It's advisable to watch the salt intake because, wherever there is salt, water is sure to follow. Also, if you curtail the high sugar intake, you can control the peak and rapid drop in your blood sugar."

She looked bewildered. "Is there is a name for this problem?"

"Yes, it's called Premenstrual Syndrome or *PMS* for short. Many women have PMS and some have it so bad it can be incapacitating in their daily activities."

"And you're pretty sure it's what I have?"

"Yes, fairly sure. Let's first do a physical exam first. Then I want to run some blood tests for any sugar and thyroid problems, but I don't think the tests will be abnormal."

"What can I do about it?"

"I'll review with you a diet to follow and some vitamins. I suggest you keep a diary of your eating habits and moods. There are medications for severe PMS, but I don't recommend them until you've tried some lifestyle changes first."

"So I'm not nuts, right?"

"No, it's unlikely, although the jury is still out on the pizza with anchovies. Just kidding! The key to controlling PMS is to recognize it, which is difficult when you're in the center of the storm. You may have to depend on your husband or cues from your kids."

"Well, that certainly won't be a problem. Jay is right back at me these days with targeted questions like *Is it getting to be that time of month again, Hon?* or, better yet, *You're starting to get weird on me.* I honestly think just hearing his comments can throw me into a bad mood. As usual, I return to my old self after my period starts, life is good again, and my family was right after all."

"Also, to help blow off steam when tension is running high, it's a good idea to get into a regular exercise pattern. Take a half-hour walk every day, swim, run, play tennis, or join a club and do some aerobics. The point is that after exercising you're more tired and relaxed and less likely to pop off at somebody. Now that you need more dinnerware, you could sign up for a community ceramics workshop and 'throw' some pots and plates constructively. Refocus you energy."

"Okay, I like those ideas. I'm psyched."

"Mrs. Long, let's meet back in one month, review your blood tests and see how making some changes affects you and your family. Any questions?"

"Yeah, just one. What'll I tell the pizza place to do with all those anchovies they special-ordered just for me?"

PREMENSTRUAL SYNDROME UNVEILED

For women in certain Native American tribes, menstruation was understood to be a time to regain spiritual energy while menstrual blood purified and cleansed the womb, removing men's dead sperm. They lived apart from their families in a separate tent during the first four days of menstruation in calm and quiet. However, for women in modern times, the menstrual cycle is anything but a time of rest. For their spouse, it may evoke shear dread.

The word is finally out. The American College of Obstetrics and Gynecology reports that 80% of women of reproductive age experience some premenstrual behavioral and physical changes. Only in about 2 to 10% of women are the symptoms severe enough to disrupt and compromise interpersonal relationships and work. For years the existence of a distinct premenstrual syndrome (PMS) has been controversial because of its overlap with atypical depression, which also manifests anxiety, emotional hypersensitivity, food cravings, and irritability.

There's more news. The term *premenstrual dysphoric disorder* (PMDD) describes women who suffer from a more severe form of PMS with functional impairment. A cyclic pattern of premenstrual symptoms for several days to two weeks with postmenstrual relief is quintessential. The woman also must have at least five of the following symptoms: anxiety or tension, appetite changes, decreased interest in activities, depressed mood, difficulty concentrating, fatigue, feeling out of control or overwhelmed, physical symptoms (bloating, breast tenderness, cramps, headaches, weight gain), or sleep disturbance. High daily symptom ratings for two consecutive menstrual cycles confirm the diagnosis. Most women are in their 30's when they seek help for the problem, but symptoms usually present in the late 20's and worsen with age. Those with PMDD are at increased risk for other mood disorders.

Is PMDD hormonal? Symptoms do correlate with the progesterone cycle, but hormonal therapies, such as hormone (GnRH) agonists or antagonists, appear to be more useful in controlling the physical than the behavioral symptoms.

Behind the mystique, what's going on in the brain? Because the selective serotonin reuptake inhibitors (SSRI's) are effective in about 60% of the cases, involvement of the serotonin system, which affects mood and behavior, has been proposed. Non-SSRI's such as alprazolam are also effective, however.

No one drug benefits all affected women, and no single SSRI has been shown to be superior. Whether the drugs can be taken intermittently or whether chronic therapy is necessary is under study. Changes in dosage or drugs should be made after observing their effect for one menstrual cycle. Manipulation of diet, exercise routine, and stress reduction also are worth trying alone and in combination with medication.

*   *   *

"You Don't Understand What It's Like"

Every so often I see a patient a couple of times before I realize that he or she is seeking help for something other than the real problem. Such was the case with Tina Rakel. The forty-one-year-old, African-American, professional woman sat in my office dressed in a black, designer pantsuit and beige, silk blouse, absent-mindedly running her hand along two, delicate gold chains around her neck. She began to address her stomachaches, headaches, trouble sleeping, and stress at work, but seemed preoccupied, trailing off and not finishing her sentences.

I noticed she was looking at a wall poster about prenatal care.

"Are you trying to get pregnant?" I asked on a hunch.

She turned toward me in surprise. A look of relief that someone had asked the question washed over her face. "I've been trying to conceive for years."

"Have you seen a fertility specialist?"

"We've seen a couple of doctors and they ran some tests." She readjusted the large black bow that held her hair tightly drawn to her head. "I took hormones, but no one seems to be able to help us. Every time I'd be hopeful and then my period would come. It was such a letdown."

"What were you told is the problem?"

"They said my husband's sperm count is okay but I have 'bad eggs.' The egg can be fertilized and starts to divide, but then it stops. The last doctor said it was hopeless." She paused. "I can remember that day vividly. That was the moment it dawned on me I wasn't going to be able to conceive."

"It's the biological clock. There's nothing wrong with you personally. I'm sure he meant that the eggs are merely too old. The biological clock for women is a quirk of nature."

"It's so unfair."

"I know. Men can procreate into old age."

"Do you know what it feels like inside to be denied something you feel you have a right to have and not be able to do anything about it? My body has failed me. I have taken care of it, watched my weight, exercised. I didn't drink or do drugs. Now all I ask is for one good egg." She blinked away tears at the thought. Then she paused and looked away. "It's hard for a person like myself who prides herself on being resourceful and a problem-solver not to be able to dig under, climb, or knock down the infertility fence. I'm frustrated and angry at myself for allowing this to happen."

"It sounds like you blame yourself."

"You know, when I was thirty-years old and just out of law school, we moved to Richmond. A gynecologist asked me if I planned to have children. I told her yes, but not right away. She warned me I'd better start soon because infertility was a problem for women over thirty-five. I remember thinking, I'm only thirty, I've got time. My husband and I were busy with our careers and could never find the right time to start a family."

Tears rolled down her flushed cheeks. I pushed the tissue box closer to her. She dabbed at the constant stream then blew her nose.

After a silence I said "I'm not making light of this, but it isn't the end of the world. Not giving birth isn't the worst thing that could happen to you, is it?"

"Yes it *is*!" she exclaimed in a hysterical crescendo. "You don't understand what it's like. I'm *barren*! I've got nothing to live for now. It's over. My life is *over*." The moment of panic in her voice was swept away by the wave of sorrow that followed. She began to sob, first softly, then uncontrollably.

I handed her a tissue and tried to reassure her, but the torrent of hurt within her gushed from a much deeper well than I could have known. Her grief needed to be released. Several minutes—a small eternity—passed before I could comfort her to the point where she was able to discuss the matter more calmly.

If there is any human condition more painful and difficult than anguish to watch another suffer, I haven't seen it in my practice. We've all experienced it at one time or another, and we know it can be revisited upon us at any time.

"I'm letting my parents down," she said, still fighting back tears. "They want grandchildren. I'm an only child, so I'm their one chance. Every cousin, friend, neighbor, or acquaintance who's had a baby I've heard about from my mother. If we go to a restaurant, she has to point out every baby in the place. It's like she doesn't think about what that's doing to me inside. Her personality has changed since she knows she's not going to get a grandchild. She's become bitter."

"Parents can put too much pressure on their children sometimes."

"It's not only my parents."

"Is your husband supportive of you?"

"Yes, I guess, but I know I'm letting him down, too. He wants a boy real badly."

"Is he saying you *must* have a child?"

"No, but every time we're out, like in the mall, he stares at all the little kids, especially the boys. He tells me he's all right and it's not a big deal, but you should see the look in his eyes. It tears a piece out of my heart every time because I know I can't give him the one thing he wants. Around holidays it's even worse. If you don't have a family of your own, there seems to be no point to them. All I can see now is babies everywhere—in the playgrounds, on TV, even on billboards. Everyone's pregnant but me."

My mind wandered to TV ads for cereals, fabric softeners, life insurance, facial soaps, and the like. It is a competitive multibillion dollar industry and babies are advertisers' aces.

"You'd be surprised at how people treat you if you're in your late thirties or early forties and you don't have kids. When you meet them, they invariably ask *Do you have children*? When you say no, it's a real conversation stopper. People look at you with pity. They don't know what to say, or they comment *That's a shame.* Men don't say that to my husband, but women say it to me. Even our friends with children at times seem to feel uncomfortable around us.

I've had perfect strangers in the ladies room ask me if I have children, and when I say no, they have the nerve to ask *Why, don't you like children?* I've also overheard women say after having children in their twenties that to be pregnant in their forties would be intolerable. I used to ignore their comments, but now I feel like crying. It seems like the only thing worse than being an atheist in this country is not having children." She became sullen.

I thought back to an anthropology class I once took in college about fertility and all the rituals and cultural rewards around it. The fertile woman is exalted and placed on a pedestal.

"Don't you think maybe you're being too hard on yourself?"

"No. I had the opportunity when I was young, but my priorities were different. I thought I had all the time in the world to get pregnant and raise a family. I've made so many wrong decisions in my life. I wish I had it to do over again."

Many patients expressed that same sentiment in so many words and under so many different circumstances.

"Mrs. Rakel, I don't want to offend you or suggest anything contrary to your religious views, but there *are* other alternatives. What about a doner egg from another woman? You would be the biological or birth mother. At least the child would have fifty-percent of your husband's genes."

"It's not the same unless it's your own flesh and blood."

"After a whole pregnancy, don't you think you'd be attached to the child?"

"It would seem like something foreign in me. And what if the donor female has very different traits? All I can think about are people telling me the child doesn't look at all like me."

"Well, I guess you could attribute it to your husband's side of the family. That could work out in your favor I suppose if it's a bad trait." I felt the need to get her to smile a little. It didn't work. She shook her head.

"How about adoption?"

"We've heard such horror stories about raising adopted children and their struggles later to find their biological parents. It can destroy a family. We're not sure yet if we want to get into that. I know how it must sound, but I can't help what I'm feeling right now. We haven't said no to it."

"You're honest about your feelings. I'm not trying to suggest that you should take any of those options, but I wanted to be sure you were aware of them."

These were some of the major philosophical questions about life, not cloaked in fancy terms or abstract principles. Here in the middle of a busy clinic, Tina Rakel was pouring out her soul to me. I was no philosopher or psychotherapist. I could feel her pain, but didn't know how I could make a difference. She'd considered many options, but also had strong feelings about what she saw as viable choices. I did know I could listen and help her make a plan.

We sat without speaking for a moment. "Where to next?" I asked.

She looked up at me. "I don't know."

"Do you want to see a counselor?"

She looked away again. "I don't know if it would help."

"Does your husband know how deeply you feel about these matters?"

She sighed. "Probably not."

"Well then, this is too big a burden for one person. A counselor won't tell you what to do, but can explore the reasons for your feelings. Understanding them might allow you to think more freely about solutions."

"Should my husband go, too?"

"Yes. Maybe not at first, but definitely at some point. You're both in this together."

I considered all the people who came to see me over the issue of fertility—either too much or too little of it; all the children abused by parents who didn't want them; the babies orphaned, damaged, and stigmatized by AIDS and substance abuse; the paucity of healthy American infants available for an ever burgeoning population wanting to adopt; the incongruities, inconsistencies, and irreconcilable points of view. Does it make sense?

I guess it's all a matter of perspective.

INFERTILITY

Gods and goddesses of fertility commanded large followings of ancient peoples. The Egyptians worshipped cow-headed Hathor and the mysterious Isis. Greek followers paid homage to Reha, and Serapis, who were also later adulated throughout the Roman Empire. Freyja, the Norse goddess of fertility—blond, blue-eyed, and lovely—traveled on a chariot drawn by cats. Almost every culture has placed a premium on fertility.

The average married woman in seventeenth century America gave birth to 13 children! Those who could not have children often were viewed as punished or cursed, at the very least unlucky. Napolean reluctantly divorced his wife Josephine because she could not bear a son, an heir, which his 18 year old second wife did for him within a year. "The pain of infertility never killed anyone," Dr. Paul Rainsbury notes, "but it's left a lot of broken hearts." Public attitudes toward infertility have evolved to recognition that it's a treatable condition with diverse causes.

The medical community's understanding and therapy of infertility and reproductive physiology have also improved greatly along with the development of new procedures and products. These trends are fortuitous because infertility clutches 10 to 25% of American couples during their childbearing years. Although only about 40% of infertile couples ever seek any care for the problem, the cost of treatment nationwide is $1 billion annually.

Who's at risk? One year of unsuccessful conception with unprotected intercourse is the usual threshold for infertility testing. Women older than 35 are at highest risk. Why? A woman is born with all the ova she will ever have. Of those 500,000 eggs, perhaps the largest cells in the human body, only 400 will mature, and their numbers diminish throughout life. Eggs decrease in reproductive viability sometimes long before menopause; hence the pronouncement: "the eggs are too old." Compare that with the 200 million sperm produced by male testes each day throughout life.

All of the following imperil fertility: alcohol, cigarettes, certain contraceptive practices, douches, excess caffeine, family history of genetic disorders, hypothyroidism, improperly timed intercourse and ovulation, low libido, prescription and recreational drugs, repeated abortions, sexually transmitted diseases, unsuccessful sex techniques, and vigorous athletic training.

STRATEGIES FOR GETTING PREGNANT

Overcoming infertility. Start with a simple chart of basal body temperature, episodes of coitus, time of menstruation, and a urine test for midcycle (LH) surge. Cervical mucus should be examined six hours after intercourse to verify its characteristics, the absence of many white blood cells, and the presence of spermatozoa. The next step may be a radiographic dye injection into the uterus (hysterosalpingography), endometrial biopsy, laparoscopy, or other procedures looking for structural abnormalities and endometriosis.

The male partner contributes to infertility in about half the cases. A semen analysis for ejaculate volume, sperm concentration, morphology, and motility is routine.

The business of treating infertility has become high-tech. Infertility treatment may be medical, surgical, or both. Antimicrobials eliminate cervicitis and prostatitis. Adhesions and endometriosis may be rectified during laparoscopy. Drugs used to induce ovulation include clomiphene and gonadotrophin-releasing hormone. Artificial insemination delivers washed, concentrated sperm directly into the uterus through a tiny catheter.

Now for some catchy acronyms. There are several assisted reproductive technologies (in order of increasing invasiveness): *in vitro* fertilization (IVF), gamete intrafallopian transfer (GIFT), and zygote intrafallopian transfer (ZIFT). All of the procedures require ovarian stimulation, oocyte retrieval by needle aspiration (trans-vaginal, ultrasound-guided), and handling of the oocytes outside the body. In 1997 alone, 12,000 IVF babies were born.

The remaining reproductive obstacles require innovative solutions. Fertilized but not unfertilized eggs can be frozen and successfully thawed for later use, provided they are kept at ultra low temperatures (below those on the planet Saturn). Some women would like to have eggs removed when they are in their twenties for use in the following decade. A technique for supplementing an older woman's egg with cytoplasm from a younger donor's egg is being tested. If successful, it may become clinically available over the next several years.

Couples must also be counseled about the rate of multiple births and risks to the infants. Some centers use fetal reduction—an ethically charged issue—to reduce four or five embyros to one or two. Better techniques for preventing unwanted multiple births caused by fertility drugs are needed.

A final word about money. Most Americans would agree that a couple's choice about infertility matters is personal; they should do what they want to do. But the decision is often financial, thanks to managed care insurance companies who limit options for infertile couples or provide no coverage at all. The costs are not trivial. For assistive reproductive technologies, a couple may spend 10 to 20 thousand dollars per attempt or cycle.

5

Chronos, Father Time

Not everyone grows to be old,
but everyone has been younger than he is now
—EVELYN WAUGH

What is the worst of woes that wait on age?...
To view each loved one blotted from life's page,
And be alone on earth, as I am now
—LORD BYRON

Every man desires to live long, but no man would be old
—JONATHAN SWIFT

Forty is the old age of youth; fifty is the youth of old age
—FRENCH PROVERB

Women, as they grow older, rely more and more on cosmetics.
Men as they grow older, rely more and more on a sense of humor
—GEORGE JEAN NATHAN

"I Walk"

"How are you, Mrs. Steuben? Are you feeling well?"

"*Ya, ya*, very good."

Gertrude Steuben *never* complained about herself; *tired, old* and *pain* weren't in her vocabulary. She was stoic and iron-willed. Although she looked her age—on the brink of ninety-six years—she had the bluest eyes, which didn't miss a trick, and keen hearing as well.

"Have you been having any new problems?"

"*Nein, nein.*" She dismissed the very thought with a quick, vigorous head shake. Here was a woman from the old country with a moderately thick German accent despite living in the United States for over forty years. She enjoyed her independence and hoped to live many more years. From time to time, she came to see me for a blood pressure checkup.

"Well, let's see how your blood pressure's been doing."

Mrs. Steuben never needed to be told when it was time to approach the examining table. When she surmised that the history interview was over, she sat on the table and began unbuttoning her dress. She always wore the same navy blue dress with a black belt at the waistline and black buttons down the front. When she sat, the dress pulled tightly over her thighs, revealing garter snaps. Her shoes, which were orthopedically designed, reminded me of my sixth grade teacher's shoes. They were black and laced, with a one inch heel. She extended her arm, waiting for the blood pressure cuff to be applied.

I pumped up the blood pressure cuff and watched the mercury fall one heart beat at a time in the manometer. After I finished, she removed the cuff. Timing and precision were important to Gertrude Steuben. She was most efficient, much like German engineering—a real piece of craftsmanship.

"I'm going to listen to your heart and lungs now."

She allowed me just enough time to auscultate her breath and heart sounds. As soon as I lifted my stethoscope off her chest, Mrs. Steuben started buttoning her dress. It was not because she was cold; she was done and ready to depart.

"Your blood pressure is fine, Mrs. Steuben. Keep taking your medicine. You are doing a good job."

Mrs. Steuben nodded.

"What transportation did you take to get to the clinic?"

"Since I was a young girl in Germany, I always relied on my own two legs," she replied with conviction.

"How far away is your home?"

"I walk uptown twenty blocks to come here." Her voice brimmed with pride.

"Did you come here with your husband?"

"Heavens, no. I buried him when I was seventy-eight years old. We were married forty-five years. We came to America together."

"Maybe you should take a bus or the subway."

"Buses and subways are for invalids and lazy people. I walk." She gathered her purse and sweater and said good-bye.

Mrs. Steuben was the antidote for some of my dependent and helpless patients. Her visits did not last long enough.

HYPERTENSION

High blood pressure or hypertension has been called a "disease of civilization." Afflicting a third of all Americans in their 50's, half of those in their 60's, and more than two-thirds over 70, hypertension is a "silent killer." Although it is a leading cause of congestive heart failure, heart attack, kidney failure, and stroke, hypertension is easy to detect and control with changes in diet, lifestyle, and medications.

What are the numbers? Hypertension is defined as a systolic blood pressure consistently at or above 140 millimeters of mercury (mm Hg), a diastolic pressure of at least 90 mm Hg, or both. The diagnosis is made after several blood pressure measurements over time unless the initial reading is extremely high.

For giraffes, high blood pressure—two to three times that of humans—is a fact of life. But they have huge hearts, 2 feet long and weighing 25 pounds, to compensate for the enormous demands of pumping blood 10 to 12 feet upward to the brain.

Weight lifters can drive up their blood pressure to a vein-popping 300/200 for brief periods. However, in humans, large, sustained elevations in blood pressure create a medical emergency (malignant hypertension), injuring the brain and retinas (hypertensive encephalopathy), heart, and kidneys. Chronic elevations of lesser magnitude, which damage by gradual increment, are no less dangerous. Hypertension thickens arteries and leaves them hardened, less elastic, and scarred. The heart must then labor more to pump blood throughout the body.

Primary or essential hypertension, which has no known cause, can be traced to risk factors such as alcohol use, family history of hypertension, increasing age, African-American descent, obesity, poor diet, sedentary life style, and smoking. Processed food harms by providing more sodium than potassium, a reversal of physiologic ratios in diets of natural foods.

A change in lifestyle may control hypertension without the need for medication. Curbing daily alcohol consumption to less than an ounce, walking for 30 to 40 minutes, losing 10 pounds, quitting smoking, and eating a reduced fat and sodium diet lower blood pressure significantly.

If medications are necessary, there are several categories to choose from, depending on the severity of hypertension and other factors. *Diuretics*, also known as "water pills," are often the first choice. *Adrenergic blockers* (alpha, beta, and alpha-beta) reduce the force and rate of heart contractions or dilate blood vessels. *Angiotensin converting enzyme (ACE) inhibitors* and angiotensin receptor blockers relax blood vessels by blocking the formation or action of angiotensin. *Calcium channel blockers*, especially the long-acting types, also relax blood vessels to control hypertension.

So treatments are out there. The *Monthly Prescribing Reference* attests to all the new ones. We just need to make the diagnosis. Only about 50% of patients with hypertension in the U.S. are being treated with prescription drugs, and blood pressure is under control in less than 25% of patients with hypertension. One-half of treatment failures are due to adverse effects of medication, complex drug regimens, cost, inadequate or inappropriate therapy, lack of patient education, and noncompliance. Truly "resistant" hypertension occurs in less than 10% or patients with hypertension.

OSTEOPOROSIS: SILENT THIEF

Gertrude Steuben was right: walking is good medicine. It's one simple measure to combat a most formidable obstacle to being healthy in old age: osteoporosis. Women comprise 80% of the 25 million Americans who have osteoporosis, which literally means *porous bone.* Osteoporosis is one of the biggest threats women face because it causes bone fractures. Women fall prey as a result of their lower bone mass than men and declining estrogen levels in their late 30's and early 40's. Consider that about 38 million women in the U.S. have gone through menopause.

Osteoporosis has been called the "silent thief," fracturing more than 200,000 bones per year and robbing people of their lives—exercise, freedom of movement, confidence to go outside, even independent living. Over a lifetime, a woman's risk of sustaining a hip fracture exceeds her combined risk of having breast, endometrial, and ovarian cancer. Fewer than 10% of people are able to walk on their own after a hip fracture due to osteoporosis. The disfiguring "dowager's hump" (kyphosis) results from vertebral compression fractures. Wrist fractures are also more common in women with osteoporosis.

According to WHO guidelines, a bone mineral density more than 2.5 standard deviations below the mean value for healthy young women signifies osteoporosis. When the abnormality is less severe the condition is called osteopenia, a warning sign of impending osteoporosis. Bone densitometry using dual-energy x-ray absorptiometry (DEXA scanning) is now state-of-the-art for assessing bone mineral density, but quantitative ultrasound scanning is also being tested. Markers of bone resorption are helpful clinically in determining the risk of bone fractures.

Calcium supplementation before bone loss starts, safe weight-bearing exercise, and estrogen replacement therapy are cornerstones to prevention and treatment. Drugs such as alendronate, calcitonin, and estrogen build bone mass by inhibiting bone resorption. Avoid alcohol consumption, excessive thinness, falling, or smoking. Our bones demineralize with disuse; use them or lose them.

"Designer estrogens" (naloxifen and tamoxifen), like natural estrogen, help prevent osteoporosis and Alzheimer's disease, reduce "bad cholesterol" (LDL), and diminish the risk of breast cancer. Unlike natural estrogens, they neither relieve the symptoms of menopause nor cause uterine cancer. Natural estrogen replacement was the most dispensed drug in the U.S. in 1996—45 million times. The new estrogens will impinge on these figures.

We must introduce preventative strategies as soon as possible—decades before they're needed. How well a young girl's bones grow may determine her quality of life in old age. Her youthful level of exercise and diet by the age of 18 contributes to 90% of the bone mass she will ever have. Planning to be healthy in old age must be a way of life from youth.

Here's an idea. Perhaps we should teach our girls a modification of the school-yard taunt:

> *Sticks and stones can break my bones,*
> *and so can osteoporosis.*

*   *   *

"I Never Want to Get That Old"

"Why did you come to the clinic today?" I asked Angela Guitterez, a plump Hispanic woman who spoke English fairly well. She wore her thick gray hair down to her shoulders and flipped up in a sixties style.

"To get the results of my tests." Mrs. Guitterez smiled. For someone getting on in years, now already sixty-six, her spirit was healthy and enjoyable. "You can look, but don't touch," she told the preschool child across the room. "I hope you don't mind," she said to me, "I had to bring my granddaughter here today to help out my daughter—she's a single mom and has to work."

"Not a problem. She's cute. What's her name?"

"Tell the lady it's Maria."

"Maria, I like the beautiful pink bow in your hair and your pretty blue dress. Look, you've got yellow and white and pink flowers on your dress." I didn't know which was cuter, Maria's dimples, her double ponytails, or the little laced white socks folded over at the top with her black patent leather shoes.

The child grew shy, put her finger near the corner of her mouth, and retreated to her grandmother's side.

"You may not think she's so cute after awhile," Mrs. Guitterez said. The paucity of lines on her full face gave the impression she didn't frown much in her life, but she had reason to: she lost her husband to heart disease.

"You had your yearly checkup?"

"Yes." She turned her head. "Maria, this is the doctor's office. You have to be good now, okay. Come here near grandma."

Mrs. Guitterez got up and retrieved the girl from the reading materials she was touching. "She tires me out, this one." The woman plunked back into the chair.

I looked through her chart. "Let's see here. The blood tests were all normal. Your cholesterol looks good." I flipped some pages. "The mammogram report was"—I paused to read down to the interpretation—"normal. And your Pap smear—I have it right here. Okay, it was normal, too."

She looked relieved. "Good."

"That's the best news I can give a person."

Mrs. Guitterez laughed; she laughed easily. Then she got serious. A mental cloud passed over her radiant equanimity. "I hope I'm never so bad physically or mentally that I want to hang it up and die."

"What makes you say that?" I hadn't expected the comment.

"When I had the blood drawn for these tests, I was sitting in the waiting room at the lab and watching people older than me. I was horrified." Her pretty eyes sparkled as she spoke. "All they did was whine, fret, and complain so much that it was getting on my nerves. I asked them what their problems were and their answers were disturbing: pain, loss of loved ones, dying. They insisted on telling me details I didn't want to know. I felt fortunate not to have those kind of problems. I'm still able to get out and visit my friends. I never want to get that old and feel that terrible."

"I don't blame you. But you know, I would guess you're the kind of person who sees the glass as half full, not half empty. You are thankful there *is* a glass."

Mrs. Guitterez laughed, wrinkling up the corners of her eyes. "Well, I try to keep a good outlook."

"I admire that. You are much younger than your years."

The woman beamed. "Thank you."

Meanwhile, Maria had pulled all the pamphlets about diseases for patient education out of their holders amidst playful, self-contented murmuring.

"Put them back," Mrs. Guitterez said.

"I want to read them," the child insisted.

"You can't read yet. Besides, you don't have arthritis or these other diseases. You don't need to read about that." Mrs. Guitterez turned to me. "See what I mean?" She said good-bye and they left.

There weren't too many people like her in the clinic. She projected unmistakable inner warmth and good will. Maybe she would consent to stay all day and try to put the other patients in a better frame of mind. An ounce of Angela Guitterez's outlook could sustain me and many of my other patients, I thought.

I guess it's true. Youth is not a time of life—it is a state of mind.

THE BATTLE AGAINST LOOKING OLD

Apparently John Davies of Hereford was wrong. Beauty's not just skin deep—it goes to the bone. For most people the effect of age on the face is a story of sagging and loss. We all lose bone mass, the thick dermis layer, overall facial support, skin integrity, and subcutaneous fat. Both skin and muscles become lax.

Never fear: plastic surgeons can transport fat, cartilage, and bone from one part of the body to another, restructuring, augmenting, or restoring at will, but it's not painless or cheap. The top ten cosmetic procedures performed on women in 1996, according to the American Academy of Cosmetic Surgery, were: chemical peel (490,416 women), sclerotherapy (488,328), liposuction (238,000), laser resurfacing (119,253), blepharoplasty (84,290), breast augmentation (76,407), rhinoplasty (71,959), facelift (42,269), dermabrasion (41,166), and hair transplantation or restoration (27,383).

But the time for strategic planning against the effects of aging is when we are young. Some say the eyes are the key to looking younger. The top eye agers are cigarette smoking, drinking less than 8 glasses of fluid a day, inadequate sunglasses, pollution, squinting, and sun exposure (photo-aging). Cut down on crow's feet and facial lines by making these few simple lifestyle changes.

*   *   *

"It's So Eloquent"

Iris Savick looked up expectantly as I opened the door. The first thing I noticed was how bright her eyes were; they seemed to illuminate the room. Her skin seemed soft, like a baby with wrinkles—not deep ones, just superficial. She appeared to be in her fifties.

"I think my toe is broken. You should have seen it yesterday, it was worse." She massaged her foot as she sat on the examining table, dressed in black, spandex pants and a loose-fitting, hot-pink shirt.

"Tell me what happened."

The words tumbled out. "My adorable grandchild—she's three years old—came running up to me to show me something and I had on my sandals. She ran into my foot with a her little, red wagon. I screamed and thought I saw stars—it was so *painful*. Then she started crying, and I felt bad I startled her. But the darned thing hurt so. It just kept throbbing."

"When did this happened?"

"A couple of days ago. First the toes swelled up, then my whole foot got black and blue. I'm here because I need something for the pain. I've got a dance rehearsal."

"What kind of dancing do you do?"

"Oh, I do ballroom dancing. It's so eloquent. Been dancing for forty years now. I love dressing up and looking pretty." She ran her hand through her thick, wavy, silver, almost shimmering hair. Most of it was pulled over the sides of her head and caught in the back under a fluffy white tie. A few strands had escaped. "Have you ever seen the gowns?"

I nodded.

"They're fabulous. And so feminine. You can see, I need my foot better so I can get back to dancing."

While I examined her foot, she continued to reminisce. "I used to weigh a-hundred-and-ten pounds. If you could have seen me when I was younger, I was so pretty—ouch, that hurt some."

"Sorry." I finished examining her foot. "You're still pretty. You don't look your age."

"Bless you." She stood and gave me a quick hug.

I ordered an x-ray because the last two toes were swollen and extremely painful. Both were fractured.

"The good news is you won't need a cast. The bad news is you do have fractures and will have to stay off your foot a few weeks. As the swelling goes down, your foot will feel better."

I buddy-taped them to the nearest normal toe, then wrapped her foot using a compression wrap. Afterwards I reviewed with her the R.I.C.E. treatment: rest, ice, compression, elevation.

She was disappointed. "Well, maybe I can spend more time with my grandchildren. I wish they were babies again. I just love taking care of babies. I miss them so much. If I could have a baby now I would."

"Really? Well, you know, there are hospitals in need of people like you to volunteer and spend time rocking and feeding abandoned and neglected babies."

"Oh, I'm interested in that." Her eyes widened.

The look on Iris Savick's face convinced me that another chapter in her life was about to open, one she would later reread and relish many times.

WELLNESS AND WHOLENESS IN THE OLDER ADULT

George Washington would have told you the truth. When he became President in 1789, life expectancy for Americans at birth was about 35 years. Now life expectancy hit a record high: 76 years. All the more reason to assure the wellness and wholeness of the aged. The U.S. Bureau of the Census reported in 1991 that of all those 65 and older, about 31% live alone, 54% live with a spouse, 12% live with relatives, and a few percent with non-relatives. Women were two and one-half times more likely than men were to be living alone. The longest-lived person was a woman 122 years old!

Ralph Waldo Emerson once penned in his journals: "All diseases run into one, old age." Today, many people are reaching old age in good health. We've all heard that as we age we need to diet to help prevent diabetes and exercise to stave off osteoporosis and heart disease, but the hardest task may be to keep the mental outlook fit.

To offset the gradual decline in vitality and increased vulnerability associated with aging, older adults must preserve the sense of self and strive toward a maximum level of functioning. Key areas are connectedness, healing, humanistic activities, and self-actualization. This is what the WHO had in mind: "Health is a state of complete physical, mental and social well-being, and not merely the absence of disease or infirmity."

Living alone doesn't necessarily mean being lonely. Getting socially active can take the form of joining civic or church groups, spending more time with family, or meeting neighbors for coffee or outings. Hobbies, such as cooking, gardening, painting, playing a musical instrument, woodworking, or anything else a person enjoys, can bring happiness. Getting regular physical exercise improves the appetite, betters health, and promotes good sleep. Traveling on a small or large scale with friends or travel groups is often exciting and memorable.

As Mae West was fond of saying, "You're never too old to become younger."

*   *   *

"I Heard It from My Husband"

When Lena Wilson came to the clinic, I knew I was in for the update of the week. The woman knew about all the recent happenings in town. She was the CD/ROM of persons, places, and things.

"Do you know if the FDA has cleared that new European drug for high blood pressure?" When she told me its name, she was surprised I hadn't heard about it. She then recited several other bits of health information before going on to news about current events, politics, gardening tips, travel, movies, and fashion trends.

"Where do you hear all this news?" I finally asked.

Mrs. Wilson laughed with satisfaction. She was a petite woman who wore little spectacles and was in the habit of peering over them. Her uncombed, short hair seemed to have no sharp boundaries—it trailed off into the air.

"From my husband."

"But I thought your husband was dead?" I was sure of my information.

"He is."

"So you remarried?"

"Heavens, no." Mrs. Wilson laughed unselfconsciously again. "My husband is my radio."

"What?"

"When my husband died, I was very lonely, particularly at night. I got in the habit of playing the radio. I would turn it on in the evening. I put it on my dresser near the head of the bed. It comforted me so I kept doing it, listening to it longer each evening. Now I play it all night long."

"Doesn't it keep you awake?"

"No. I turn down the volume. When I wake up in the morning, the radio is on. I hear familiar voices talking. It comforts me then, too."

"Have you had a chance to get out and try any of those social activities we talked about last time?"

"Yes, and I am more active that way; but nothing takes the place of my radio."

I nodded, almost understanding. I tried not to see the dark side Lena Wilson's life. Whatever kind of companion the radio could be, for now at least, it was working for her.

"Keep it up, Mrs. Wilson," I said lightheartedly. "I depend on you for the news."

SUPPORT FOR WIDOWS AND WIDOWERS

Loss of spouse and family members is a major cause of depression in the aged. Depression can make you feel all alone in the world. Leave it to holidays to intensify feelings of boredom, isolation, and loss. For these reasons, social support from family and friends may foster the adjustment to a successful new life.

The message is clear. If the newly bereaved have only a small social network, they should be encouraged to contact the Senior Citizen Center for meals, social events, and trips. Senior centers usually serve a hot meal on weekdays and provide a free shuttle service or other means of transportation.

Persons who have been involved in volunteer activities that provide social contact should resume those activities as soon as possible. A job can promote feelings of self-worth and usefulness. Employment services are resources for full-time or part-time jobs.

Bereavement support groups do exist, especially for individuals who have cared for a spouse with Alzheimer's disease or other disorders. Nurses can also provide support by maintaining contact with the surviving spouse.

Education is a remedy for those who are bored but have an active mind. Local civic groups, colleges, high schools, libraries, museums, religious organizations, universities, and the YMCA provide continuing education courses as well as seminars. In their absence, home-study or correspondence offers a viable alternative.

*   *   *

"Your Hands Are Freezing"

"My son-in-law said I have tendinitis." Gwendolyn Sparks, a slight, well-groomed, gray-haired woman, rubbed her left shoulder.

"Oh," I said, "Why does he say that?"

"His doctor told him his own shoulder problem was tendinitis from a tennis injury."

"I see. Is your shoulder the only joint that hurts?"

"They all ache at times—especially my knees and elbows—but the shoulder's the one that's acting up now." She rubbed her knees in a circling motion.

"Does your shoulder ever get red or swollen?"

"Sometimes, not usually."

"And do you tend to have more problems in the morning when you wake up or at the end of the day?"

"I'm pretty stiff in the morning. My joints sometimes make a crackling sound—I don't know how else to describe it. It takes me a while to get going."

"Do you do any exercises?"

"I'm not much of an exercise person."

"What have you taken to relieve your shoulder pain?"

"I've been using over-the-counter medications, but they don't help enough. I'm afraid I'm taking more than I should."

After completing the history, I told her I wanted to examine her. Her problem sounded like arthritis not tendinitis. I wanted to determine what type it was and what could be done for it. When I touched her on her bare arm, she jumped.

"Child, your hands are freezing. It's cold enough in this room as it is."

"Oh, I'm sorry. I guess they *are* kind of cold. You know what they say: *Cold hands, warm heart.*" I quickly rubbed my hands together like I was standing in front of a fireplace.

"Dirty feet and no sweetheart!"

"What?"

"That's the rest of the saying. Didn't you know that?"

"No."

"You're not from the South, are you?"

"Well, no."

"Everyone knows that saying down there."

"But my feet *aren't* dirty and I *do* have a sweetheart," I teased. She giggled.

I always feel better when I get a patient to laugh.

ARTHRITIS

We're tough on our bones and joints. Running exerts pressures of 5,000 pounds per square inch. Jumping's even worse—some 20,000 pounds of pressure. When the joints are normal and youthful we are unaware of these feats. But for people with arthritis, even minimal activity can trigger disabling pain. No wonder: our skeletons contain 206 bones, half of which are in the feet and hands.

At least 55 million adults in the U.S. suffer from osteoarthritis, the most common form of joint disease. After spending $2.4 billion yearly on anti-inflammatory drugs, hydrocortisone injections, or surgery, only one-third report relief, and little more than one-sixth show improved function. Symptomatic or not, 90% of all people over the age of 40 will have radiographic evidence of osteoarthritis in weight-bearing joints.

Osteoarthritis is a degenerative disorder of cartilage, which normally should be glassy smooth and lubricated by synovial fluid, one of the most remarkable fluids in the human body. In patients with osteoarthritis, the articular bone becomes hypertrophic and minimally inflamed. A coarse crackling sound (crepitus) may be felt in the joint. Rest relieves the pain and activity makes it worse. The pattern of joint involvement and absence of systemic symptoms help confirm the diagnosis. Obesity and competitive contact sports, but not recreational running, raise the risk of degenerative joint disease.

There are many other kinds of arthritis. Infectious types are due to gonococcus or other bacteria (septic arthritis) and viruses, including HIV infection. Arthritic disorders with systemic involvement include autoimmune diseases, like connective tissue disease, lupus (systemic lupus erythematous), psoriasis, rheumatoid arthritis, various cancers, and others. Gout, inflammatory bowel diseases, and several lung diseases also produce arthritis.

Rheumatoid arthritis severely deformed the hands of the French Impressionist painter Pierre August Renoir. He had to painstakingly mix colors and place the brush in his more severely affected hand with the other hand. To change colors or clean the brush, the painful process had to be reversed, then repeated. How he was able to produce masterpieces under those conditions is a testimonial to his character.

Thomas Jefferson and Theodore Roosevelt were also among the countless millions who suffer from rheumatoid arthritis. Half of the patients with rheumatoid arthritis cannot function at their jobs within 10 years after the diagnosis and have a mildly shortened life span. Because joint destruction occurs early in the disease, modern immunotherapy for rheumatoid arthritis is aggressive.

The management of arthritis should provide symptomatic relief and treat the underlying cause where possible. The non-drug management entails application of heat and cold, education about arthritis, exercise, joint rest, splints, sufficient bed rest, and weight loss. Assistive devices, such as a cane, crutches, gripping bar, raised toilet seat, or a walker, benefit patients with severe knee or hip arthritis.

The principal drug treatments for osteoarthritis are nonsteroidal anti-inflammatory drugs. Because these drugs must be taken chronically and often in high doses, their gastrointestinal side effects should be kept in mind. Almost one-quarter of all hospitalizations and deaths from peptic ulcer disease are caused by nonsteroidal anti-inflammatory drugs, but only one in five victims has warning symptoms. Antimalarials, chemotherapy, corticosteroids, gold salts, are other drugs for rheumatoid arthritis.

*   *   *

"I Used to Have Very Reddish Hair"

William T. Robinson—fragile, wizen, stooped, white-haired—was ancient-looking even for being ninety-seven-years old. An L-shaped, pewter-colored handle topped his cane. After I obtained his history, I said I needed to examine him. "Please take off your undershirt."

"I'm too cold."

The room actually felt excessively warm to me. Sometimes the older patients complained about being so cold that I would give them a blanket, even in summertime.

"Would you rather put on a gown?"

"No, no."

"Okay. Leave your undershirt on and I'll pull it up when I listen to your heart and lungs."

When Mr. Robinson removed his outer shirt, I could see that his clothes were unwashed. He had body odor, and a brown ring lined the inside of his collar. The hair at his nape was continuous with that of his back.

"You know, you should go to a dermatologist, Mr. Robinson. These bumps on you face could be removed easily." His face was covered by raised skin plaques.

"No, I've had them for years.They're not going anywhere."

I looked closer to make sure the lesions were not cancerous. "Okay, it's your face."

"I used to have very reddish hair," he said abruptly. His hands shook a little. His wide eyes watered.

"Is that right?"

"Yeah, I was in WW I and WW II."

"I know."

Mr. Robinson liked to tell tales about the war, mostly WW I, because he was active in that war. To me, WW I was merely a dark chapter in a book, but Mr. Robinson actually lived it. What an experience it was to talk to him.

"Me and my buddies were in German-occupied France. We got separated from our unit and found a French *underground* restaurant that took in allies for shelter and food. I spoke pretty good French because my mother spoke French and my ancestors were French. My buddies would always take me to the restaurant because I could order food for them. They did not speak much French." He paused to see if I was following the story.

"And you could go to the restaurant without being detected?"

"We were disguised," he whispered throatily.

"Okay."

"One time, evidently, my buddies went to the restaurant without me. They wanted to order two eggs. The word for eggs in French is *oeuf.* One guy held up two fingers and said *oeuf, oeuf.* He pronounced it like a dog's bark. The waiter didn't understand the Englishman's French, so he replied *comment,* which means *what.* My buddy said again, *oeuf, oeuf.* Finally the waiter said *Ah* and went back to the kitchen. When he returned, he brought two hot-dogs because he thought the guy said *oeuf, oeuf* to mean two dogs."

William Robinson rewarded himself for his storytelling with a hearty laugh. Still quite amused at his own story, he stopped laughing and squinted at me to see if I got it.

I smiled. "That's a good one, Mr. Robinson. I'll have to remember that. Well, you look good. Things are going well for you."

"You bet'cha. I'm doing great. I'm feeling one-hundred-percent today."

"I guess I can't beat that."

"I'd like to see you try."

His sense of humor was as healthy as he was. Quiet a nonagenarian. I would have liked to talk to him longer, but I had another patient to see. I finished his examination, renewed his medications, and sent him home.

SKIN SURVEILLANCE

Sun worship has thrived over the centuries. Native Americans of North and South America, from the Iroquois to the Incas, paid homage to the sun as a deity or a symbol of the Almighty. The sun was also a god to the Babylonians, Egyptians, Greeks, Hindu, and Persians, who called it Apollo, Helios, Phoebus, Ra or other names. Only the Dravidians of southern India regarded the sun as evil.

But now sun worship has changed. Modern peoples worship the sun for its tanning rays—incredibly powerful for having traveled 93 million miles to reach earth—penetrating rays with far-reaching implications.

Popular wisdom has it that the sun is good for us. We view tans as healthy, sexy, even youthful, yet accumulated sun exposure is a principal risk factor for skin cancer. Most people are unaware that they may have received 80% of their lifetime exposure to UV light prior to the age of 18. Cumulative lifetime exposure to the sun, inability to tan, and number of sunburns are important skin cancer risk factors. People who work outdoors, have fair skin or a family history of skin cancers, or harbor more than 50 moles are most vulnerable. As Jane E. Brody wrote for the *The New York Times*, "The time to start protecting against the sun is the moment when we first can see it."

Skin cancers, the most common of all carcinomas, are on the increase. Over the last ten years, the incidence of melanoma rose by 20% and other skin cancers soared by about 60%. Although basal cell and squamous cell carcinomas constitute about 95% of all skin cancers, melanomas account for 75% of all deaths from skin cancer. Scientists warn about ultraviolet B (UVB) and a gradual reduction in the atmosphere's protective ozone layer. According to estimates, a 5% decrease in the ozone layer will increase melanoma by an equal amount and superficial skin cancers by 30%. Why? Ultraviolet light mutates our DNA.

The U.S. Public Health Service set a goal of annual skin examination for 40% of adults aged 50 and older by the year 2000. Because only about one third of skin malignancies are discovered first by the patient, total skin examination is a crucial tool in the fight against skin cancers. A skin survey can be combined easily with a physical examination.

A useful mnemonic is *A,B,C,D*: *A*symmetry, *B*order irregularity, nonuniform *C*olor, and *D*iameter more than 6 millimeters (about 0.25 inches). Moles fitting this description deserve attention and follow-up, possibly removal. Body maps or simple sketches in the chart document the lesions.

Basal cell carcinoma, the most common skin cancer, increases in incidence with age. It assumes many forms, some nodular, others crusted, fibrosing, pigmented, superficial, translucent, or ulcerated. It spreads slowly, rarely metastasizes, but can disfigure and cause functional impairment by local extension. The cure rate is very high.

Squamous cell carcinoma, the second most common skin cancer, is a pearly, telangiectatic papule. Actinic keratosis, a premalignant condition affecting millions of Americans, may progress to squamous cell carcinoma. With early detection and excision, a cure is likely.

Malignant melanoma, the third most common skin cancer, is an irregular multi-colored lesion, greater than 5 mm in diameter, which forms nodules or papules. Because it metastasizes and survival rates are inversely proportional to the depth of skin penetration, early recognition and surgical excision are important. Melanoma affects people of all ages, especially women, and about one-quarter of patients are younger than 40.

Treatments for skin cancer include cryosurgery, curettage, electrodesiccation, radiation therapy, and surgical excision. Advanced malignant melanoma requires adjuvant immunotherapy or chemotherapy.

Many skin cancers could be prevented by education about safe sun exposure. Broad spectrum sunscreens are preferable. A chemical that blocks both UVA and UVB (parsol 1789) has just become available over-the-counter. We should use protective sunscreen lotion liberally (sun-protection factor [SPF] rating of at least 15), avoid sun exposure between 10 AM and 2 PM (when UV radiation is strongest), cover exposed areas with loose-fitting clothes, note the Ultraviolet Index, avoid tanning salons, and read educational materials about skin cancer.

Don't be modest. Everyone should do self-examinations with hand-held or full-length mirrors and with the assistance of their partner for difficult-to-visualize areas.

*   *   *

"I Want Some Earrings"

I heard a knock on my partially open door. A tall, heavyset woman and a younger, slimmer woman entered.

"Hello, I'm Dorothy Scandler from Nursing Administration. Maybe you've heard of me?"

"Oh, yes, nice to meet you." Of course I was clueless.

The tall, gray-haired woman coddled the young woman almost maternally. Her reading glasses hung around her neck on a gold-link chain. "I have a nurse practitioner student here who needs a preceptor for six months. Her name is Marlena Lesner. Her previous arrangement fell through at the last minute and we noticed that you haven't precepted a student this year yet, so we thought it was your turn."

The student stood at the door, looking the way kids in school do while selections for softball teams are being made. She was a petite brunette with shoulder-length hair, fair complexion, small, fine features, and blue eyes. I guessed she was probably in her mid-twenties.

I thought about the extra work involved in mentoring a student, but it wouldn't be every day; students also had classes. I glanced over at her. She seemed to be a presentable enough young woman. I consented reluctantly.

"When does she start?"

"Now."

I looked at my watch. It was three-thirty P.M, a strange time to begin. "Okay."

"Thank you," the administrator said. "You won't regret it. I'll send you the evaluation forms through the interoffice mail later this week."

Marlena thanked me profusely for agreeing to take her on. I almost preferred she wouldn't turn out to be nice. That way I might not feel as guilty if I couldn't spend lots of time with her because of the clinic schedule. She asked me what I wanted her to do.

"Do you know where the bathroom is?" I asked.

"Yes."

"How about the cafeteria?"

"Yes."

"Good. Those are two of the most important things," I said with a smile. "Right now I'm returning phone calls from patients. You can listen to me or read some of the pamphlets on the table over there about the common diseases that you will see here in the clinic. I'm on walk-ins, so when a patient comes in, they'll call me and I'll take you with me to see them."

"Okay."

Marlena's lab coat looked folded, like it just came out of the package. As I watched her scan the room, all of a sudden I saw the room for what it was. The old green curtain, used to draw around the patients while they undressed, had been replaced by a new orange one. What it matched in the room wasn't apparent to me. The brown carpet on the floor was utilitarian and threadbare. The desk and the examining table looked like they had been obtained from a used office furniture store. Artificial ceiling lighting did not make up for the lack of a window.

Thelma walked into the room. "Ready for another one?"

I held out my hand for the chart. "Thelma this is Marlena. She's a nurse practitioner student who will be with us for six months."

"Nice to meet you." Thelma turned to me. "Can she see her own walk-ins?"

"No, she has to see them with me. Nice try."

"Too bad. Anyway, this should be the last one for today."

"Good," I said. Thelma left. "Well, Marlena, let's go find your first patient."

Lucille Foster, a black woman in her eighties, wore a wig in the style of the Motown Supremes with a hot pink bandanna tied at the top. Her face was actually pretty through the excessive rouge and the furrows between her eyebrows and at the sides of her mouth. Adorn-ed with her false eyelashes and brilliant, pink-red lipstick painted be-yond the edges of her lips, she didn't look her age. Ms. Foster liked very bright, almost garish colors and large print dresses.

I introduced the student, alerting her that the patient was hearing-impaired.

"How are you doing, Ms. Foster?" Marlena broadcasted through-out the clinic.

It was difficult to tell if the patient understood. I asked Ms. Foster to repeat what Marlena said so I could be sure she comprehended.

"I'm okay," Ms. Foster answered. When she spoke, some of the lipstick got on her front teeth.

As I was taking a history, Ms. Foster kept glancing over her shoulder at her female home attendant, putting her hand to her right ear lobe and tugging on it. I thought that Ms. Foster couldn't hear and was signaling the attendant to tell her what I was saying.

"Can you hear me?" I asked.

"Yes," Ms. Foster replied, but continued to pull her ear lobe.

After this went on for about five minutes, I finally wrote her a note: *Ms. Foster, why do you keep pulling on your right ear lobe?*

She yelled back to me, "'Cause I want some earrings on myself. I left them at home and I dons't feel dressed up without my earrings." She pointed to the home attendant. "I want *her* earrings to wear."

The home attendant laughed and good-naturedly took off her own clip-on earrings.

Ms. Foster immediately snatched the earrings from her hand and attached them. With a look of relief she exclaimed, "I feel much better. *Now* I can continue talking to you."

"After that, I'll make a habit of writing her messages," I remarked to the student.

The visit was for a routine history and physical examination. I showed Marlena the ropes and gave her an opportunity to see the whole process. After the patient and her attendant left I said, "When you've seen a few patients with me, I'll send you in first."

"Good."

"What did you think of her?"

"She's an amazing lady. Did you see the jewelry she wore on all her fingers except the thumbs—the big rhinestone kind—like period pieces? They looked surprisingly well on her long tapered fingers."

"Yes, she's quite a character."

"The veins on the back of her hand were gnarled," Marlena added while rubbing her own hand.

"Yes, she used to be a cleaning woman. Well, that should be all for today. I'm going to finish my notes. You can head home."

"Okay."

I could tell Marlena wasn't ready to leave. She sat down and we ended up talking frankly about age.

"I see what age does to people," she said. "I notice the women particularly. You imagine what they looked like when they were young."

"Some of them tell you. They make comparisons. You see how they try to cover their age, or minimize it, or ignore it. Too much make-up or not enough make-up, or none at all. I see vestiges of youth in their faces. For some women it's the eyes. The brightest, warmest eyes look out at you, unfettered by a ravaged face. Others have young mouths and their aging affects the upper face more. I have a few ladies whose ears don't have an extra wrinkle. I notice those are the ones who like to wear earrings. But the most revealing sign of age is the spirit."

"What do you mean?" Marlena changed positions in the chair. She seemed to like to remove her shoes and sit with one leg under her.

"Well, a person's spirit—that's what I call it—shines through the face. The face is transparent; what they are inside comes out. The young-hearted patients—you can tell them apart. I don't want to say glow or aura, but it's something I pick up on as soon as they walk in the room.

I have patients in their nineties who are still young. If I talked to them behind a screen, adjusting for voice if necessary, I'd envisage someone younger. They're animated and they still care about something. Maybe it's a son or daughter or a grandchild, but often it's a pet, a friend, getting the morning newspaper, or walking down the street on a clear day. You hear it in their voices: they are excited to be alive. They enjoy having another day to live. I am taken back by the incongruity of their attitude and their bodies sometimes. I take care of women with rheumatoid arthritis who manage to keep active despite chronic and severe physical pain."

"What about the other extreme: people who are aged by their lack of spirit?" Marlena leaned forward a bit.

"Some old people are cut flowers, sustaining themselves for a while solely on the memory of what life used to be when they had roots. Inevitably, they wither and fade. They have given up. The reason is sometimes apparent—the death of a loved one, a chronic disease, inability to fulfill their dreams—or it may be unknown to them or kept hidden from me. Seeing them bothers me."

I glanced at my watch. "Look, why don't you do a write-up on this patient. Then you can present her to me and I'll go over your write-up with you. Now go on. Get out of here already."

I pondered those same issues as a student. Marlena would make me remember.

HEARING IMPAIRMENT

Alexander Graham Bell was trying to develop a hearing aid when he accidentally invented the telephone in the 1880's. Although he never got back to it, years later he did invent the audiometer, a device which measures hearing acuity.

The quest to restore hearing and overcome deafness is centuries old. Ear trumpets to gather sounds and funnel them into the ear were used before the 17th century. Some wealthy old rulers went to extremes to have elaborate devices built to overcome their failing hearing.

Presbyacusis, the hearing loss of aging, is the fourth most prevalent chronic disability in people older than 65, men out-numbering women. About 40% of individuals over the age of 75 have significant hearing impairment, and in nursing homes the prevalence approaches 70%. The problem may be a reduction in hearing threshold sensitivity, impaired brain processing, or both. Each cause requires a different approach and treatment.

Only 20% of physicians routinely screen their older patients for hearing loss. Screening by whispers or watch-ticking is inadequate. An audiologist will document the extent and nature of the problem. Pure tone audiometry measures hearing sensitivity. In normal aging, sensitivity to high-frequency sounds declines first, becoming clinically significant when at or below the 4,000 to 8,000 Hz range. Ordinary conversation covers a range of frequencies from 250 to 3,000 Hz, but clear enunciation of certain consonants involves higher frequencies. As a result, hearing-impaired older adults may have difficulty discerning "b," "f," "p," "s," "sh," "t," or "v."

First the good news: some causes of hearing loss are reversible. Cerumen may impact the outer ear canal. Hearing loss also may be the consequence of middle ear disease, drugs, and tumors. Early treatment can prevent further impairment. The appropriate specialist for initial referral is the otolaryngologist.

The bad news is that a lifetime of excessive noise exposure rather than the aging process is a leading cause of ear damage. Noise is a more formidable hazard than it seems because it does not produce any external evidence of injury. A noise-damaged ear cannot be repaired. One sound blast of 85 decibels (dB) or more can rip apart the ear's inner tissues and cause scarring. Every 10-decibel increase in noise causes ten times more ear-battering. Incapable of regeneration, the hair cells of the inner ear die. A noisy video arcade (110 dB), subway platform (100 dB), power drill (100 dB), and screaming child (90 dB), each tolerable for short periods, are noxious to the ear.

Here's the paradox: hearing aids help most older people with hearing impairment, but only about 20% of the 28 million Americans with hearing loss wear them. New digital hearing aids are superior to tradition ones, which amplify background noise and require adjustment of volume when moving from room to room. Though pricey (about $3,000), they offer higher customer satisfaction. An assistive-listening device, utilizing remote microphone technology, is another alternative. New technology promises dramatic improvements in the future.

6

Memories Lost, a Broken Mind

We forget all too soon the things we thought we could never forget
—JOAN DIDION

*Memory is a net; one finds it full of fish when he takes it from the
brook; but a dozen miles of water have run through it without
sticking*
—OLIVER WENDELL HOLMES, SR.

She was losing her mind in handfuls
—MARION ROACH

*I want to smell the roses now, because I may not be able to recognize
them later on*
—SALLY WEINPER

Those whose illness is a loss of self
—ANITA DESAI

"She Was So Young Then"

The Fritzes were in their seventies. Nelly was the wife of Henry Fritz, who brought her to the clinic. Mr. Fritz did most of the talking—at least the talking that made sense.

"Are you my daughter?" Nelly asked me. She seemed genuinely perplexed.

"No." I looked to Mr. Fritz for help.

"It's her mind," he sighed. "Nelly's losing her mind." He appeared disgraced and disgusted.

"No, I'm not," she retorted. "My mind's as sound as it ever was."

Mr. Fritz shook his head. "She doesn't see what's been happening to her. A year ago, it was subtle. I tried to convince myself nothing was wrong."

"What did you notice?" I was a little uncomfortable with Mr. Fritz talking about his wife as though she were not present.

"She became more argumentative and irritable. I thought it was something I was doing, but I wasn't doing anything different. We've been married fifty-two years. I couldn't explain the change until she started forgetting things—not just anything, but recent things. She could tell you a story about twenty years ago like it was yesterday, but if you asked her what she did last night, she couldn't recall."

"That's not true," Nelly protested. "He's lying."

"Shut up, Nelly," Mr. Fritz flashed. His face became plethoric and the vein on his temple stood out momentarily. Then he reached over, took her hand and held it. After a deep sigh, he continued.

"Anyway, she's gotten worse. One day she was very confused and thought I was her father. She's unsafe with an iron because she doesn't remember she left it on. Same thing with cooking. Last month, she almost burned down the house because she forgot the pots on the stove. I rushed into the kitchen when the smoke alarm went off to find flames leaping from the pans. She was outside watching the birds." Turning to Nelly, he asked, "Do you remember that?"

"Nope," she said while staring at her feet.

"Of course, you don't," he said.

Mr. Fritz turned to me. "She's losing her mind. This is not the woman I married." He paused. "We had such plans. Now, what's the point. I'm going to be spending my last days taking care of a vegetable."

"Quit talking about me," Nelly Fritz yelled.

Mr. Fritz leaned his elbow on the corner of my desk and rested his head on his hand. He had the demeanor of a man who has hit rock bottom. The frown lines on his forehead revealed his chronic frustration. "I don't know what to do."

I was concerned about the level of tension between the two. With this much conflict apparent in the office, who knew what was going on at home.

"We need to do several things, Mr. Fritz. I'll want to ask you some more questions and then examine your wife. After that, we'll make a plan."

"It's Alzheimer's disease, isn't it?" he said fatalistically.

"Maybe. We'll need to rule out some other treatable causes of dementia before we can make that diagnosis."

"That's what her mother died of. She ended up in a nursing home."

I refocused Mr. Fritz on helping me assess his wife. The rest of Nelly's evaluation revealed no physical evidence for other causes of dementia, such as head injury, tumor, or thyroid problems. Her short-term memory was wiped out, but her long-term memory remained intact, just as her husband had noticed.

After discussing the case with my attending, I ordered blood tests and a head MRI scan, but did not expect to find any reversible cause of Nelly's problem.

"Once the diagnosis is confirmed," I explained to Mr. Fritz, "I'll refer you to an Alzheimer's support group. I think you might find it helpful to talk with spouses of patients with Alzheimer's who have gone through this."

He shook his head in agreement.

"I'd like to arrange for a home attendant to help you," I added cautiously. People reacted differently to the suggestion that a stranger should come into their home on a regular basis. "How does that sound?"

"It sounds great, if they'll do it." He looked surprised and eager at the prospect. A smile appeared.

This is going to work out all right, I thought. "I'll refer you to social services to make the arrangements." I turned to Nelly. "Wouldn't that be nice, to have someone help out with your work at home?" Involuntarily, my voice had taken the soft tones of a parent coaxing and reassuring a small child.

Mrs. Fritz looked up from her stare as if first noticing me in the room. "You look so familiar," she said. "I can't place you. Are you one of my daughters?"

"No, I'm not, Mrs. Fritz. I'm a nurse practitioner."

"Why am I here, Henry? Why are we at this place. I want to go home."

Annoyed, Mr. Fritz replied, "We're going home now, Nelly." Then he reached over and patted her knee affectionately. To me he said, "When can that attendant start and will my insurance cover it?"

"I'll ask social services to work on that. As to when the attendant starts, they'll give you a better idea about that, too."

Mr. Fritz helped up his befuddled wife and stopped by the doorway on their way out. "We never thought anything like this would happen to us when we got married. She was so young then. You should have seen her. She was a beauty." His clear, blue-green eyes moistened before he turned away.

I felt that knife blade of empathy beginning to slice through me again. "Try to remember that same person in the times ahead, Mr. Fritz. She can't help it."

"I know. That's what makes it so damned difficult. I want to blame someone and there's no one to blame. It's just life."

After the Fritzs left, I sat down at my desk and thought about my own parents. I hoped this wasn't in store for them. I thought about myself becoming that age. Losing my mind was not a way I wanted to go. Soon my attention returned to the paperwork involved in making the referral.

Months later, Sally Buchanan, Nelly's home attendant, approached me in the clinic hallway. Tall and robust, she had the ideal physique for being able to assist those who could not care for themselves. "I want to talk with you privately about Nelly Fritz," she began.

Sally had taken care of another patient of mine, so I knew she did't usually feel the need to speak in hushed tones. I motioned her toward my office.

"You know how Nelly's husband has been at his wit's end with her?"

"Yes."

"Well, I've gradually noticed small bruises on her arms and buttocks when I bathe her, particularly over the past few weeks. I figured Nelly injured herself accidentally. Recently, when I dressed her, I saw larger bruises on her neck and stomach. I asked Nelly how she got those marks, but she wouldn't tell me. It's strange, too, that Nelly's husband always seems to take off the moment I arrive for my eight hour shift. I brought Nelly in to see you today because, when she opened the door, she was crying and had a beefy-red, swollen cheek. If you want my personal opinion, I think Nelly's husband is beating her."

"Did you confront him?"

"No. I never saw him do anything, but I don't know of anyone else who might have done it."

"I see. Why don't you bring her back here and I'll talk to her."

When Sally returned with Nelly, I asked, "What happened to your face, Nelly?" No answer. When I pressed her about it, she broke into tears. "I'm not supposed to say."

"Say what, Nelly? You can tell us."

"I didn't mean to make him mad," she blurted. "I didn't mean to. Why did he get so mad at me? I tried, didn't I?" She put her head down.

Sally looked at me as if to say *See, I told you.* Home attendants were of a varied background and quality. Some were lackadaisical; others were like Sally, skilled and devoted.

I asked Nelly to sit on the examining table and took a closer look at her left cheek. The bruise was fresh and swollen enough to compress her lower eyelid and partially occlude vision in her left eye. Other bruises on her body were the yellow-green or purple of older injuries. Worried about the possibility of a fracture, I ordered facial x-rays.

An hour later, the radiologist called back. "Is your patient a heavyweight boxer or what?"

"What do you mean?"

"She has a cheekbone fracture in two places."

"I was afraid of that."

"How'd it happen?"

"We're not sure yet. We think she went a few rounds in the ring with someone she knew." Because of confidentiality, I couldn't reveal the specifics.

"Well, that person nailed her pretty well. I can see soft tissue swelling, too. Doesn't it make you sick?"

"At least you don't see all the colors on x-ray."

"It's none too pretty in black-and-white either."

When I related the history and physical findings to Dr. David Morrell, the Fritz's primary doctor, he suggested we do the difficult thing: take the bull by the horns.

"Nelly, I need to ask a social worker to investigate what happened to you," I said. "You know we can't leave you alone with your husband right now."

"Do you have to? It's going to get him mad."

"You've got fractures of the cheekbone. We need to admit you to the hospital. Once you're discharged, social services will place you in an assisted living home and help your husband get counseling if he's the one who did this."

The news made Nelly cry. Sally put her arm around her. "It's going to be okay, Nelly. No one's going to hurt you anymore."

While we were waiting for Nelly to be admitted, Sally said to me, "The sad thing is her husband probably deep down still loves her, but he's so angry. Poor Nelly will be more confused than ever."

"Yeah. She will be taken away from someone she has known for over fifty years, be placed in an unfamiliar environment, and will lose you, her advocate, too."

"I feel bad I had to bring her in," Sally said.

"No. You may have saved her life."

Sally and I exchanged glances as the irony of my words hit us. What life?

Although I never saw Nelly or Henry again and would like to have found out what happened to them, I didn't have to. Over the years, I have seen many other patients like Nelly. The names and the circumstances begin to blur and fade, and I am left with a composite: eyes grown vacant, a face no longer illuminated from within, a voice lacking conviction and personality, a shadow of a former self, and lengthening stares into the void of dissolution. All of life's sweet and happy times, its struggles, ironies and absurdities—but for this one—vanished. I can only hope that they have found peace.

DOMESTIC VIOLENCE

Some points can not be overemphasized: domestic violence targets women 10 times more commonly than it targets men. It signifies any assault, criminal offense, or sexual battery by one member of a household or family on another resulting in physical injury or death. More than 2.5 million women in the U.S. experience violence each year. Unfortunately, only half of them report the crime to the police; the others consider the matter private or of minor importance. About 4% of the seniors in this country are emotionally, financially, or physically abused by caretakers or relatives.

It's nothing to be ashamed of. Sometimes a woman won't tell her health care provider she's been battered, but may give cues. Physical cues include vague complaints, bruises, human bites, or burns. Depression or self-deprecating comments from the battered woman, anxiety in the presence of her partner, and a partner who controls or hovers are important behavioral cues. A pattern of frequent, unexplained moves, missed appointments, or social isolation provide vital social cues. Children's behavioral and physical ailments also may signal a problem.

The pattern of violence is characteristic. A tension phase, with yelling, criticism and threats, leads to violence, which is followed by apologies, promises to change, even gifts.

There is no one cause for domestic violence, but rather many contributing psychological and social factors, such as male dominance, the need to maintain personal control, and a history of parental childhood abuse. Substance abuse places the batterer at a higher risk for domestic violence. The abuser controls the victim through financial control, isolation from family and friends, psychological manipulation, physical abuse or threats, sexual abuse, and threats to harm the children.

Why don't women just leave an abusive relationship? Women who leave their batterers are at a 75% greater risk of being killed by them than those who don't leave. The goal of successful intervention is to identify, refer, and treat abused patients. Make an organized plan for a safe escape. Simply asking a patient about abuse and listening to her can be as important as providing physical care and resources. Many dozens of local, state, and national domestic violence resources are available.

*   *   *

"Peetee Came Back to Me"

My next patient, Delilah Anthus, forgot her false teeth again. It wasn't a surprise considering her dementia. Her speech was understandable with effort on my part.

Dementia does strange things to people. It had stripped Ms. Anthus of her adulthood and the independence it afforded, but it gave her a second childhood. How peculiar to see a woman in her eighties with an innocent, childlike demeanor. She laughs, and sings, and talks to herself contentedly. Her mouth is covered with ruby red lipstick.

"I went out to a ballroom dance last night," she said lightheartedly. "All the men wanted to dance with me. I wore a beautiful white gown and had a yellow flower in my hair. A young man danced with me nearly all night. He was a handsome gentleman." She smiled sweetly, absorbed in her reverie.

The home attendant who was sitting behind her wheelchair made a cuckoo sign behind her back and mouthed *no*. "You were home with me last night, Delilah. Don't you remember?"

Ms. Anthus waved her hand with annoyance at her for bringing back the voice of reality. "I was afraid of getting in trouble with my mother for staying out all night," she continued with the mannerisms and voice inflections of a child. "I was very, very good."

I glanced at the home attendant who was shaking her head.

"Peetee came back to me," Ms. Anthus said without prompting. She arranged her brightly colored print dress over her legs.

Am I hearing her right?

"Peetee? Who's he?"

"Peetee is her favorite pigeon who comes to her window sill every day," the attendant explained.

"How do you know it's the same pigeon?" I asked innocently.

"Because I know his markings, that's why." She implied *of course*. "One day he didn't come to my window. I watched all day for him to come. But he didn't. I thought he got killed." Her gaze became momentarily intent.

"She was very upset. I had a hard time getting her to eat," the home attendant added. "I was as relieved as she was when the bird did return."

"I'm glad he came back to you, too, Ms. Anthus."

"Thank you, dear. You're very nice. Your mother would be proud of you."

I thought to myself that my mother probably *would* be proud to see me spending time with people in their old age.

"Would you check her backside," the home attendant asked. "It's been getting red in a couple places."

"Sure, if you'll give me a hand getting her onto the examining table."

We hoisted her without too much trouble. She was quite thin and frail now, delicate looking, though, with her little pierced earrings. She could be a nice grandmother, I thought. You can imagine my surprise when I examined her buttocks.

"What's this?" On her left buttock, faded but still readable, was a tattooed rose and the words: *My heart belongs to daddy but my ass belongs to John.*

The home attendant smiled and shrugged. I felt like laughing and crying at the same time. There are many unexpected twists and turns. Tattooed on young women, I'd seen flowers, butterflies, coiled dragons, even arrows on inner thighs pointing to the vagina—but this? I wondered, had she not been demented, would Ms. Anthus have been embarrassed. Perhaps she might have felt the same way about John today. At least there were no signs of skin breakdown or decubiti, and I went over with the attendant some steps she could take to prevent them. After a quick checkup, I sent her home.

"Good-bye, Ms. Anthus," I said as the home attendant wheeled her away.

"Good-bye!" she rejoined cheerfully. "I'll tell little Peetee I saw you."

I smiled and waved. There yet remained a fragment of something special about her. I imagined her as a young lady, dancing with a lover, eyes closed, holding each other tightly, swaying, turning, spinning. That's the way she probably would like to be remembered.

I made a fundamental observation long ago. You can lose your mind in two ways: one leaves a person happy and the other, angry and scared. Delilah Anthus was lucky to be a happy one.

THE BURDEN OF ALZHEIMER'S DISEASE

Nov. 5, 1994

My Fellow Americans,

I have recently been told that I am one of the millions of Americans who will be afflicted with Alzheimer's disease .... In opening our hearts, we hope this might promote greater awareness of this condition .... At the moment I feel just fine .... Unfortunately, as Alzheimer's Disease progresses, the family often bears a heavy burden .... I now begin the journey that will lead me into the sunset of my life ....

Sincerely,
Ronald Reagan

So wrote our former president in a two-page, widely reprinted, open letter to the public.

Alzheimer's disease—a national burden. It causes about half of all cases of dementia, which is a loss of at least two of the following capacities: judgment, language, memory, or spatial and visual abilities. The decline in cognition begins gradually, but is progressive. Behavior and mood swing erratically. About 72% of those with the disease are apathetic and 36% are disinhibited. Social skills are so well preserved that the early symptoms of Alzheimer's disease may be overlooked or excused as part of normal aging for 2 to 4 years. About 50% of those with Alzheimer's disease remain undiagnosed.

As the disease progresses, management becomes more problematic. Sixty percent of the afflicted become agitated and aggressive, cursing, shouting, shoving, striking, and resisting caregivers. Some patients deny that a family member or friend is who they claim to be (Capgras syndrome). Alzheimer's disease ranks second only to schizophrenia as a leading psychotic illness in the U.S. The burden most often falls on the normal spouse, but sometimes the afflicted patient is abused. The emotional, physical, and financial impact on family, friends, and society is enormous.

This much we know: four million individuals have dementia, the fourth ranking cause of death in this country and the primary disease of nursing home patients. About 100 billion dollars a year are spent on it. Experts say that a person who lives to be 80 will have a 1 in 4 chance of getting Alzheimer's or a related disease. By the year 2040, an estimated 14 million Americans will have Alzheimer's disease. These figures were reported as a consensus statement by the American Association for Geriatric Psychiatry, the Alzheimer's Association, and the American Geriatrics Society in 1997.

Alzheimer's disease is certainly not new. The Assyrians, Greeks, and Romans all knew of dementing diseases. But it was the German neuropathologist Dr. Alois Alzheimer in 1906 who identified the cellular "fingerprint" of the disease (neurofibrillary tangles) in the brain of a demented patient using a silver stain technique.

Because Alzheimer's disease is not the cause of all dementias, the demented patient should have a medical evaluation for other disorders such as endocrine and metabolic problems, infections, inflammation, trauma, tumors, or vascular insults (multi-infarct dementia).

Many conditions look alike. Dementia must be differentiated from confusion or delirium, which is more common, affecting as many as one fourth of persons over age 65. Confusion is caused by a physiologic disturbance and develops over a short period of time. Once the underlying cause is corrected, the confusion improves. A patient with dementia may have episodes of confusion, but the confused patient need not have dementia. Depression also causes a syndrome that resembles Alzheimer's disease (pseudodementia), but responds to antidepressants.

Having said all this, most slips of memory are *not* Alzheimer's disease. It has been estimated that Americans spend a year of their lives looking for misplaced objects. Some forgetfulness is the nature of the beast.

DEVELOPING NEW TREATMENTS

New insights about the diagnosis and treatment of Alzheimer's disease offer hope. A genetic risk factor for familial Alzheimer's is apolipoprotein E-4 (Apo E-4). Positron emission (PET) scans show a loss of activity in the parietal-occipital region of the brain cortex. In those suffering delusions the frontal cortex is involved, too. The goal of researchers is to recognize the disease in asymptomatic patients so that preventative measures can be instituted.

The cholinesterase inhibitors donepezil and tacrine, the only drugs currently approved by the Food and Drug Administration (FDA) for the treatment of Alzheimer's disease, are effective only in mild or moderate cases. They increase the availability of the brain neurotransmitter acetylcholine, which is lost as brain cells die. A-typical antipsychotic drugs like risperidone treat the psychosis, and the depression responds to antidepressants. In agitated, non-psychotic patients, anticonvulsants such as lorazepam reduce agitation.

Although the findings are not definitive, estrogen may play a role in delaying or preventing Alzheimer's disease. Other drugs being evaluated for Alzheimer's disease include the antioxidants selegiline and vitamin E; botanical agents, such as ginkgo biloba; calcium channel blockers that reduce excess calcium levels in nerve cells; and nonsteroidal anti-inflammatory drugs.

The prinins are exciting new compounds in clinical trials for Alzheimer's disease. Unlike other treatments which merely reduce symptoms, prinins regulate the production of cell growth factors in the brain. Restoring or promoting these neurotrophic factors may be an important therapy for neurodegenerative diseases. Prinins can be taken orally, but other ways of delivering drugs only to injured areas of the brain are being developed.

7

The War Zone

I believe that man will not merely endure. He will prevail. He is immortal, not because he alone among creatures has an inexhaustible voice, but because he has a soul, a spirit capable of compassion and sacrifice and endurance

—WILLIAM FAULKNER

From a single crime know the nation

—VIRGIL

The face of "evil" is always the face of total need

—WILLIAM BURROUGHS

Anger is momentary madness, so control your passion or it will control you

—HORACE

The city is not a concrete jungle, it is a human zoo

—DESMOND MORRIS

"Like Hawks after Baby Sparrows"

Harold Pitts, at the age of ninety-three, was as smart as a whip. He always wore clean, long-sleeve shirts, even in the summer, and fresh-smelling cologne. You could tell that he polished his shoes before he came to the clinic, something you don't see much nowadays. Harold would sometimes leave tissue paper on his face from shaving cuts.

"Nobody saw those on you?" I asked as I removed them.

"Nobody looks at nobody in the subway," he said with a laugh.

"Do you always take the subway?"

"You bet. I know this city like the palm of my hand. I found out when meal times are at senior citizens centers and make a practice of going around for my meals. I also ride the subway to cash my social security checks. Do you know the best way to get social security checks cashed in the city without being robbed, beaten or mauled?" He waited patiently for my reply. The lines across his forehead were deep and he had bags under his eyes.

"No, I don't, Mr. Pitts."

"First of all, you arrange to have your check mailed to a post office box, which I rent for a small fee. On the day the check is to arrive, I go to pick it up with a young man who is built pretty big, if you know what I mean. This guy escorts me to a store that cashes checks on the spot. He and I go right to my landlord and pay my rent. I reward my bodyguard with some cash."

I nodded, thinking about his life. What an idea. Was the story true?

"You'd be surprised," he confided. "I've seen thugs—black, white, Asian, and Hispanic—standing on the corners where old people get their social security checks cashed. They go after them like hawks after baby sparrows." He made a clawing motion for emphasis.

One day, Harold brought in his bodyguard. I was a little awed. The guy was built like a refrigerator with the muscles and face of a human pit bull. He stood ready to launch into attack mode at the slightest nonverbal cue. "I'll stay outside while you see pops," his gruff voice announced.

I let out a little laugh of relief. After meeting the bodyguard that day, I didn't worry about Mr. Pitts again.

Nobody messes with Harold Pitts.

IMPACT OF CRIME AND VIOLENCE

A national disgrace. According to the 1991 Uniform Crime Reports, one violent crime is committed in the U.S. every 17 seconds: a burglary every 10 seconds, an aggravated assault every 29 seconds, a robbery every 46 seconds, one forcible rape every 5 minutes, one murder every 21 minutes. The result is more than 40 million personal crime victimizations annually.

Too often seniors are victims. Some possess a will or spirit that will not be broken and adapt to their violent environment. Others become isolated; they suffer emotional, financial, and lifestyle victimization. Those who live in inner-city projects or poor urban areas are reluctant to leave their apartments to attend even the hot lunch program out of fear. Many speak of crime and violence in their neighborhood with acceptance and resignation in their voices. Physical vulnerability and compromised health further predispose them to victimization. They live with perpetual apprehension.

Survivors change their habits. They stop carrying large sums of money on their person when it is time to pay their bills or when social security checks arrive. Utilizing teenagers to help with escorting and shopping fosters their self-esteem and responsibility while assisting seniors. Despite efforts of formal agencies to help the aged, many rely on informal social support from family and friends.

*   *   *

"Mugger's Bait"

It doesn't always go that way. Another man's luck was different.

Lee Whitfield, an active member of a local Baptist church in the Bronx, came to see me because he was feeling anxious. He said that the minister wanted to announce his upcoming one-hundredth birthday to the congregation. Instead of being excited about stepping into the limelight, Mr. Whitfield was horrified.

"Mr. Whitfield, you're a centenarian! That's great."

"I don't want to stand in front of everybody. He wants me to take a bow."

"Why are you afraid?" I asked. "How often does a person turn one-hundred?"

"I don't want people to know I'm so old. I'm worried about being mugger's bait?"

"What?"

"I don't want to get beaten to a pulp."

The idea was hard to comprehend. Who could assault a meek man like Mr. Whitfield? I wasn't able to dissuade him from his preoccupation.

Two weeks later, I heard from his family that he'd been admitted to the hospital for five days because a gang found out where he lived and attacked him.

"How did they find out?" I asked his nephew.

"The boys in the gang happened to be at church when his age was announced and they got a good look at him."

"The muggers went to church?"

"Yes," his nephew said. "That's weird in itself."

Lee Whitfield was right. Unfortunately, his premonition came true. Now I understood too well the significance of "mugger's bait."

CENTENARIANS

"Dare to be 100" is now a common expression and goal of many baby boomers. Centenarians constitute the fastest-growing segment of the U.S. population, numbering about 60,000 today. The Census Bureau projects that one in 26 baby boomers will reach 100 and one in nine will survive into the 90's. The number of centenarians in this country is expected to reach 500,000 by the year 2020. They would agree with Cicero: "Old age alone has no precise and determinant boundary."

Chronic illness is not an inevitable consequence of aging, but rather of lifestyle choices, bad genes, or bad luck. The oldest of the old enjoy better health than those in their 70's do. Although diet, exercise, and use of the mind are all factors in longevity, it is very important to choose your parents well. Successful aging is also a psychological feat, as loneliness speeds our demise. Staying connected and engaged is vital. When centenarians die, they don't linger; they fulfill the motto, "Live long, die fast."

*   *   *

"I Had to Put Him Away"

Shattering thunderclaps drew me to the clinic window. Torrents of rain transformed the window into a lens that distorted the shapes of cars and passers-by. A frenzy of lightning momentarily bathed the buildings in an eerie light. The sky was gray enough with November as it was; the storm presaged nightfall.

Wilma Washew stopped by unexpectedly. She slowly discarded her long, black raincoat and untied the scarf over her head. She attempted to close her umbrella, but it had been sprung by gusts of wind.

Hers was a complicated life. She lost her sister six months ago and her mother the year before. Her brother, having had two major heart attacks, was hospitalized and most likely won't survive the next one. Although she said she wanted a check-up, that wasn't the crux of the matter.

"What's really troubling you, Mrs. Washew?"

"I had to put him away," she said remorsefully. Another violent crack of thunder.

"I don't understand."

"I had to admit my own son Ronald to a mental institution."

"Why?"

"For paranoia and thoughts of harming himself and others. Ronald's been having problems controlling his behavior since he was a teen-ager. Now he's thirty. He lived with me in my second-story apartment when he couldn't hold a job no more. The doctors put him on medication, and it did help, but he stopped taking it and flipped out. The whole thing scared me terribly. I called the authorities. I feel *so* bad about it."

"What did he do?"

She hesitated. "He took a knife to his own mother's throat." She shook her head and remained silent for some time. "The world's crashing in on me." Wilma Washew cradled her head in her hands.

I was startled by the sustained thunder. It sounded like the keel and hull of the mighty *Titanic* had ripped through the roof of the building.

After I talked to Mrs. Washew awhile, I referred her for some grief counseling. In the face of her persistent streak of bad luck, she needed professional help.

When I stepped outside my door, I was ready for a breath of fresh air. That's when I saw Jerry. Jerry Klein stood at the front desk waiting for me. Drug representatives are the most patient people, I thought.

In his late twenties and dressed in a sharp-looking, navy blue suit, Jerry had the broad shoulders and assured manner of a former athlete. He did enjoy talking football with the doctors and managed to promote his pharmaceutical company's drugs at the same time. The doctors sifted through the puffery and got some great tickets to sports events out of it.

"Have you been using our products?"

"I need a product that cures poverty and human misery."

He thought I was kidding. "I don't have anything like that just yet, but if something is developed I can assure you our company will be the first to get it." He smiled broadly. Smiling came easy for him and he wielded a vigorous laugh—a natural salesman. "If you're nice, I'll show you what's new." He unzipped his leather portfolio. His eyes twinkled and his clean-shaven, wide, full face had a sheen.

"What's that?"

"It's my Slim-Jim."

"What?"

"You know, *Slim-Jims*. They have all the information about our products on a laminated narrow strip. You probably already know this, but I'm going to review it with you."

I have to admit, my mind wasn't on what he was saying. Thoughts of Mrs. Washew's story intruded. I guess my face showed it.

"Look, I know you're busy, so I'll leave you some stuff."

I knew the motivation wasn't altruistic, but drug samples served a purpose in our clinic. Some patients couldn't afford to pay for medication. Being able to put free medication into their hands made it more likely they would actually take it.

"Thanks, Jerry. Those samples come in handy."

"Okay, well, let me know how your patients are doing on them." Another winsome smile.

He's obviously use to being around people.

After saying good-bye, he departed.

A while later, I happened by the front desk to ask Thelma about another patient. I saw Jerry again, this time looking frazzled.

"Do you believe someone stole the airbag out of my car while I was in here talking to you?"

"You're not serious."

"I wish I weren't. And it's pouring out there; I got soaked. Then I tried to call on my cell phone, but the battery died." No more smiles. "Next time I visit this neighborhood I'm taking a cab."

VIOLENCE IN PSYCHIATRIC PATIENTS

The NYC "ferryboat slasher" drew tremendous public interest in part because he was being treated for mental illness. The idea of such individuals at large escalates already rampant fears about violence at the hands of the mentally unstable. In reality, only a minority of murderers are psychiatric patients. Those patients usually can be medicated.

In violent patients who are mentally ill, mood disorders (depression, mania), personality disorders (antisocial, borderline, and intermittent explosive), paranoid schizophrenia, and other disorders may be at play. Aggression and violence, symptoms rather than diseases, are usually not due to an underlying medical condition.

Contrary to popular belief, most schizophrenic people do not commit violent crimes unless there is a record of criminal violence before hospitalization. Of the 12 to 15% who are violent, most are paranoid and 90% show positive symptoms. Violent outbursts require treatment. Schizophrenics are much more likely to commit suicide than homicide.

The seriously agitated or violent psychotic patient, like "Wilma Washew's" son, requires a sedative. Haloperidol has the advantage of being potent and injectable. Sedative benzodiazepines handle mild to moderate cases. For intermittent, explosive outbursts, the anticonvulsants carbamazepine and valproic acid, or lithium and selective serotonin reuptake inhibitors are recommended. Propranolol and pindolol have a role in the treatment of chronic aggressive states.

*   *   *

"How They Found Out About It, God Only Knows"

"You better come over here right away." Thelma, the clinic receptionist-secretary, startled me as she swept into my office.

I looked up doubly surprised. Who was this person? The Thelma I knew was a heavyset, middle-aged woman who'd learned years before how to adjust her activity level for long-term survival as a hospital employee: when the pace got too fast, she moved slower. Thelma always seemed to be conserving her energy for some future disaster. For her to be moving and talking fast, something was terribly awry.

"What's the problem, Thelma?"

"Hurry up! They're on the floor."

In the background, I heard people shouting. I jumped up and ran down the hallway close behind Thelma. As I rounded the corner, to my considerable surprise, I saw two men wrestling on the floor in the waiting room. The one on top punched the man below him. His fist made a sickening thud.

An old woman next to them, obviously distraught, was trying to move away. "Help, help!" she screamed. A small crowd gathered at the raw display of violence.

"Call security, STAT," I hollered to Thelma.

Thelma stood motionless amidst the pandemonium, like a scared rabbit in the headlights of an oncoming vehicle.

"Thelma! *Now.*" I turned to the men and hollered, "Stop fighting! This is a hospital. You *must* stop at once. You're frightening the patients."

The men ignored me. One had a bloody nose and blood oozed from the corner of the other's mouth. They were yelling at each other in Spanish, but I couldn't understand what they were saying. I wasn't good at translating swear words.

Gripped by the immediacy of the situation, the thought of getting between the two men crossed my mind, but I was worried about being punched myself. Besides, I knew I would not be able physically to separate them. I escorted the crying woman out of the waiting room.

"I'm going home," she protested. "I don't want to stay here a minute longer!" She jerked her elbow from me and made a beeline for the exit.

With that, two large security guards shot out of the stairwell. They strong-armed the pugilists and whisked them away from the patient area with alacrity and surgical precision. The rapidity of the scene change was uncanny. Soon, it was back to business as usual.

I turned to Thelma. "What was all *that* about? Any idea?"

"If my Spanish is good, one man was sleeping with the other man's wife. How they found out about it, God only knows."

Thelma's remark reminded me of a German proverb I once heard:

The eyes believe themselves;
the ears believe other people.

What a perfect ending to the day. Nurse, doctor, social worker, and now—referee.

PROFILE OF AGGRESSION AND VIOLENCE

The problem of violence is pervasive. The typical demographic profile of a violent aggressor is an inner-city, socioeconomically deprived male under age 25. Males commit nearly 90% of all homicides, making them 10 times more likely than women to kill. About 20 to 50% of murders in the U.S. occur within the family, and police are called for more domestic disputes than for all other criminal activities. Violent individuals often have been abused themselves.

A significant portion of all violent deaths in this country are related to alcohol and drugs like amphetamines, crack cocaine, and other stimulants. Phencyclidine (PCP), which lowers the pain threshold, triggers bizarre, violent behavior. Violent acts take place in half-way houses, hospitals, nursing homes, outpatient clinics, prisons, and many other settings besides the home.

We can't predict what we don't understand. Dangerous aggressive behavior directed toward others is no more predictable by clinicians than by lay people. "Talk down" a violent individual or defuse an acute situation by creating a non-threatening environment, moving slowly, talking plainly and reassuringly. Don't crowd or talk loudly, threaten abuse, or make false promises.

When physical measures are necessary, the presence of several personnel reinforces the idea that further violent behavior is futile. Otherwise, actual physical restraint is needed to control the situation—something best left to security.

*   *   *

"Remember That Boy?"

It promised to be a wonderful fall morning. The clarity and blueness of the sky were spectacular. I was in a super mood.

Thelma opened the hallway window because the clinic was too warm. "Thought I'd air out this stuffy old place today," she said.

"Just what I need more of, New York's fine clean air." I smiled.

"We'll close it if it gets too cold in here. By the way, your first patient canceled for this morning so you're a free woman until 9:15."

"All right! I'm off to grab some coffee and maybe a donut if there are any left. If you need me, I'll be over talking with Susan in her office."

I noticed a tall adolescent boy. I didn't give him much thought as he headed for the bathroom, which was near my office. He must be with a relative, I surmised.

On the way I stopped in my office, reached down, and unlocked my left bottom desk drawer to get some change from my purse. I closed the drawer and walked out of my office leaving the door open as I always did. Then I breezed over to the conference room where the physicians held their financial meeting. I was in luck. There were several donuts left from the meeting. I took a few minutes to talk with my colleagues.

"Your patient just arrived," Thelma said afterwards as she handed me a medical chart.

"Thanks." I motioned for Claire Wooster to follow me from the waiting room. "First, let's get your weight," I said as we passed the scales.

The visit with Mrs. Wooster was a routine follow-up appointment for congestive heart failure. She was very compliant with her new diuretic and responded nicely with minimal side effects. On examination, her lungs sounded drier and her legs were less edematous.

"I'm able to sleep on one pillow at night instead of two," she said.

"I can believe it. You're weight has come down. I think you lost some of that excess water." I reached down into the right bottom drawer of my desk to give her some educational pamphlets on her heart condition. I noticed the left drawer was open and so was my purse.

In a flash it dawned on me that I'd been robbed. Stopping in mid-sentence, I quickly opened my purse all the way. My wallet was missing! I riffled through the rest of the drawers as the patient looked on.

"What's wrong?" she asked.

"My wallet is missing, someone took my wallet!"

"*I* didn't do it," she exclaimed.

I looked at the startled, seventy-two-year-old woman, her hair more white than gray. "No, no. Mrs. Wooster," I said with a wave of the hand. Excusing myself, I dashed down the hallway toward Thelma.

"Thelma, call security. Someone stole my wallet."

"You're kidding me."

"No, I'm *serious*." All I could think about were which credit cards I had in my wallet. *How much cash did I carry in my purse? It had to have been taken when I went over to get some coffee and— that boy!*

"Thelma, remember that boy who was kind of hanging around this morning by my office?"

"Yeah, he was acting edgy or something. He went to the bathroom then left."

"Was he with one of our patients?"

"I don't know, I never saw him before. All the doctors were in the conference room and I stepped away from my desk after you left. He must of been watching and waited for the best moment. I'm so sorry."

"It's not your fault. I let my guard down. I must not have locked the desk drawer. What a stupid mistake! At least I only lost forty dollars in cash. If the robber thought I was wealthy, boy did he get the short end of the stick."

Just then, two hospital uniformed security officers approached. I recounted the events of the morning. The guns they wore reminded me I worked at an inner-city hospital where drugs were sold openly on street corners. There was always an armed guard stationed at the entrance of the emergency room day and night.

"Well, it's unlikely you'll ever get your wallet back," one officer said, "but we'll look around and see if he tossed it into a trash can in the building. Most of them run fast and hard and ditch it in some alley out in the neighborhood."

The other officer took notes and handed me a report. "If I were *you*, I'd start calling to cancel those cards 'cause he sure as hell will try to use them right away. Were there any spare keys to your apartment in your wallet since he knows where you live by your driver's license?"

"No, but now I feel really unsafe knowing a thief has my address."

"These types are going for quick cash and credit cards. They don't usually head for the owner's place to steal from them there."

"If you have two locks on your door, one being a dead bolt, then I'd say that you'll be safe," the first officer added nonchalantly.

In the excitement, I forgot all about the patient in my office. I ran back and apologized profusely to her for the interruption.

"Don't worry, I understand," she said. "Do you need a subway token to get home tonight, dear?"

"How sweet of you, thank you, but I have a couple of spares ones." Her display of compassion and concern for my welfare touched me.

"Just count you blessings you weren't here when he tried to take it. I've been mugged four times in my own neighborhood for cash. I'm an old pro at being a victim," Mrs. Wooster said.

I escorted the patient out to Thelma, who, still upset by the crime, was telling everybody about it. Fortunately, my next patient was late, so I spent the following fifteen minutes canceling my credit cards through an automatic credit card protection service. I found out I wasn't liable for anything that was charged since I called within one hour of the incident.

When it came time for lunch, I went downstairs and grabbed a quick bite. I was absorbed in thoughts about the robbery. It seemed like a personal affront. For all I knew, the crime was perpetrated by a patient, someone who'd seen my office and knew where I kept my purse. Maybe the man was a relative of one of my patients. How could my patients do this to me, I asked myself. It's easy to jump to conclusions.

Two weeks after the robbery in the clinic, I received a four-hundred dollar American Express bill. I knew I canceled the card and couldn't have made purchases. One item was listed: a gold chain necklace from a jewelry store in the neighborhood of the hospital. I didn't end up having to pay the bill, but I was disappointed. If someone needed to steal my wallet, I hoped they needed the money for food.

8

Insatiable Cravings

There is no sincerer love than the love of food
—GEORGE BERNARD SHAW

Thou shouldst eat to live; not live to eat
—MARCUS TULLIUS CICERO

Alcoholism isn't a spectator sport. Eventually the whole family gets
to play
—JOYCE REBETA-BURDITT

What three things does drink especially provoke?
Marry, sir, nose painting, sleep, and urine.
Lechery sir, it provokes, and unprovokes;
it provokes the desire,
but it takes away the performance
—WILLIAM SHAKESPEARE

Only the opium eater truly understands the pain of death
—JOHN CHEEVER

"You Caught Me Red-Handed"

"Thelma. I'm starving and in desperate need of sugar and a stimulant. If Amy Katz comes in, tell her I'll be back in a jiff. Don't tell her I stopped for a donut. She's diabetic and is not compliant with her diet."

"Pick up a glazed one for me, too," Thelma called after me as I zipped down the hallway. "I'm not a happy camper today either."

"You got it, Thelma Louise." I headed for the snack shop. Because I woke up late, I missed breakfast. I barely made it under the wire for my first patient's appointment. Now my second patient was not on time, affording me the luxury of a cinnamon-sugared donut and a regular coffee.

At the entrance of the snack shop, I got a paper tray and entered into the queue. Instantly I knew why Mrs. Katz was late for her appointment. There she was in line waiting to pay the cashier for *three* chocolate donuts and a *large* orange juice. So much for the forty-five minutes I spent with her last week about diabetes and her twelve-hundred-calorie ADA diet.

I deliberated about marching up and reminding Mrs. Katz of her diet. *If I wait until I see her back in the clinic, I can do a finger-stick to measure her blood sugar. When the level of glucose comes back sky-high, I'll confront her.*

No, why make her stick herself when I know she's been cheating; she's already taken a few bites of the chocolate donut. I can't force her to put back all three donuts, but... I can make her feel guilty enough to return the other two donuts and get a small orange juice...

The moment was too felicitous to ignore. When I walked up to her, she immediately registered primal fear and guilt. Incriminating donut crumbs dusted her lips. "Oh, my, what a surprise. I was just on my way to see you." She was painfully self-conscious as she tried to laugh through a weak smile.

"Well since you were late, Mrs. Katz, I thought I'd grab a healthy *apple* for a mid-morning snack, how about you?"

"You caught me red-handed. These two donuts are for my grandchildren at home and I got one for myself. I just get so hungry with that insulin that I crave something sweet." She was talking too rapidly and with more excitement than usual.

"Why don't you turn in those two donuts for some fruit for the *grandkids* and trade your *large* orange juice for a *small* orange juice. We'll talk about your exchange list upstairs, okay?"

She realized resistance was futile. I had her best interest in mind.

I resumed my place at the end of the line and watched Mrs. Katz buy two bananas and a small orange juice. I waved her on and gave her the thumbs up signal. After my impromptu lecture, I felt it would be inappropriate to buy donuts, so I opted for apples. Thelma would have to understand.

As I walked into the office, Thelma said, "Your patient, Mrs. Katz, is here and I'm ready for my—" She looked stunned as I pressed a shiny red apple into her hand.

"I'll explain later," I whispered forcibly.

While walking back to the clinic, I'd taken a few bites of my apple and gobbled the rest of it in my office. I called in Mrs. Katz, weighed her on the office scales, and then escorted her back to my room.

"I have to be honest with you," she said. "Those two other donuts weren't for my grandchildren. They were for me."

I smiled. "I know, but thanks for admitting it."

"Nobody understands what it's like. I enjoyed having a big stack of pancakes with lots of maple syrup or a couple of donuts and coffee for the past thirty-five years. Then my body betrays me. I'm suddenly told I have diabetes and must limit the amount I eat and how often I eat. I have to check my blood glucose fasting before breakfast, two hours after breakfast, at dinner and at bedtime. It's too much.

I want my old life back. My fingers feel like pin cushions. I have to worry when I go out to a restaurant about what I can order. I get fewer invitations to eat at friends' homes because they don't know what to make for me. It's not fair. Sometimes I just want to stop at a hot dog stand on the sidewalk and order the works. I use to enjoy that when I went on walks in Central Park." Mrs. Katz started to cry.

I reached over her desk and offered her some tissues. "I can appreciate that being diabetic is difficult. It's easy for me to preach. The good news is that diabetes, although it's not curable, is treatable *if* you have the discipline and will power to stay on top of it. I get the impression you're feeling isolated and abandoned."

Mrs. Katz nodded.

"There are diabetes support groups all over the city. They welcome new members, and it's a chance to make new friends who understand what you're going through. This is not the time to be an ostrich and stick your head in the sand, hoping the problem will go away. I want you to be honest with me and tell me what's not working for you. Perhaps you're too strict with the diet. We could increase you to a fifteen-hundred-calorie ADA diet. So far you've lost fifteen pounds over two months. That's great. Your walking exercise program is good. Maybe you need some friends to call when you feel tempted to stray. Anybody who has seriously tried to lose weight knows what it's like to count calories, exercise daily, and watch what they eat all the time."

Mrs. Katz blew her nose on the tissues. "I feel better already getting all that off my chest. It's time I start taking control of my life and stop acting like a big baby." She offered her left third finger for the finger-stick routine.

"Let's forego that today. We both know it's going to be high from the donut. Instead, let's talk about the exchange list so that once a week you can have a donut for breakfast. Today you'll have to stick your finger when you get home before lunch to see if you'll need regular insulin to cover you. Is that agreeable?"

"Yes!" Mrs. Katz said appreciatively.

I gave her the number of the local chapter of the American Diabetes Association. We agreed on another visit in two weeks.

When Amy Katz left, I reflected on how badly I wanted that donut earlier, just like she must have felt. Will power is hard to sustain. Had I not seen my patient in the snack shop, I would have routinely gone over diet, checked her blood glucose and adjusted her insulin. She would have agreed to everything, gone home and eaten those three donuts, felt physically terrible later, then added more insulin to counteract the high sugar. The more insulin, the more the hunger. It's a vicious cycle. I had to be more insightful about my patients' plight.

DIABETES, THE SILENT ENEMY

Hindu physicians recognized the symptoms of diabetes as early as the sixth century B.C. The disease that caused excessive thirst and urination was named *diabetes*, meaning "a passing through," in the second century by Aretaeus. Before glucose could be measured in the blood, the sweet, honey-like taste of the urine was used to make the diagnosis, hence the added name *mellitus*.

Diabetes mellitus is serious. The International Diabetes Foundation predicts it will become one of the major killers of the 21st century. The WHO estimates it will affect some 300 million persons by the year 2025. Diabetes presents a tremendous challenge, demanding immediate changes in diet, exercise, health monitoring, and often medication.

But the biggest problem is its stealth. Sixteen million Americans have diabetes, but many don't realize it—diabetes is silent. Because it's a risk factor for other diseases, such as cardiovascular and renal disease, the price of failing to control diabetes is high: amputation of the legs, blindness, damage to peripheral nerves, heart attack, kidney failure, susceptibility to infections, and stroke.

Ninety percent of those with the disease have Type II diabetes, the form approaching epidemic proportions as the country's fourth deadliest disease. An individual may have the disease for 8 years with little or no symptoms before the diagnosis is made. Sometimes only a catastrophe or complication brings it to light. The lowered cutoff for fasting blood glucose (110 mg per dL) makes it easier to diagnosis diabetes early.

Type II diabetes presents in adult life when pancreatic cells produce insulin but the body cannot use it. The cells have fewer insulin receptors and a number of those receptors are blocked. Exercise and weight loss increase the number of insulin receptors. Exercising 4 to 5 times a week for 40 minutes a session hastens weight loss and enhances blood sugar control. For patients with complications of diabetes or high blood sugar levels, these guidelines need to be tempered.

A "diabetic diet" no longer exists. New nutrition guidelines provide many food choices, allowing for food preferences and ethnic and cultural influences on diet. All food intake must be accounted for in the day's total caloric intake as well as the proportion of protein, fat, and carbohydrates. By making adjustments and substitutions within food groups, occasional desserts can be worked into the menu. Non-nutritive sweeteners (aspartame, saccharin) are alternatives to sucrose. A caloric intake of 10 to 20% protein, no more than 30% fat (at least 90% should be unsaturated), carbohydrates, and 20 to 35 grams of fiber is desirable.

FIGHTING BACK WITH DRUGS

When diet and exercise fail to control blood sugar, oral glucose-lowering (antihyperglycemic) drugs are the next step. Sulfonylureas, which stimulate the pancreas to secrete more insulin, remain the most widely prescribed oral antidiabetic drugs. The biguanide metformin, which works by a different mechanism, has been advocated as a first-line drug for obese, insulin-resistant diabetics. Acarbose, a representative competitive inhibitor of intestinal brush-border α-glucosidase, reduces the rate of carbohydrate absorption after meals. Troglitazone is a prototype of a new class of agents that sensitize tissues to insulin.

The leap to insulin has many implications. For the patient, it may signify failure and serious risks, which must be worked through emotionally. For the health care provider and patient, the need to start insulin is the beginning of an extensive education. The patient needs to learn to draw up and inject insulin, understand the different types of insulin (lente, regular, NPH), make adjustments in diet and exercise, monitor his or her own blood sugar with a glucose monitor, keep careful daily records of all blood testing, and recognize the warning signs of dangerously low blood sugar (insulin reaction) and how to treat it. The frequency of blood testing depends on the type and severity of diabetes, but may include a finger-stick before meals and at bedtime, more often with a change in exercise or illness.

For emergencies, keep a glucagon kit nearby, as the hormone glucagon reverses the action of insulin. A ready sugar source, such as a piece of hard candy or orange juice, also should be available.

*   *   *

"So Don't Preach to Me"

I asked Marlena Lesner, the student nurse practitioner, to see Regina Boulez, a Hispanic woman in her fifties who routinely came to the clinic for diabetes. Because I felt I knew Ms. Boulez well and would be able to evaluate the adequacy of the student's assessment, I let Marlena start with her. Ms. Boulez could be difficult, but would make an impression. Forty minutes later, Marlena returned.

"I don't understand," Marlena began. "She acts like she doesn't have diabetes. She eats all types of desserts and takes second helpings, ingests large amounts of alcohol, smokes a pack a day of cigarettes, and is gaining weight. She already has high blood pressure, high cholesterol, an enlarged heart, vision problems from the high sugars, and is heading toward renal failure."

"You've got the picture, Marlena. Ms. Boulez is determined that diabetes is not going to affect her lifestyle. She couldn't care less about what she eats or when she eats it and continues her dangerous habits. Nothing I do motivates her to comply with measures that could save her life."

"What are you going to do?"

"What would you suggest?"

Marlena had no answer.

"Let's go see her together."

In the clinic room, I found Ms. Boulez sitting in a wheelchair with her home attendant at her side. She wore a loose, shapeless, patterned dress, and a simple metal barrette held her hair at the back of her head. She was confined a wheelchair because she had bilateral AKA, an acronym for above-knee-amputation of both legs, due to uncontrolled diabetes. Grossly obese, with a protuberant belly, Ms. Boulez's hands looked very small. The rings on her fingers had the appearance of being embedded in her flesh. Because she ran such high blood sugars, with daily ranges of four-hundred to five-hundred instead of the normal seventy to one-hundred-ten or so, her skin was constantly warm and moist from sweating. Her self-destructive debauchery had literally whittled her away.

"What are we going to do, Mrs. Boulez? I'm hearing that you are not taking your diet seriously."

Ms. Boulez merely laughed, imperturbably unblinking. Her face was frozen in a perpetual grimace.

"Are you doing finger sticks?"

"Yes."

"Can you show me the numbers in your record book?"

"I didn't bring it with me."

She *never* brought the book. Quick to nod and say *yes* all the time, she refused to learn to do her own finger-sticks. She let herself have blood drawn from her vein for a fasting blood sugar, but never fasted. I often got the impression that Ms. Boulez was mocking me every time we had a session together. In my mind I was reviewing remaining treatment options.

"Ms. Boulez," the student interjected, "I forgot to ask you if anyone else in your family has diabetes?"

The patient looked at Marlena with thoughtful penetration, never taking her eyes off her. Her once complacent voice now bristled with raw anger. "My parents both died of diabetes when they were in their early sixties. I'm fifty-five now. They passed on this disease and they expect me to suffer, too. I hated them when they were alive. I ran away from home when I was sixteen. Don't you see their revenge on me from the grave?

Well, *I* won't suffer. I live and enjoy my life like I always have, and that includes good food and booze. So I lost my legs, *so what!* This wheel chair and that girl who helps me out at home are all I need. I tell her what to buy at the food store and liquor store, and she does what I say 'cause I pay her to."

Regina Boulez glared at Marlena then turned her attention to me. Her face was plethoric. Pointing her finger as if to skewer me, she exclaimed, "So don't preach to me. *You* didn't grow up with my parents. *You* don't have this curse."

Stunned to hear all this revealed in response to one simple question, I looked over at Marlena whose mouth dropped open in disbelief. So, behind that comfortable persona lurked demons Ms. Boulez had never shared with me before. I wanted to be sure she didn't misconstrue my aversion to her attitude as a condemnation of her as a person.

"No one is saying things have been easy for you," I said. "But why do you come here to see me and listen to all my teaching about taking care of yourself when you have no intention of doing so? It's a complete waste of your time and mine. I'd say that to anyone who did what you're doing. Are you trying to *kill* yourself?"

Then the lid closed on her jack-in-the-box emotions. Ms. Boulez's frozen smile returned and with it her congeniality. "Because it's a chance to get out of my apartment, take a free cab ride to the hospital, and see lots of people. Just remember, don't judge a person before you've walked a mile in their shoes. I read that once somewhere. I believe it's true."

"I am not judging you. I'm just trying to—"

"Oh," she sneered, "and I don't go in for that psychotherapy *crap* either. Believe me, my doctor tried that on me. Now, I better be going because I have an appointment with the eye and kidney doctors today, too." She then pulled out of her canvas tote bag a two-pound box of Godiva's dark chocolate pieces. "I love to munch on these between meals. Would you care to have a few pieces?"

I watched in disgust as the patient and the home attendant helped themselves to two pieces before she packed them away in the tote bag. Annoyed by the affront, I decided I wasn't going to take this.

"Ms. Boulez, I can't in good faith keep taking care of you. I am having no impact on your health care and I cannot in good conscience continue our sessions. You're on the path of self-destruction. I acknowledge your right to choose freely, but I can only help you if you *want* my help. I'll give you an appointment with your primary doctor next week and will explain the reason why. I am very sorry, but you are not letting me help you."

Ms. Boulez merely shrugged her shoulders indifferently.

The student looked shocked at what I said.

The home attendant got up and backed Ms. Boulez out of the doorway. She told her how good the chocolate was and Ms. Boulez agreed.

Ms. Boulez's final words to me were, "Have a nice day, hon."

I walked over to Thelma, the appointment receptionist, and explained that Ms. Boulez needed an appointment with her primary doctor, not me. Thelma looked up surprised, but, after studying my face, she decided not to ask why.

Although it was over quickly, the moment had been so intense that it took a while to come down from the supercharged heights.

Back in my office, Marlena was upset. Her normally reserved manner vanished. "How could you get angry with that patient?"

"I just put my foot down."

"But she's a patient. She can't help the way she feels. Diabetes is a terrible disease."

"No, wait, Marlena. Diabetes is a responsibility. What's terrible is that she doesn't take care of herself. By denying she has diabetes, she's allowed the disease to ruin her life. She thinks she's ignoring it. A person cannot *ignore* diabetes. You *have* to deal with it. If you don't, you'll end up like her."

"I think we shouldn't give up on her."

"I know it must seem strange to you," I said. "But if you have a patient who won't follow your advice and who continues to self-destruct, you need to send a strong message that you don't condone the behavior. If she wants to change her ways, she knows where I am. I gave her that option. You cannot help a person who does not want your help." Immediately I thought back to people telling me those same words.

"But shouldn't you have kept trying to make her see reason?'

"This is the first time you've seen her. I have seen her many times over the last few years. Believe me, I have hit my head against the wall over this lady. She hasn't changed one iota. I haven't made any difference. Maybe someone else can. I've recommended that she see a therapist about dealing with chronic disease. She won't go. She won't do anything to help herself."

Marlena looked unconvinced. "I feel like we failed her."

Having a student around was somewhat like having a teen-ager at home challenging you all the time. The experience could be vexing. On the other hand, I knew that students rejuvenated the conscience.

"Nursing school doesn't train you for the unexpected situations you will find yourself in. You can't apply the usual approaches. Ms. Boulez is not your failure. Most patients try to help themselves more than she does. Realize just how extraordinary she is and deal with her accordingly. I know I'm not always attentive, insightful, or politically correct, but I'm trying to do what I think is right."

Marlena and I exchanged views for awhile. I kept alluding to my experience and the student referred to what she had been taught in the classroom. When all was said and done, I imagined she thought I was calloused.

Although I saw other patients before I left work that day, thoughts of Regina Boulez trickled back on my way home. Soon, the trickle became a stream and carried me toward unsettling, turbulent, philosophical waters. Was the student right?

Should I have stuck with Ms. Boulez no matter what? Had the system failed a person like Regina Boulez? Years ago, the need for tight control of blood sugar was not appreciated. I realized that not all diabetics could be controlled even with insulin and had Ms. Boulez followed her diet, she might have lost her legs anyway. But in most cases, diet and exercise, as well as careful foot care, could prevent such problems. When had Ms. Boulez given up the fight? Did she really believe she was doomed because her parents died young? Had she, feeling overwhelmed and hopeless, much like an alcoholic, chosen to drown her sorrows, but with sugar instead?

I was left with the thought that Regina Boulez was trapped not by her dead parents, but by her living and perpetual anger toward them, she, her only jailer, judge, and executioner.

Understanding Treatment Failure

Failure to control diabetes has catastrophic consequences. The highest recorded blood sugar level in a conscious person was 1,791 milligrams per deciliter—at least 12 times normal. The tissue damage may be irreversible. Compared with people who do not have diabetes, diabetics carry a 2 to 4 times higher long-term risk of heart disease and stroke, according to the Center for Disease Control (CDC). About 60 to 65% have high blood pressure and nerve disease (stocking-glove neuropathy). Diabetes is the leading cause of new blindness, end-stage kidney disease, and amputation in adult Americans.

Take care: diabetics are more prone to develop foot problems because diabetes injures blood vessels and nerves and deforms the feet. They can injure their feet without feeling it and the injuries become infected easily. Never soak the foot. About 85% of foot and leg amputations could be prevented by early detection and appropriate treatment of skin ulcers. Diabetic patients must be participants not spectators in their own management and understand proper foot hygiene, footwear, and nail care. Major problems can be minimized if caught early.

Denial about the diagnosis stands behind the scenes together with divorce, drinking, financial difficulties, and other personal problems, undermining compliance and control. Failure to learn how food groups can be varied may lock a patient into an unpalatable diet and reduce compliance. Seeing the disease progress due to failed treatment can also be demoralizing. The push for good control must be made early in the course of treatment. Referrals to a certified diabetes educator, dentist, dietician, ophthalmologist, podiatrist, psychologist, psychiatrist, or social worker, as indicated, should be prompt.

For many patients, fingersticking is the worst aspect of monitoring. Warming the finger in warm, running water for a few minutes before lancing, massaging blood to the fingertip, and rotating the finger sites all help.

Systematic monitoring three to four times a day for several consecutive days provides more useful information than sporadic testing done over a longer period of time does. Infrequent and improper blood testing paints the wrong picture and may give the false illusion of good control. Recently, researchers have found that post-lunch glucose measurements are better markers of glycemic control than fasting glucose is.

The gold standard for determining long-term diabetic control is glycosylated hemoglobin (HbA1C). Bringing the test results down to the normal range of 3.8 to 6% is the goal.

Successful management of diabetes requires clear, two-way communication, explanations of how actions impact on diabetic control, short- and long-term goals, and individualized care in collaboration with the patient. A simple understanding of the biology of diabetes will help the patient realize how treatment works and the importance of good control of blood glucose. Patients need resources to contact when they can't solve a management problem.

*   *   *

"I Need You to Fill This Out"

When I returned from lunch, I found a chart stuffed in the box outside my door. The patient was left-over from the morning walk-in clinic. Annoyed at first that Susan Crawley, another nurse practitioner, was dumping on me, I quickly realized she was overloaded.

"Daniel White," I called out in the waiting room.

A black, obese man stood up and walked toward me, boom box in hand. Rolls of fat on his trunk heaved and pitched, colliding together with the impact of each lumbering step. The friction of his pant legs as his thighs rubbed together sounded like sandpapering, one slow, deliberate stroke after another.

Good heavens, I said to myself. Obesity had to be one of the most difficult medical problems to deal with. As we came to the scales, I stopped. "Please step up, Mr. White."

He shifted his weight from side to side as he climbed on. The scales shook violently like they would crumble under his weight. I slid the metal counterweight until it clicked at three-hundred-thirty pounds or about one-hundred-fifty kilograms! His weight was almost off the scale. His height was only five-and-one-half feet or one-hundred-sixty-five centimeters.

As Mr. White entered my office, swaying side-to-side, I looked at his body habitus. He fit the stereotype that men are apples and women are pears. Obese men and postmenopausal women store fat in the upper body, particularly the abdomen and around abdominal viscera, giving them an apple shape. Most obese premenopausal women store fat in the lower body, especially the buttocks, hips, and thighs, or "saddle-bag" area, conferring on them a pear shape.

When I searched through his chart to see his last weight, I saw that Daniel White missed his last several appointments for weight checks. He was supposed to lose ten pounds on a new diet. Instead, he *gained* fourteen more pounds! Most people who seriously diet will lose weight in seven days from water loss alone. He stepped down off the scale like a boy who's gotten a bad report card and trailed me into my room.

"What brings you to the clinic today?"

"I need you to fill this out." He presented me with a piece of paper that he unfolded from his shirt pocket. Out of breath, he wiped the perspiration from his brow and shaved head. Some drops of sweat ran down his cheeks until they were trapped by his short beard.

It was a form. I spotted the dreaded word at the top. "Disability?"

"Yes." He looked sheepish. His features seemed small as they floated on his full face.

"What disability?"

"My high blood pressure." He made intermittent, vocalized expirations, like a steam locomotive come to the last stop.

"But your blood pressure is completely stable and controlled with medication."

"I feel that I needs this to help me survive and pay for my medication till I gets a job."

I knew that in the current system, he wouldn't receive disability for hypertension unless he was chronically compromised or unstable and it affected everyday lifestyle. "Have you been looking for a job?"

"Sure, I've been trying real hard, but with my high blood pressure, I can't do nothin'." He mopped his brow again.

"How so?" I wondered how he was going to make his case.

"I can't breathe and physical labor makes me get short of breath."

"Well, Mr. White, I think that has more to do with your weight. Every pound of fat is an extra mile of blood vessels your heart has to pump blood through. It's an enormous burden."

Mr. White opened his mouth, but no words came out. His head

seemed dwarfed by his gargantuan body.

"How about an office job, sitting doing paperwork or filing?" I asked.

Mr. White's impatience mounted. He grew tired of pretenses. "Can't you help me out with the disability?"

As I looked at the morbidly obese, thirty-five-year-old man, galvanized by a strong sense of denial, I realized that the real problem was motivation. Without superior motivation on the part of everyone concerned, nothing could be accomplished. It was clear to me that this patient was malingering.

"I don't think you really need this. I will leave the form with a note for your primary doctor. He can decide if he wants to sign it. Do you think you'd feel better if you could lose some weight?"

"Maybe," Mr. White said indifferently with a shrug of his shoulders.

"Are you sticking to your diet?"

"I try to."

I worked out the incriminating math. His weight in pounds multiplied times twelve gave the total calories he consumed each day to maintain his weight:

$$330 \times 12 = 3,960$$

The result was impressive, but did not surprise me. Leaving aside his weight gain, he was ingesting at least three-thousand-nine-hundred-sixty calories a day. Some diet!!

Then I calculated his body mass index (BMI)—his weight in kilograms divided by his height in meters (1.69) squared:

$$150 \div 2.86 = 53$$

BMI is more reliable than the standard, height-weight insurance tables are. A BMI of nineteen to twenty-five is considered healthful. A BMI above twenty-seven in a person who does not have lean body composition poses significant health risks. His was almost *twice* that—grade III obesity with astronomically increased health risk! At that level, drug treatment is necessary, but it would not be successful without dieting. If Mr. White didn't take the matter seriously, he might be facing surgery.

"I don't think you're sticking to your diet. I calculate that you are eating two or three times more than you should be eating."

He sat with his arms folded and looked straight ahead, avoiding my eyes. His face turned expressionless.

"If you eat right—plenty of whole grains, fruits, and vegetables—you can still eat pretty well and it won't seem like a diet. Do you want to talk to the dietitian again?"

He thought for a moment. That face again. "No."

"Okay, then. Let's start over and set a weight management goal. If you could lose five pounds in a month, that would be something we can work with. If you could lose any weight, you'd feel good that you are doing something about this."

My inner voice was less optimistic. I wondered why I bothered going through the motions. We both knew that nothing was going to happen. "Are you getting much exercise?"

"I walk some."

"Good. For how long?"

"I walk mostly around the house."

That would explain it, I thought. "Anything else?"

"No, not really."

"Do you have any outside activities?"

"Like what?"

"You know, like shooting hoops with friends or taking a walk with your girlfriend?"

"Lady, in my neighborhood, no one goes for walks, even if I did have a girlfriend."

"Okay, I can see your point, but exercise is important if you want to lose weight. It burns calories and helps your heart. It also puts you in a frame of mind to eat the right foods. Even if you walk thirty minutes every day, that's something. That will help eventually. We have to make a change in your way of living. You will also need to go on medication."

He shrugged noncommittally. I didn't help him with his disability claim, so now he wasn't going to cooperate with me. Such was the unwritten law of the clinic.

Like a mother trying to coax a recalcitrant child, I felt foolish.

Without warning, Daniel White stood up. The chair creaked and groaned as if in pain as he did so. He grabbed his boom box and snatched the disability form from my desk. His parting words were to the point: "Dieting sucks."

I had to agree with him. But I hoped maybe he'd meet a woman who might motivate him to lose weight. Sometimes what we can't do for ourselves we'll do for others we hold close to our heart.

The Epidemic of Obesity

The Guinness Book of World Records documents just how much weight the human body can gain. The heaviest male was 1400 pounds, gaining about 300 pounds in six months. The heaviest female weighed 1200 pounds. For most people weight gain is not as dramatic, but it is no less serious. Are we the same creatures who could survive without consuming anything but water for a month?

At a time when half a billion individuals, about one out of every eight, are suffering from chronic malnutrition worldwide, the prevalence of obesity is rising at an alarming rate in all affluent countries. In the U.S., 59 percent of the adult population meets the current definition of clinical obesity, easily qualifying the disease for epidemic status. Minority populations, especially African-American women, are disproportionately affected.

A typical American gains about 20 pounds between the ages of 25 and 55, manifesting in men as the all too familiar ballooning potbelly. Although Americans today consume about the same number of calories as those living in 1910 did, we exercise much less. Only one-fifth of the population exercises enough to help control weight! The U.S. is the fourth largest calorie-consuming country in the world—3,732 calories daily per capita.

Obesity now threatens the health of many citizens of the U.S. where obesity-related illnesses kill 300,000 persons each year. Sadly, the deaths are preventable. Excessive weight consorts with cancer (breast, colon, endometrium, and prostate), coronary artery disease, diabetes, gallbladder disease, gout, hyperlipidemia, hypertension, osteoarthritis, and premature death.

At the center of many syndromes lies obesity. Most are endocrine or inherited disorders. *Syndrome X* is the cluster of diabetes, obesity, and hypertension. The acronym *CHAOS* stands for coronary artery disease, hypertension, atherosclerosis, obesity, and stroke.

Treating obesity and diseases associated with it costs more than $100 billion in annual health care expenses. Many primary health care providers are disillusioned by the paucity of effective treatments, and many patients who mistakenly believe their obesity is caused by a metabolic problem lack motivation to make the necessary lifestyle changes.

GENES, DIETS, AND DRUGS

As the epidemic of obesity spreads throughout the industrial world, scientists are grappling with its biology. Obesity is an imbalance between caloric intake and energy expenditure. The problem is complex, regulated by multiple feedback loops. The healthy body stores only a few tenths of a percent of ingested calories. Fat, a type of endocrine tissue, is in a dynamic network involving brain, digestive tract, and muscle. Although the number of fat cells may be genetic, how large they become has everything to do with our lifestyle.

Why do we eat so much? Genetics, behavior, and environment conspire against us. It comes as no surprise: genes influence our body mass, eating habits, metabolism, and physical activity. Several "fat genes," like the *ob* gene, have been cloned in animals, but have not been found in humans. Insensitivity of the brain to leptin, a protein secreted by fat cells when fat is stored that squelches the appetite and revs the metabolism, may be a problem in obesity. Perhaps multiple genes interact with each other under the influence of economic and psychological factors to trigger obesity.

Americans lavish more than $32 billion dollars on fad diet and lose-weight-quick schemes, but 90% do not maintain the weight loss over a 3 year period, according to a recent study. The body is not easily fooled by would-be dieters: weight loss reduces the body's rate of burning fat. According to the set-point hypothesis, the brain maintains a target body weight by adjusting our metabolism and eating behaviors. Another, more optimistic view, the settling-point hypothesis, instead posits that achieving an equilibrium between our environment and our gene-governed metabolism allows us to maintain our weight. Ingesting more energy than can be burned results in obesity.

Science has come to the rescue with information about dietary fat. We constantly hear about "good" and "bad" fats and oils. Polyunsaturated (corn and soybean oils) and monounsaturated (olive and canola oils) fats are healthier than saturated and trans fatty acids are. Because the FDA does not yet require that trans fats be listed on food labels, it is best to avoid partially hydrogenated oils, which often contain trans oil. Nuts rich in monounsaturated fats and vitamin E are almonds, cashews, hazelnuts, macadamia nuts, and pecans—not peanuts and pine nuts. Remember that even "good" oils pack calories. Eating fruit, garlic (if your friends tolerate it), legumes, soluble fiber, and soy products also helps lower cholesterol. Olestra, an artificial fat that tastes like ordinary fat, is not digested by the body and has been approved by the FDA as a fat-substituting food additive.

Some researchers propose that the treatment philosophy of the last 40 or 50 years, which has focused on dieting, should be supplanted by a drug-oriented approach. They recommend drug treatment for BMI's over 30. Dexfenfluramine is the first weight-loss drug approved in the U.S. in a couple of dozen years. The popular "phen-fen," a combination of phenteramine and fenfluramine, was discontinued due to fatalities.

Regardless of the treatment approach, it is easier to deal with the problem of weight gain before it escalates to massive or morbid obesity. Otherwise, drastic measures may be necessary. Gastroplasy, an operation that reduces the size of the stomach, is effective, but may cause digestive problems and carries the risk of major surgery.

As obesity has no cure, prevention would be better. Good dietary and exercise habits are a life-long commitment to weight control and good health. Eating right becomes a way of life. It's true that snack attacks can strike more quickly than a lightning storm can. How can you protect yourself? Some overweight people misread their own emotions, interpreting troubled feelings as hunger. Insight into this habit, together with support groups or therapy, can modify the behavior. So the next time your hand is poised on the refrigerator door handle, ask yourself: *Am I sure I'm really hungry?*

*   *   *

"You Were Hurting Me"

"Don't *ever* do that to me again," Lawrence Burns yelled belligerently. "What the hell's wrong with you, squeezing a man like that?" He was a big man with salt-and-pepper hair. He wore a soiled, baseball T-shirt and dark blue workman's pants.

"I was only taking your blood pressure," I explained.

"You were hurting me," he insisted, ripping off the blood pressure cuff and throwing it down. His gut hung over his belt and shook with his motion. He had a wild look in his eyes.

"You've had your blood pressure taken before."

"I thought my arm was going to explode." He looked contentious and eager to quarrel.

I stared at him in disbelief.

"This is all a bunch of crap anyway," he complained. "I don't need your tests or your pills. There's nothing wrong with me." His gray eyes were red-rimmed and his skin was flushed.

"You have high blood pressure. You *need* your medication."

"It's none of your goddamned business." As his irritation mounted, he let loose one obscenity-laced denunciation after another.

At first I didn't know how to answer. "You've been drinking quite a bit, haven't you." I was thinking out loud as I moved toward the door. This was all I could say?

"Just leave me alone!"

No argument. I left the room to find Dr. Gary Montrose, an attending physician in the clinic.

I'm a nurse practitioner at a major NYC medical clinic, I said to myself; *I should be ready for anything. When I smelled alcohol on his breath, I should have refused to see him. Be more careful. Do you want to get assaulted?*

But I didn't want to make him mad by sending him out unseen either. What was I supposed to do?

Part of me was still shaking inside. Perhaps it was the eternal child who emerged during such situations. Or perhaps it was the woman who was still abhorrent from time to time at yet another of the big city's vicissitudes.

At that moment, Dr. Montrose walked by. "What's all the commotion?" he asked with a hint of annoyance.

Dr. Montrose was a tall man of average build with a studious, nonathletic appearance; slightly disheveled, layered, brown hair; and dark eyes. The bow tie was his signature.

"Gary, your patient is giving me a hard time."

"Who?"

"Mr. Burns."

"Is he drinking again?"

"Yes."

"I'll go in with you this time."

We went back into my room and found Mr. Burns pacing around

the room muttering to himself. I was worried that he was too agitated, but Dr. Montrose knew him from previous visits.

"What's going on, Larry?" Dr. Montrose queried.

"Ask *her*." He jabbed his thumb toward me in the air. *"She's* the one causing the trouble."

"Let's all calm down and talk this through. She is only trying to help you. We need to check your blood pressure. Your blood pressure runs high."

"So what."

"It's important. High blood pressure damages the body. It can kill you."

Mr. Burns made a disgruntled sound.

"Are you taking your medication?"

"No. I don't need it."

"Look, Larry, have you started drinking again?"

"What if I have."

"You need your medication not alcohol. The two don't mix."

Mr. Burns waved him off with his right hand.

Dr. Montrose looked over at me. "I think Larry should come back to the clinic to see us when he's sober. He won't let us do anything for him today."

I agreed. How do you convince people about the risks of hypertension, the silent killer, especially when they've been drinking?

Lawrence Burns, who had been staring at the floor, suddenly spoke with emotion. "You'd drink, too, if your wife left you and took the children. I lost my job and my family this week—my whole damn life." The look in his eyes was no longer one of defiance.

Silence hung in the room like a nerve gas that left it's victims paralyzed but for the darting movements of their eyes at one another. Finally, Dr. Montrose stepped forward.

"Come on, Larry, I have a gap between patients. Let's go into my office. I'll get you some coffee and we'll talk." He placed his hand on Mr. Burn's back as he coaxed him out my door and down the hall.

I should know by now. It never turns out to be what you think it is.

ALCOHOLISM

Alcohol consumption is an integral part of society, dating from the beginnings of recorded history. Used in ancient Egypt for religious

ceremonies long before it was available as a beverage, wine supplanted beer as the main alcoholic beverage by 3000 B.C. in Meso-
potamia. Cultivation of grapes by the Greeks and Romans lead to a
profusion of vineyards into this century. Gods like Bacchus seemed
to smile on those who imbibed. The distillation of alcoholic liquor
from grain, an art newer than the fermentation of beers and wines,
dates back to eleventh century Europe. About that time, the monks
were developing liqueurs. Today there's an alcoholic beverage for
every social occasion in every country.

Problems controlling alcohol use did not take long to emerge.
Alexander the Great, alleged to be one of the greatest generals of all
time, may have been alcoholic. In a drunken fury he slew his friend
Clitus, later deeply regretting his action. Alcoholism also claimed the
Mongolian conqueror, Attila the Hun, whose name meant "scourge
of the gods." When he married the last of his many wives, he drank
excessively at the wedding feast, had a nose bleed—as he often did
after drinking—and drowned in his own blood while he slept. He
was too drunk to get up. The list of modern-day alcoholic celebrities
is too long to recount.

The statistics are sobering. About 10% of adult American drink-
ers or 14 million persons are probably alcoholics. Alcoholism, on the
rise worldwide, is a chronic and usually progressive illness linked to
excessive consumption of ethyl alcohol. Drinking alcohol contributes
to approximately 40% of unintentional injuries, the leading cause of
death for adolescents, and a substantial number of suicides and homicides, the second and third leading causes of death in this group.
Each year, alcohol abuse kills about 100,000 individuals and costs
the economy $136 billion dollars. Alcoholism is one of the hidden
conditions, underdiagnosed and underreported.

Whatever else it may be, alcohol is a toxin. With excessive consumption, it damages the brain, nerves, and muscles. Its toxic effects
on the liver result in cirrhosis, esophageal varices, and bleeding. Alcoholism causes adverse reactions to medications, anger outbursts,
dementia, depression, diarrhea, falling, fractures, incontinence, insomnia, liver disease, memory lapses, peripheral neuropathy, poor
self-care, and sleeping problems. Male alcoholics manifest femini-
zation by breast enlargement (gynecomastia), loss of body hair, and
testicular atrophy; the facial features of female alcoholics mascu-
linize. Alcoholic patients with Korsakoff's syndrome confabulate
elaborate stories because they've lost their recent memory. No won-

der Bertrand Russell called drunkenness "temporary suicide."

Who is alcoholic? Have you ever: felt you ought to *cut* down on your drinking, had people *annoy* you by criticizing your drinking, felt bad or *guilty* about your drinking, or had a drink as an *eye opener* first thing in the morning to steady your nerves, get rid of a hangover, or to get the day started? These four screening questions comprise the "CAGE" screen for alcohol dependency. If you answered yes, you may be alcoholic and should seek help. Drinking before a medical appointment, sometimes incompletely masked by a breath mint, is a strong indicator of alcoholism. Frequent bruises, emergency room visits, and falls may be clues to an alcohol problem in the aged, who develop more difficulties than young persons do with consumption of less alcohol.

The success rate for rehabilitating alcoholics is about 50%. Alcoholics Anonymous (AA) is known for its 12-step motivational therapy. Psychotherapy has not been highly effective. Drugs to treat alcoholism must be taken daily. Disulfiram prevents alcohol use in detoxified patients by inducing severe vomiting when they drink, but compliance is poor. Naltrexone blocks some rewarding effects of drinking and reduces craving. Clinical trials of acamprosate, a drug that decreases the desire for alcohol possibly by altering the gene expression of excitatory amino acids in the brain, are underway in the U.S.

According to a report of the U.S. Depression Panel, between 10 and 30% of alcoholics suffer from depression, which alcoholics are twice as likely as non-alcoholics to develop. The depressive symptoms usually resolve several weeks after the patient becomes sober and the alcoholism has been treated.

9

When the Computer Crashes

Man is still the most extraordinary computer of all
—JOHN FITZGERALD KENNEDY

When the mind is thinking, it is talking to itself
—PLATO

The mind is capable of anything—because everything is in it, all the
past as well as all the future
—JOSEPH CONRAD

The feeling of sleepiness when you are not in bed, and can't get
there, is the meanest feeling in the world
—EDGAR WATSON HOWE

"I Feel I'm Slipping"

Salvadore Dominguez was a rather attractive fifty-five-year-old man from Puerto Rico. His lean and muscular physique—strong forearms and biceps, narrow hips, flat stomach—and deep tan exuded masculinity. His face could have garnished a *Gentlemen's Quarterly* advertisement for blue jeans: strong jaw, full lips, dark brown eyes, a sculpted nose, and wavy black hair, which was short in front and laid over his shirt's collar in the back. What could be the problem with this guy? He looked *too* good for his age.

"So, Mr. Dominguez, what can I do to help you today?"

His voice instantly revealed the whole story. With a very flat affect, he admitted softly, "I see no purpose to my life nor a reason to continue it."

"Why?"

"I am in good health physically, but I take no pride in that. I am a man without a cause. It took a lot of will power to get myself showered and dressed just to make this appointment today. I feel I'm slipping. A friend told me I should see a doctor."

"Have you been feeling this way for a long time or only recently?

"It's been like this for a couple of months. I don't call my friends. Sex is boring. I just don't care anymore."

"Did anything happen to you that might have triggered these feelings?"

"It seems to have started about when I got the pink slip at my job after the company I worked at for twenty years went belly up. I was in senior management and made some good dough. I use to wake up every morning Monday through Friday at five-thirty. I worked out in the gym for an hour. I was at the top of my game. Now I don't care if I ever brush my teeth again." He sighed deeply. "What is it with me?"

I questioned him about his medical history, but came up with no other clues. He denied he had any plans to kill himself. He just wanted his old self back again, even without the job, so he could enjoy life again.

"How is your appetite?"

"Not good."

"Have you lost weight?"

"Yes. I am six feet tall and used to weigh one-hundred-seventy pounds."

"Your weight today was one-hundred-sixty-three," I noted.

"I eat, but quite honestly, food doesn't have any flavor. I used to have a penchant for cookies and sweets. A friend told me I need to take an antidepressant drug. What do you think?"

"I think we need to make sure nothing else is wrong with you first." Depression *was* my preliminary diagnosis as I told him to disrobe and put on a gown. I'd gone over the review of systems with him carefully and found nothing except for depression. Possibly this was the first time he'd taken a look inside himself. He seemed depressed at losing his job. Without a long-term relationship, children, or his work, perhaps his life felt empty to him. We'll see what the physical examination shows up, I thought as I pulled back the curtain and laid out my instruments.

I started the neurological examination at the head and worked my way down. "Mr. Dominguez, I want you to look straight at my nose and tell me when you first see my finger wiggle in your peripheral vision, but don't move your eyes to see it, okay?"

After a few minutes of doing this to each eye, a yellow flag went up. The patient had significant visual field cuts. He could not see my wiggling finger in a large area of each visual field. I asked him again if he had troubles with his vision. The patient said that he bumped into objects he swore weren't there. He thought he was turning clumsy the past few weeks.

"I want to look inside your eyes." With the ceiling light off and the door to my room opened only enough to allow a sliver of light into the room, I peered into his right eye with my opthalmoscope and couldn't believe what I saw. The optic disc was blurred on the edges and the veins from the disc were engorged. The other eye looked the same.

I turned on the room light. Once we both accommodated to the light, I asked Mr. Dominguez if he was sure he wasn't having any headaches.

"Well, I was thinking about that since you asked me earlier. I do wake up with bad headaches during the night now and then and have to take something for the pain. Sometimes the headaches are so bad I take two kinds of pills. I meant to ask you for something stronger for the headaches because those medicines don't cut it anymore."

"Let's go over these headaches. Describe them to me in detail." I could hear the alarm in my own voice.

"A month ago, I got headaches occasionally. I figured it was because I wasn't sleeping great. The pain is deep and intense behind my eyes. It doesn't throb and I usually don't feel sick to my stomach, although the other night I did. My vision is okay, except when I'm tired, I see two of things. I figure I'm just tired and go lie down, and then I'm okay."

I nodded and finished my neurological examination, which was otherwise normal. I knew what test needed to be ordered ASAP and which consultant to call. The depression was not from losing his job; a coincidence, yes. This could be a brain tumor. I felt concerned for Mr. Dominguez.

I excused myself while he got dressed. Knocking a little too loudly on Dr. Mike Conley's door, I said, "Mike, I need you for a moment."

"I'm with a patient. It'll have to wait a minute," he said apologetically.

I backed away when he opened his door and escorted his patient to the receptionist. After he returned, I presented my patient to him.

"Let me confirm that it's papilledema you're seeing before we order a scan. I'll use my own opthalmoscope. It's better than the ones in the clinic. What's his name again?"

"Salvadore Dominguez."

Dr. Conley introduced himself and reviewed the history with the patient, focusing on headaches and visual problems. He examined the patient's eyes carefully, spending a good two minutes on each one. Mr. Dominguez began to suspect that something was wrong.

"What do you guys see in there that's so interesting?"

Dr. Conley explained. "The swelling of the optic nerve and its veins as well as your decreased vision may be linked to your depression. We need to do an important test to rule out one very serious possible cause: a mass."

"A *mass*? What kind of mass?"

"We don't know yet. It could be an abscess, a blood clot, or a tumor."

"A tumor! A brain tumor! I thought I was feeling the blues because my life sucks since I lost my job. What should I do?"

"The nurse practitioner is going to order a CT scan of your brain right away and we're going to have a neurologist see you today. The neurologist may want to do other tests depending on the outcome of the CT scan. You may end up getting admitted to the hospital today.

I want you to be aware of that possibility."

I glanced at my watch and noticed an hour had elapsed. There was still a lot do to. Thelma agreed to page the neurologist on call and arrange an emergency scan.

I instructed Mr. Dominguez to wait in the waiting room until someone came for him. Looking slightly bewildered and overwhelmed, he nodded. Thelma promised to keep an eye on him and call me if anything seemed wrong.

The neurology resident, Dr. Leah Wright, called back promptly and I briefed her. "I'll call the neuroradiologist and okay an emergency scan," she said. That meant delaying everyone else's scan. "Bring the patient down to the ER and I will meet you both there. I want to see Mr. Dominguez quickly before he goes for the scan."

I was able to secure only an ancient wheelchair with adhesive tape holding the armrests together. Then I called to prepare the ER and proceeded to wheel over the patient. There, after introductions were made, I handed Dr. Wright the chart with my notes and said good-bye to Mr. Dominguez.

"Please call me with follow up on the patient," I said. "Here's my beeper number."

Dr. Wright was preoccupied, but agreed to call later.

After a quick lunch, I saw some patients with allergies and colds, filled out some medical permission slips for worked missed, and gave one man a routine PPD screen for tuberculosis. For the time being, there were no walk-in patients to see, so I added details to the patient charts for the day. Then my beeper went off. The four digit extension was the Radiology Department.

Dr. Wright picked up on the first ring. "I'm looking at your patient's head CT scan right now. He has a brain tumor the size of a golf ball. It's unclear at this point what kind of tumor it is, whether it's primary or metastatic, malignant or non-malignant. We'll be admitting him, of course. I haven't told him the news. Feel free to follow him in the hospital; he'll be in the Neurology Unit. Gotta go. By the way, nice work up."

I took pride in making the diagnosis, but was worried about my patient's prognosis. It also gave me a chill to think what might have happened had I hurried through the examination and missed the papilledema. I thanked my lucky stars I hadn't merely sent him home with an antidepressant. Here was the one depressed patient in a hundred to have a brain tumor. Just a careful examination made all the difference.

A week or so later, Dr. Wright called to tell me that Salvadore Dominguez's brain tumor was not malignant and he was doing well after surgery. When I heard he was making passes at all the nurses, I knew he was on the road to recovery.

THE CHRONIC HEADACHE

Ancient peoples used to chisel holes in the skull to vent pain and release demons or any other evil humors at the root of headaches. That's got to hurt! Many died. Headaches tormented us even then. Julius Caesar, Lewis Carroll, Sigmund Freud, Thomas Jefferson, Alfred Nobel, St. Paul, and Virginia Wolff were among the celebs believed to suffer from migraine headaches. Lewis Carroll is supposed to have taken some of his characters for *Alice in Wonderland* from apparitions he saw before migraine attacks.

The enormity is staggering. Headache is the dominant pain problem in medical practice, affecting over 90% of the population. Most individuals admit to at least one significant headache a month. About 20% of them have recurrent or chronic headaches. Because people look normal between headaches, the impact of headaches on the quality of life probably has been underestimated. The level of mental, physical, and social functioning in headache sufferers may drop as low as in some serious chronic medical diseases.

Be comprehensive; get to know the patient. Even though most headaches are not caused by underlying disease, possible medical problems must be eliminated in arriving at the correct diagnosis. In addition to the usual examination, the head and neck should be checked with extra care. Secondary causes of headache include infections (illnesses with fever, meningitis, sinusitis), neurological problems (hemorrhage, hydrocephalus, tumors), musculoskeletal abnormalities (arthritis, congenital abnormalities), vascular disease (stroke), medications, and many other conditions. Fever, muscle tenderness and guarding, neck stiffness (nuchal rigidity), and swelling of the optic disks (papilledema) are important signs of pressure or irritation due to hydrocephalus, intracranial hemorrhage, meningitis, or tumors.

The International Headache Society devised 13 classifications of headache with subtypes. Tension and migraine headaches are the most common types of primary headaches, although controversy persists as to the biological distinction between the two. In their extremes, both types can be differentiated easily.

Tension-type headaches, the most prevalent headache, do not throb, but exert constant, dull, tightening pain or pressure behind the eyes. They cause no other neurological symptoms.

Migraines, which are genetic, conscript about 10% of the population; 75% of those affected are women. Migraine headaches usually produce nausea, sensitivity to light and sound, and a throbbing quality. Besides these "common" migraines, which account for 85 to 90% of all migraines, there are also "classic" migraines with visual problems, such as the experiencing of flashing lights or sparkling (scintillations) and missing areas of vision (scotoma). The headaches are hemicranial, but different headache episodes will involve either side of the head.

The most involved type is the "complicated" migraine, which may be accompanied by paralysis or weakness on one side of the body (hemiplegia), inability to speak (aphasia), or loss of consciousness and convulsions. About 15% of all migraines are these more complicated or "uncommon" types.

Cluster headaches are severe seasonal headaches over one side of the head. Irritability runs high as the pain is quite intense.

STRATEGIZING AGAINST HEADACHES

What should be done? Individuals with mild, simple, or infrequent headaches usually do not need any laboratory tests if they have a normal examination. An MRI scan or CT scan with contrast is indicated in patients with an abnormal examination, complicated migraines, a suspect history or age, or worrisome characteristics to the headache. A spinal tap (lumbar puncture) may be necessary to rule out infections such as meningitis or other causes of increased intracranial pressure (pseudotumor) once a scan has been done to eliminate the possibility of an intracranial mass.

The majority of chronic headache sufferers *can* be helped. Headache-prone individuals need to avoid and be aware of provocative factors such as bright lights, missed and non-nutritious meals, sleep deprivation, various foods and food additives (alcohol, avocados, bean curd, caffeine, cheese, chocolate, monosodium glutamate, soy sauce, tyramine), menstruation, stress, and weather changes. Non-drug therapies include acupuncture, biofeedback, manipulation, and relaxation techniques.

Use drugs in two ways: *prevent* the headaches or *abort* them in progress. With more than 30 non-habituating drugs available for use, potentially habituating medications should be avoided. The main preventative drugs are antidepressants (tricyclics or SSRI's), beta-adrenergic blockers, calcium channel antagonists, ergot derivatives, and other agents. In the case of migraines with warning symptoms and known triggers, prevention is far easier than stopping an established headache.

Not all headaches can be prevented. Most abortive headache treatments are analgesics like nonsteroidal anti-inflammatory drugs. For patients with nausea and vomiting due to migraines, triptans or ergotamine derivatives have the advantage of being injectable. Sumatriptan and DHE-45, serotonin receptor agonists, can be taken intraasally. A combined preparation of caffeine and ergotamine tartrate is particularly helpful.

BRAIN TUMORS

The brain provides clues to its maladies for the careful observer. Sometimes the clues are misleading—take "Salvadore Dominguez" who thinks he's depressed because he lost his job. We ignore the symptoms or do not recognize the warning signs. George Gershwin's life might have been saved by a simple neurological examination, which could have detected the earliest signs of his brain tumor.

About 17,000 primary brain tumors crop up yearly in the U.S., and about 12,000 patients die of them. Epidemiological data suggest that more brain tumors are coming to medical attention in recent years than in the past. Early detection often depends on the health care provider's awareness of risk factors: a positive family history of cancer or conditions associated with brain tumors, significant exposure to radiation, and controversial factors such as head injury or chemical solvents.

Another caveat: one-half of brain tumors produce no headache. They may cause behavioral changes like apathy or disinhibition, impaired vision or speech, loss of mental faculties, numbness, seizures, and weakness. Although there may be nothing special about a brain tumor headache, headaches that always involve only one area of the head, interrupt sleep, or worsen in the morning should spell danger.

Brain tumors come in dozens of types, some benign, others malignant. Gliomas (malignant) account for about half of adult primary brain tumors, followed by meningiomas (benign). Tumors differ in the region of the brain or head they affect, their propensity to spread and invade, and their resistance or vulnerability to treatment. Although not all tumors are malignant, they may cause serious problems by compressing vital structures.

Given this unnerving scenario, what can be done? The treatment options must weigh the advantages of removing the tumor against the neurological impairment that may result. Metastatic brain tumors from another diagnosed source need not be biopsied, but a pathological diagnosis is extremely useful for selecting the proper diagnosis and treatment for primary brain tumors.

Chemotherapy, radiation, steroids, and surgery are the mainstay of conventional treatment. Among other newer unproven treatments, radiosurgery (gamma knife) is promising for selected tumors. Gene-transfer therapy already is being evaluated and a vaccine for brain tumors is coming to clinical trials soon.

*   *   *

"Just to Walk Ten Feet"

"I was fine," Linda Allen explained languidly, "until one day, I collapsed. I felt weak, like I had the flu. It dragged on for a couple of weeks. Then I realized it was my legs. Just to walk ten feet to the bathroom exhausted me. My legs tingled, too." She was a middle-aged woman of average height, with brown, stringy hair and a prominent nose. Her pasty complexion was startling.

"When you saw your doctor two weeks ago for this problem, did he order some blood tests?"

"Yes. He said the results weren't back yet." She kept raking her hands through her hair and looked scared.

"And how are things now?"

"Worse. There's another problem. I found out I'm not going to get a neurology appointment for several weeks. I wondered if it could be moved up. I'm feeling weaker. I don't want to wait that long." Her tone sounded desperate.

I imagined waking up one day to find myself having to use a cane to get around. Ms. Allen was a little too close to my age for comfort. How she had to drag herself was pathetic. I examined her and got on the phone. "I'll call and see what I can do," I told her.

To my surprise, I was having no better luck in getting her an earlier appointment. "I have a patient here in my office who really needs to be seen," I pleaded.

"We're booked solid," the clinic receptionist insisted.

"What am I supposed to do?"

"I don't know. I can call her if there's a cancellation."

"That won't do," I retorted.

"I'm sorry."

That was that. What were the patient's options? She needed to be seen by a specialist. There might be something going on that required immediate attention, particularly a lesion pressing on the spinal cord. "I have an idea, if you don't mind waiting around the hospital today."

"If it gets me seen sooner, I'm willing."

I contacted the Rapid Assessment Unit of the ER. "I have a patient in my office with deteriorating leg weakness. She needs to be evaluated today by neurology. They won't take her in their clinic for several weeks."

"We're not a dumping ground for your clinic. No one called to clear it with *us*. You can't just bring someone down without *our* approval."

"That's why I'm calling you now."

"Does she *really* need to be seen?"

"Yes," I persisted. "Her problem won't wait."

Finally, the ER capitulated. I was enormously relieved. They agreed to evaluate Ms. Allen only if I personally escorted her with her chart in hand.

"Thanks." Linda Allen smiled halfheartedly, gathering up her things. I brought her a wheelchair. "It's scary," she said. "You don't know when your health is going to be taken away from you. I never appreciated it while I had it."

As I wheeled her to the ER, I reflected on those words. I didn't appreciate my health either. I took for granted all the mornings I woke up and felt okay, not having to take medications, and not spending my life going to the hospital to be treated for an illness.

Later I learned from the neurologist that multiple sclerosis was a strong possibility in her case, but the diagnosis could not yet be proven. Although finding demyelination on a MRI scan of the brain would support the diagnosis, a viral illness, even Lyme disease from a tick bite, could cause the same findings. MS is a disorder of multiple lesions in space and time; an infection is usually a one-time event. We must wait to see if the disease remits and then reappears. I hoped it wouldn't return.

THE CHALLENGE OF WEAKNESS

According to the *Old Testament*, when Delilah shaved Samson's head, he lost the supernatural strength with which his hair had endowed him. The betrayal lead to his eventual demise and hers. The hair had enabled his legendary feats.

For the rest of us, strength is controlled by the nervous system: the brain, spinal cord, 12 pairs of cranial nerves at the base of the brain, 31 pairs of nerve roots connected to either side of the spinal cord, peripheral nerves, the junction of nerves and muscles, and the muscles themselves. People may feel weak due to fatigue, depression, and systemic illnesses such as the flu, but have normal strength (pseudo-weakness). The diverse causes of acquired muscle weakness would fill a few pages. Weakness is most serious when it compromises the muscles of breathing, as with the high spinal trauma suffered by actor Christopher Reeve.

Some simple guidelines. Weakness on one entire side of the body (unilateral) most likely originates from the brain, and the weakness is opposite the side of the brain injury (contralateral). Complicated migraine headaches, seizures, strokes (blood vessel clots or hemorrhages), or tumors may cause unilateral weakness. Multiple sclerosis, a progressive immunological disease of white matter, can produce such unusual patterns of weakness and sensory loss they are sometimes misdiagnosed as hysterical. The symptoms, such as double vision, are episodic, relapsing, and remitting.

Weakness involving just the legs more likely emanates from the lower spinal cord. Abscesses, hemorrhages, or tumors compressing the spinal cord are medical emergencies because they may cause permanent damage. Abnormal sensation below a certain level on the trunk, an abnormal toe reflex (Babinski sign), and loss of bowel and bladder function commonly accompany spinal cord disorders. High level spinal cord injuries prevent breathing.

When a solitary limb is affected, suspect a peripheral nerve problem (neuropathy), especially when deep tendon reflexes in the limb are decreased or absent. Diseases like diabetes are important causes of peripheral neuropathies, but occupational or recreational injuries are also common. Weakness of the whole body beginning with the legs may be a sign of Guillain-Barre syndrome, a transient, post-infectious disorder of nerve roots (ascending polyradiculopathy); it can jeopardize breathing.

Now to the muscles—46 to 54% of our body mass. Myasthenia gravis, an immunological disorder of the nerve-muscle junction, and myositis, an inflammation of the muscle, sap muscles of their strength. So can a low blood potassium level.

Treatment of weakness begins with considering the correct diagnostic possibilities, ordering the proper tests, and intervening effectively. The range of treatments is wide. Supportive care, even a ventilator, may be needed until the underlying condition improves spontaneously or with drug treatment. High doses of steroids and radiation therapy shrink many tumors. Early intensive immunotherapy is also the preferred treatment for myasthenia gravis, myositis, and multiple sclerosis. Surgery may be necessary to evacuate a blood clot from a hemorrhage or tumor. Treatment of diabetes and other metabolic disorders often improves the neuropathy they caused.

BRAIN MATTERS

The brain—10 billion nerve cells, 3 pounds of pink-gray tissue, the nexus of emotions, memory, movement, sleep, thirst, thought, and virtually all other vital activities—is nothing less than an elaborate computer. The exquisite, cellular, bioelectrical cortex or "gray matter" is thinner than a computer's motherboard. More complex than any other organ, the brain inherits its mainframe, but life provides the software. We take it for granted until it crashes.

More than 50 million persons in the U.S. or one-fifth of the population will experience neurological problems at some time in their lives. The spectrum of brain dysfunction is phenomenal: coma, confusion, dementia, dizziness, headaches, incoordination, involuntary movements, loss of consciousness, memory loss, seizures, weakness, and visual problems. Sometimes the glitch is a simple "power outage," caused by diseases or events elsewhere in the body. When the power is restored, the brain usually comes back on-line—perhaps some files were lost. If the trouble is a "hardware" problem, the patient may have Alzheimer's disease, a brain tumor, epilepsy, a movement disorder like Parkinson's disease, meningitis, multiple sclerosis, or stroke.

The period of 1990 to 2000 has been designated as the "decade of the brain," an era that has seen the greatest push to conquer brain diseases to date. Exciting new advances pave the way for the tough challenges ahead.

*   *   *

"My Hand Feels Thick"

John Flagger and his wife hung their heavy winter coats on the door hook and sat in chairs next to the examining table. The damp cold seemed to radiate from their coats—I knew it wasn't so—enough to give a person chilblains. Mr. Flagger, a tall man whose nose and cheeks were still wind-chill-reddened, had the habitus of a once lean and sinewy manual laborer. He spoke slowly and deliberately when I asked him to describe his problem.

"My hand feels thick."

The word *thick* didn't register with me. "What do you mean by *thick?*"

He looked down at his left hand as he wiggled his fingers. "I don't know what I mean exactly. My arm just isn't right. It doesn't do what I want it to do."

That was worrisome. Now the problem involved the whole arm? Having heard patients describe weakness in such a manner, I wanted to know if the entire left side of the body was affected.

"Does your leg also seem strange or only your arm?"

"No, not my leg, just my arm."

"When did this happen?"

"Oh, 'bout two weeks ago," he answered dryly.

"Have things changed since then? Are you getting better or worse or no different?"

He looked at his sharp-faced wife. She returned his gaze and offered a noncommittal shrug. "Some better, I'd say."

She agreed. The disparity of their sizes was striking: she was diminutive.

"All right, what were you doing when it happened?" I watched as he searched his memory.

"Nothing really. I woke up with it."

"Think carefully now. Tell me what you did the night before." I hoped he was precise regarding details.

"We watched TV. I took out the garbage like I always do and went to bed."

"Then what?"

"I went to sleep."

"Did you get up during the night?"

Mr. Flagger's facial expression asked: *Why on earth would anyone in their right mind want to know what I did during the night.* He was too polite to object. "I got up to pass my water once, I guess. I usually do."

"Okay, then what?" I knew that ninety-percent of a neurological evaluation was in the history taking. There were always clues; I had only to find them.

"I woke up at five o'clock as usual."

"Did anything seem to be wrong with you then?"

There was a pause. His answer was no.

I nodded. "Tell me about your morning routine."

"Well, I ate breakfast."

"I mean in detail. How did you get out of bed?"

"The regular way." He suggested with a laugh that it was a silly question. "What do you mean?"

"No, I mean did you jump up right away or sit at the edge of the bed first?"

"I got right up."

Here was a clue. In older patients like Mr. Flagger, hopping out of bed was bad for the brain. After all, the blood vessels, heart, and brain had acclimated to being horizontal. Abruptly, they became vertical. That was often enough to trigger a stroke in a susceptible individual.

"Did you go to the bathroom again?"

"Yes. I had a bowel movement."

The trail is definitely hot. "Were you straining to have it?"

"Yes. I've been irregular lately."

A major clue. Straining at stool increases venous pressure and dilates blood vessels in the head. An abrupt change in pressure after a night of sleep could precipitate a stroke.

"Did you feel funny after that?"

"Now that you mention it, I did have a little headache."

"Then what did you do?"

"After I ate, I laid back down in bed for an hour and a half until our cats came in and jumped on the bed."

"Then what?"

He paused to recollect the crucial detail. "When I got up again, that's when I noticed things weren't right in my arm."

"And has anything like this ever happened to you before?"

"Nope."

In taking the rest of the history, I learned that Mr. Flagger was right-handed, meaning the left side of his brain was probably dominant for language. He was a smoker and was not restricting his fat intake. He drank some, but had no other medical problems. I was reassured to find he had a normal blood pressure.

The neurological examination revealed weakness of the left arm. There was some reduction in sensation as well. Reflexes in the affected arm were somewhat brisker than normal.

"I think you've had a stroke," I said as I walked over to my desk chair.

"A stroke?" He and his wife exchanged a look.

"Yes. The *right* side of the brain controls the *left* side of the body, so the stroke is in the right half of the brain. Straining at moving your bowels in the morning might have triggered it. Maybe getting out of bed hastily made you more vulnerable."

"How?" his wife asked. The idea must have seemed unorthodox to her. What had the bowels possibly to do with the brain?

"It puts pressure on the blood vessels in the brain and starts a series of events that choke the arteries or cause bleeding."

I could see the wheels turning as Mrs. Flagger contemplated what she just heard.

"I have to ask why you waited two weeks at home before seeking help, Mr. Flagger?"

"Well," he said nonchalantly, "I didn't think anything could be done. It's just something a person has to get over."

"We didn't know it was a stroke," the wife added.

"You were lucky. This could have been much worse."

They both looked unimpressed. After all, hadn't time proved them right: he *did* recover on his own.

I ordered a head MRI scan and made a referral to neurology clinic. When I spoke with the neurology resident on the phone, he commented that so much time had passed, there was nothing to be done acutely. He did tell me to order several tests looking for any clotting disorders, blood vessel diseases, heart problems, or other causes of strokes. He would make the evaluation for possible physical therapy or drug treatments to prevent another episode when he saw the patient in his clinic.

I later found out that the scan showed a small area of infarction, which looked to the radiologist to be a couple of weeks old, in the part of the brain supplied by the right middle cerebral artery. There was no hemorrhage or tumor.

John Flagger's prognosis for continued recovery was good. Because he was still at risk to have other strokes in the future, I made sure he understood not to wait to be seen if it happened again. The next stroke could be the big one.

STROKE

PRESIDENT HARDING DIES SUDDENLY; STROKE OF APOPLEXY AT 7:30 P.M.; CALVIN COOLIDGE IS PRESIDENT

Those were the headlines of *The New York Times* on Friday, August 3, 1923. Other U.S. presidents to suffer strokes while in office include John Quincy Adams, Chester A. Arthur, Millard Fillmore, Woodrow Wilson, Franklin Delanore Roosevelt, and Dwight Eisenhower. Notable foreign heads of state, such as Winston Churchill, Nikolai Lenin, Joseph Stalin, and Paul von Hindenburg, also had significant strokes, but the problem is not confined to politicians. Louis Pasteur made his most famous discoveries after his stroke, whereas Maurice Ravel lost the ability to compose music after his. Mention of stroke is made even in the *Bible*.

According to the American Heart Association, a stroke occurs every minute in the U.S. and a person dies of a stroke every 3.5 minutes. As we approach the new millennium, an estimated 1.5 million persons a year will have a stroke. The third leading cause of death in the U.S., stroke kills about 30% of its victims. Arriving too late at the hospital is the single biggest reason that strokes are not treated more effectively. One major reason for the delay is that most people don't know the warning symptoms of stroke: difficulty speaking, dizziness, headache, loss of balance or vision, or weakness.

Why does it occur? Stroke is a sudden compromise of the blood supply to the brain due to occlusive blood clots (infarction) or hemorrhage (intracerebral or subarachnoid), resulting in a neurologic deficit. About 400,000 ischemic strokes, 75% of which are first-time events, and 100,000 hemorrhagic strokes occur each year. The blood vessels may be thrombosed by atherosclerotic disease or by a shower of clots (emboli) from the heart.

Risk factors for stroke are AIDS, alcoholism, atherosclerosis, cardiac arrhythmia (atrial fibrillation), cigarette smoking, diabetes, drug abuse, excessive nocturnal sleeping (>8 hours) with daytime napping, a family history of stroke, hyperlipidemia, hypertension, migraines, and valvular heart disease. Individuals who have had stroke symptoms that disappear within 24 hours (transient ischemic attack or TIA) are particularly prone to stroke.

The site of brain injury gives stroke its distinctive pattern. Infarction of the cerebrum (the largest part of the brain, some 85% of its weight), which usually occurs on one side of the brain, may cause weakness or paralysis and loss of sensation on the other side of the body. Involvement of the left side of the brain, where speech is controlled in most people, destroys speech (aphasia). When the stroke involves large blood vessels, such as the internal carotid artery or middle cerebral artery, and the damage is massive, many brain cells die, causing brain swelling, seizures, coma, and death.

Small strokes (less than 5 mm in diameter) involving tiny vessels in deep brain areas (lacunar infarcts) may produce few or no deficits. "Silent" strokes cause symptoms only with multiple events over time. Some areas of the brain receive blood from multiple sources (collateral circulation), optimizing the chances of recovery.

What happens to stroke survivors? As many as 25% recover fully. About 55% have varying degrees of disability one year following the stroke. The rest die. What does that mean in human terms? Almost 70% of disabled stroke victims report that they can't read, enjoy hobbies, or help out with the gardening or shopping. They are no longer mobile. The burden to the individual can be immense.

Drugs *do* make a difference. Several agents, taken alone or in combination, depending on the circumstances, prevent stroke: aspi-rin, dipyridamole, ticlopidine, and heparin or warfarin. Other drugs also are being studied.

Exciting new treatment options emphasize the importance of seeking medical attention immediately after a stroke. Tissue plasmin-ogen activator (TPA) and pro-urokinase provide thrombolytic thera-py for acute stroke. Clinical trials of glutamate (NMDA) blockers also are underway because neurons can be protected experimentally by blocking the excitatory chemical glutamate in the brain. Calcium channel blocking drugs like timodipine are under evaluation, too. When the carotid arteries are maximally stenosed and the patient has recovered with little disability from a stroke, surgical removal of plaques (carotid endarterectomy) reduces the risk of further strokes.

We can do better. A recent national symposium on stroke reset therapeutic goals. A full 70% of stroke patients should be engaged in activities of daily living 3 months after stroke. The overall death rate should fall to 40%. All this is possible with current means. Bottom line: if you have a stroke, get to the hospital immediately.

*   *   *

"It Was a Pretty Ordinary Sunday"

"I'm not going to forgive you until you call me by my middle name."

"Okay, Anita, what's up?"

"I'm here to see you because I had a dizzy spell over the week-end. I debated whether to go to the ER, but since I felt better, I de-cided to wait and come into the clinic today." Ruth Anita Deville, a tanned, athletic blonde, was approaching thirty gracefully. She brushed back rivulets of her long hair.

"Have you had any more spells?"

"No, it hasn't happened since."

"Do you feel back to normal?"

"Totally." Her eyes were a cool gray-blue. Her complexion was flawless.

"Okay, if you don't mind me asking a lot of questions, I need to understand exactly what happened."

"That's perfectly all right."

"Did you pass out?"

"I guess I must have because I woke up on the floor."

"Did anyone witness the episode?"

"No. My husband was outside in the backyard trimming the hedges."

"And do you remember going down?"

The instantaneous look of recollection. "Yes, I recall my arms and legs getting very heavy and then starting to fall." She dropped her arms into her lap, re-enacting the scene. "That's about it."

"How long were you out?"

"I'm not sure exactly. It couldn't have been too long." She adjusted the shoulder strap of her V-necked, casual black dress.

"Okay, good. Now let's go over how you felt just before you fell. Did you experience any unusual sensations?"

"What kind?"

"I mean smelling something unpleasant or burning, seeing bright or flashing lights, or have any strange feelings like something bad was about to happen?"

"No." She wrinkled her nose. "Why are you asking about that?"

"Because seizures may start that way."

She raised her eyebrows, alarmed at the thought that she might have had a seizure.

But a seizure became more unlikely when she denied losing control of her bowels or bladder and she hadn't injured herself when she fell. Patients with seizures also do not usually recall events during the episode.

"Did you have any unusual sensations in your chest—like your heart was doing flip-flops—or any chest pains?"

"No. Now you're worried about my heart?"

"Not really, but we have to ask about all possibilities." I pursued the heart as the possible culprit, but came up empty-handed. Getting the information I needed always seemed like an interrogation. A momentary thought of the patient perspiring under a spotlight fueled the illusion.

"Do you have migraine headaches?" I knew that some migraines could result in loss of consciousness, particularly in women.

"No."

"Did you wake up with a headache after you fell that day?"

"No."

"Fine. Did you feel hot or sweaty?"

"No."

"Did you see any spots before your eyes, like the TV screen when a station's off the air?"

"Ah, something like that. I saw some big spots."

"Were they bright or dark?"

"It's hard to remember. I think they were dark."

"Did your vision narrow like a tunnel?"

"Yeah, a little."

"And did you feel like you were going to faint?"

"Well, I don't usually pass out. The last time I fainted was when I was just a kid standing in a long line at the amusement park. I remember it because that was also the first time I tasted cotton candy. That's funny—I just recalled—it was summer, too."

"Okay, now let's talk about what you were doing the day before this happened."

She tipped her head up and rested her chin on her hand. "It was a pretty ordinary Sunday. We woke up at about eight A.M., got dressed, and went biking for about three hours."

"Sunday was blistering hot as I recall."

"Yes, it was. We were out in the sun, but had water bottles with us."

"Did you wear a hat?"

"Yeah, I have a cap."

"And what else did you do?"

"Then we went to the gym and worked out for a couple more hours. After that, we came home, got cleaned up, and grabbed a sandwich."

"That sounds like quite a workout. Do you usually exercise that vigorously?"

She laughed. "That was an *easy* day. When I trained to run in the NYC Marathon I really pushed the distance on the weekends. I still hope to do a biathlon."

Some ordinary Sunday.

"Anita, take me up to the time of the spell."

"Well, I sat on the floor and read for a while, maybe about an hour. When I stood up, I walked over to the window to see what my husband was up to, and I started to feel the way I told you. Then I ended up on the floor."

We covered the rest of the history, but I came up with nothing to suggest a serious cause of the episode. Anita Deville denied pregnancy, taking medications, fad diets, or megavitamin therapies. Her physical examination was normal. I took her blood pressure in three positions to make sure she was not orthostatic and at risk for passing out again.

"I would call this a simple fainting spell, Anita. I think it happened because you stood up quickly after sitting for so long. Maybe you were a little dehydrated from your outdoor exercise, I don't know. It sounds like you worked out pretty hard; getting behind on your fluids is easy to do. Sometimes we can't pinpoint the combination of factors that occurred that day. But everything else checks out okay now. I'll run a few blood tests to make sure you aren't anemic or having other problems, but I suspect the results will be normal. I'm not going to do an electrocardiogram unless this happens again because you're not having heart symptoms and your heart examination is normal."

"*Will* it happen again?"

"It may. But the key is to get up *slowly* after you've been sitting awhile. If you get warning symptoms again, sit with your head down or lie flat. If you don't, you probably *will* faint."

"Well, I got scared later because I thought I could have broken bones when I fell."

"Yes, but that doesn't usually happen because the muscles relax when a person faints. Don't prove me wrong."

"My husband wanted me to ask you if fainting damages the brain. He's always teasing me about getting brain damage from watching too much TV or talking too long on the telephone."

"No, no," I laughed. "During fainting, the heart rate slows and the brain doesn't get enough blood, but as soon as you're down, your pulse quickens. The whole process takes seconds. Your brain can survive several minutes without injury. But as far as TV goes, the word's still out!"

DIZZY SPELLS

Dizziness, a catch-all term, means different things to different people. To some, it's the light-headed feeling one gets just before passing out (presyncope). To others, dizziness means motion—either they are spinning or the room is rotating around them (vertigo). Some individuals use the term to indicate loss of balance (dysequilibrium), loss of control (anxiety, panic, or stress), or just a peculiar, non-specific sensation (cloudiness, floating, fogginess, giddiness, swimming) associated with emotional factors, taking sedating medications, or trauma. Many people merely refer to episodes of such symptoms as "spells."

Dizzy patients are common visitors to family and internal medicine practices. Although many will be referred to a neurologist or to an ENT specialist or both, medical causes of dizziness should be ruled out first. Dizziness can be the presenting symptom of something as serious and permanent as a heart attack or stroke or as minor and transient as certain anemias, fatigue, hyperventilation, motion sickness, or the flu.

The cause of dizziness is sometimes age-related. The history is telling. Young patients are more likely to experience dizziness as a presyncopal sensation resulting from changing body position too fast, skipping meals, sleep deprivation, or prolonged standing in hot close surroundings without sufficient airflow. If they do not correct the situation, they may lose consciousness (syncope), or in common parlance, "black out," faint, or "pass out." Presyncope is associated with clamminess, cold sweats, faintness, light-headedness, pallor, seeing blue or black dots, and tunnel-vision. Even the patient who loses consciousness remembers the prodromal events.

Syncope accounts for 3% of all ER visits. A specific cause is initially apparent in only about 50% of the cases. One-third of adults have at least one syncopal episode. A common error made by people who observe such an event is to hold or prop the syncopal patient to a sitting position, a maneuver that further starves the brain of blood and may precipitate a brief convulsion (syncope with tonic-clonic seizure).

Inner ear disorders such as labyrinthitis and Meniere's disease, or even impacted cerumen, cause vertigo. Labyrinthitis, a very common viral illness, induces nausea and vomiting with changes in head position. Rhythmic jerking of the eyes (nystagmus) is typical. An audiogram, electronystagmography (ENG), and rotational testing further identify and pinpoint the source of the problem from the ear through pathways to the brain.

Migraine headaches and complex partial seizures (formerly called temporal lobe epilepsy) may cause episodes of dizziness or vertigo. In one form of migraine, the headache occurs after the dizziness if at all and may not be severe. Unless followed by losing consciousness, dizziness or vertigo alone are usually not indicative of a seizure.

Dizziness may be a symptom of a cardiac arrhythmia. In the presence of a heart murmur and click, mitral valve prolapse should be considered.

In the older patient, combined impairment of position sense, tactile sensation, and vision—multisensory deficits—aggravates dizziness. The problem is extremely common in this population.

Is there any remedy? When the cause of dizziness or vertigo is vestibular and attacks are frequent and severe, drugs to suppress vestibular responses can be tried. Antihistamines are mild suppressants that can be taken chronically, but benzodiazepines and neuroleptics drugs, which are more sedating, are appropriate only for short-term management. Antiemetics can be used for attacks associated with vomiting.

*   *   *

"I'm Afraid to Go to Bed at Night"

"I know how this must sound, but I'm afraid to go to bed at night." Ed Grogan rubbed his left eye and yawned. Despite his well-groomed, clean-shaven appearance, he had dark circles under both insipid eyes.

Is this a big kid scared of long-armed monsters lying in wait beneath the bed? With graying temples, sitting bent over, elbows on his knees, he doesn't fit that bill.

"Why?" I asked.

"Because I know what's going to happen."

"What happens?"

He sighed like a man weary of his own story. "Well, I lie down. I'm tired. I fall to sleep right away. Then I'll wake up with a start, maybe thirty minutes later or in an hour or so. And that's it. I'm sweating and worrying about things. Everything seems bleak. It's like peering down a long corridor into the future and things don't look too good. I see each thing I've done wrong in my life. I feel like I screwed up my life and there's nothing I can do about it. I think about my parents and friends dying. I tell myself to think about something pleasant and relax. I know this isn't the way things seem during the day, but I can't shake the feeling at night."

"What do you do when this happens?"

"You mean what *haven't* I tried." He stroked his hair from his forehead. "I've done everything I can think of and then some—warm milk before bed, a light snack, relaxation tapes, window shades. I've tried lying there. One night I was awake in bed for three hours. You can imagine how I felt the next day. In a magazine I read you're supposed to get up and do something until you get sleepy. I tried that, too. I started reading a book. I've also listened to the radio. Nothing much happens on TV at that hour except old movies or people selling jewelry." He shrugged it away as incredulous. "I looked outside and found out some of my neighbors must have insomnia, too. One time I got sleepy in an hour or two. Another time I never went back to bed. It's an ordeal."

"How long has this been going on?"

"Months."

"Why are you seeking help for it now?"

"Because I'm at my wit's end. I need to get some rest."

"Have you fallen asleep at work?"

"Yes. It's embarrassing. I dose off at meetings. My boss noticed. Fortunately, he has a sense of humor. He'll call out my name to wake me and watch me flounder as I try to figure out what the group was talking about. But the worst of it is what happened on the road. I travel a lot, being in sales and all. For the past six months I've been on the road. Late at night I was driving down back-roads to get to the next town and find a motel. The next thing I knew, I was riding off the road, heading for a tree. Only the roughness of the shoulder jarred me awake and I veered back on the road at the last moment."

"That's frightening."

"Not enough." He shifted in his seat, now more animated. "You know, I lowered my window and turned on the radio, but I was still drowsy. Here my heart was beating fast from the adrenaline and I was already starting to get sleepy again. I had all I could do to get to the motel. That's what prompted me to finally come here for help. I could have gotten killed, for God's sake." He raised his hands in frustration.

"Have you taken any medications for sleep?"

"Just about everything you can purchase without a prescription. Nothing works for me. Some of them gave me headaches or upset my stomach, so I stopped."

"Mr. Grogan, is your job more stressful lately?"

"There's always stress with that job. I told you about all the traveling."

I tapped my pen point on the chart while I thought. "Can you tell me a little about your life?"

"What do you want to know?" He yawned again.

I was amazed how sleep deprivation could make a person appear physically ill. He looked down a quart on some mysterious, vital body fluid. "Whatever you want to tell me. Anything that would give me an idea about the kind of person you are."

"Well, not much to tell. I live alone. I date, but there's no one steady. I'm divorced—I guess you probably figured that out by now. Things didn't end too well with her. She figured I wasn't making enough of myself."

"When did that happen?"

"About two years ago. Just as well. I had a lot to give her, but she didn't see it." He winced. "I'm glad to be done with all the problems."

How the past is full of nightmares, I thought. *For many, a time of frustration, decisions made unconsciously and later regretted—a career chosen hastily, a marriage or family formed unwisely. Ed Grogan is only one of the multitude of travelers in the eerie light that illuminates the dark caverns of memory and reveals the many things along the way we never saw or heeded. Now it is time to notice and to understand...*

"Do you have family for support."

"No, none of my family—siblings, cousins, aunts, or uncles—lives here in the East. We're not real close-knit anyway."

I was back to pen tapping. "What do you do to relax?"

"I like sports, so I go to games when I can."

"But that's not every day. What do you do most of the time?"

He looked down. "I've never been good at relaxing. I'm a type-A person. I'm not good at vacations for that reason. That was one of my ex's complaints. I don't play games; they're not serious." He paused on the verge of further self-deprecating candor. "I guess I'm kind of boring." He made an unconvincing attempt to laugh it off.

"So, you're pretty much a loner?"

"Yeah."

"You turned forty recently?"

Mr. Grogan looked face-slapped as though I'd spoken the forbidden word, apparently not realizing his date of birth was stamped on the top of his clinic record. "This past June."

"Was it a rough one?"

"The worst. I didn't want to celebrate, but they threw me a party at work. The birthday card had *40* written all over it. So did the birthday cake. They gave me a shirt with the big *4-0* pressed on it. It was like a sword being driven into me. I know they all meant well, but I could have done without the whole scene." He sat back and folded his hands in his lap. "I work for a company, but always hoped I'd have my own business by now. I guess I feel like a failure. I haven't gone as far in the company as I could either." He nodded a few times as he appeared to be thinking about what he said.

I had pulled on a thread and now the whole garment was unraveling. It wasn't necessary that he say more. "How's your appetite been?"

"*Too* good. I've been hitting the snacks pretty hard. The next day, I can't believe I ate that crap. When I'm out on the road I have too much access to junk food. I squirrel away snacks in my car so I won't have to stop as often."

"Have you lost weight?"

"Nope. Put on fifteen pounds in five months. I'm always taking people out to restaurants. Sitting in the car so much doesn't help either."

"Are you getting any exercise?"

"I used to jog, but I don't do that anymore. I have to leave for work pretty early in the morning, and in the evening I don't feel like doing anything besides vegging out in front of the tube."

"Do you nap?"

"I often fall asleep in the evening. I can't help it. I'm dog-tired."

"Do you drink?"

"Alcohol?"

I nodded.

"Social drinking. You can't sell to clients if you don't drink with them."

"How much?" I looked at him closely.

"Not that much," he said a little defensively. "I don't get drunk, but I drink more than I would usually drink—maybe a coupla beers, sometimes more."

"Do you have any medical problems?"

"No. I've been pretty healthy."

Almost everything I asked had turned up a positive. This unfortunate man broke all the taboos that protect sleep. He admitted to drinking too much alcohol, an inadequate diet, isolation, job dissatisfaction, poor sex life, sedentary lifestyle, and stress. I took the rest of his history and examined him carefully. He passed everything. We returned to my desk to make a plan.

"What do you think is going on here, Mr. Grogan? What would you tell a friend who told you what you've told me?"

"Well, I'm not stupid—I mean I *know* things are troubling me. I'm not happy with my life. Nothing ever seems to make me happy. I think that's why I was always critical of my ex. I was unhappy and I made her unhappy, too. I can keep a lid on it during the day, but at night, all hell breaks loose. I put a magnifying glass on everything that's ever gone wrong in my life. I'm defenseless."

"Have you thought about seeing someone over what's troubling you?"

"You mean a shrink?"

"Or a counselor. Some objective stranger to hear you out."

"I haven't done that. I guess I've never thought I would be the kind of person who needed to." He felt the need to avert his eyes.

"There's no special kind of person. It can happen to *anyone*. I'm of the opinion that unless you start to get a handle on what's bothering you, I could throw all the medication at you I have to offer and you still wouldn't be able to regain a natural night's sleep."

"Is it confidential?"

"Absolutely."

Ed Grogan sighed again. This time it was a sigh of resignation. "I'm willing to give it a try. I'll do anything."

THE SLEEP PHENOMENON

Charles A. Lindbergh had flown 28 hours when the desire to sleep almost overcame his determination to complete the first non-stop, trans-Atlantic flight. With no one to relieve him, his lightweight plane stripped of any diversions, and five and one-half more hours to go over the ocean, he tried whatever he could to stay awake, including sniffing ammonia capsules. The night before his historic May 20, 1927 flight, "Lucky Lindy" slept only a few hours. Lack of sleep almost cost him the cheers of 100,000 spectators when he landed in Paris, medals, prize money, a place in history—and his life.

Shakespeare knew the meaning of a bad night's sleep of a different sort:

> *To sleep! perchance to dream;*
> *ay, there's the rub.*

For centuries the restful sleep of a baby has been the envy of many an adult. Spending a walloping 90% of their time in la-la-land, most babies can fall asleep anywhere, in any position.

Now the rub. More than 100 million adults in the U.S. are chronically sleep deprived. Maybe growing up isn't such a good thing. In a 1995 Gallup poll, almost 50% of Americans admitted having insomnia or other sleep-related disorders. Sleeplessness is now the number one complaint of patients. The total direct and indirect costs on productivity and rate of accidents in 1990 was estimated at a walloping $166 billion.

The National Highway Traffic Safety Administration estimates that lack of sleep contributes to 100,000 automobile crashes each year, causing about 70,000 injuries and 1,500 fatalities. The worst day?—the first work day after the change to daylight savings.

It's a mystery. First a yawn. Then we lie down with our eyes closed for periods of time roughly totaling a third of our lives. Our creativity, immunity, mental faculties, personalities, physical health, even sanity, depend on it. Parts of the brain become exceedingly active, blood flow to them increases dramatically, and our brain waves transform, while we play "movies" of our own design to ourselves, remembering bits and pieces or whole sections the next day. And while this mental projector runs, revealing vivid colors and surrealistic plot twists, our muscles remain flaccid and our eyes roll around under our eyelids like we're trying to scan the horizon, a time called rapid eye movement sleep (REM). The brain's as active while we sleep as when awake, but in a different way.

The pituitary gland's release of growth hormone (GH) during non-REM (NREM) sleep, especially after exercise, is associated with a deeper sleep. The hormone may slow aging—another perk of a good night's rest.

If you're a dolphin, no problem. Only half of a dolphin's brain sleeps at any one time. The other half can keep tabs on the environment and take care of business. But for humans, sleep is all-or-nothing. Even losing 30 to 60 minutes of sleep a day accrues a "sleep debt." According to sleep researchers, about one-third of healthy adults suffer from sleep deprivation. Some call it the price of modern society.

Just how much sleep does a person need? It varies between individuals, but most adults require 6 to 8 hours a day. Regularly sleeping more may shortened life span and predispose to strokes. Sleeping less leads to excessive daytime sleeping. The sleepy brain cannot perform well. Unless you're prone to insomnia, which napping tends to aggravate, a 30 minute nap can improve mental sharpness. Cats do it!

Insomnia includes trouble falling to sleep or staying asleep. Taking a half hour or more to fall asleep is considered abnormal. Most people normally wake up 15 to 20 times a night, but remembering 5 or more such episodes and being unable to drift back to sleep for at least 30 minutes is outside the norm.

Poor sleep hygiene and negative conditioning are the usual reasons for primary insomnia. Abuse of alcohol, depression, excessive napping, heavy smoking, medical illnesses, "jet lag," a "night owl" biorhythm, sedative-hypnotic drugs, and too much coffee or other stimulants are other causes. Researchers have discovered that insomnia due to mental disorders, such as anxiety, depression, and personality disorder, is far more prevalent than primary insomnia.

BATTLING SLEEP DISORDERS

Here's what you can do: try natural, sensory sleep inducers. Cover your eyes (sight); experience aromatherapy with chamomile, lavender, or orange blossom (smell); listen to a calming CD or tape (sound); eat legumes or turkey at dinner, or have a glass of warm milk, rich in tryptophan at bedtime (taste); massage your face, neck, or shoulders, or relax in a hot bath for 30 minutes at least two hours before bed (touch). Sleeping in a cool room, as low as 60 to 65 degrees, is optimal.

Avoid arguments before bed, changing bedtime or time of getting up by more than two hours, clock-watching, eating or exercising too late in the evening—especially foods that cause gastric distress—late evening naps, lying in bed trying to force sleep, and restless bed partners. If you can do without medications for sleep, all the better. If not, antihistamines, triazolam, or zolpidem often are prescribed. Sedative antidepressants do the trick when depression is the cause of insomnia. Many people self-medicate with melatonin, but its long-term safety has not been established. Recently, researchers have reset the internal "time clock" by exposure to light behind the knees during sleep.

Who dares to stop breathing 30 times a night for 10 seconds each time? About 30 million Americans with sleep apnea do, but they don't know it. They habitually snore and wake up gasping. The results are depression, excessive daytime sleepiness, memory impairment, restless sleep, and sleeping too much (hypersomnia). Most people with apnea do not have an airway obstruction, but obstructive apnea can be life-threatening. Other causes of hypersomnia are narcolepsy, a precipitous falling off to sleep during any activity (even driving or having sex), one of a tetrad of disturbances during REM sleep, and making abnormal movements during sleep known as periodic movements.

The third kind of sleep disorder is what Shakespeare was getting at in *Hamlet*: parasomnias. Nightmares usually occur during REM sleep. Night terrors, in which a person appears to wake up terrified but is actually in deep sleep and doesn't remember the episodes, occur in NREM sleep. Sleepwalking (somnambulism), usually a phenomenon of young children, may return in adults with dementia or seizures, or who take drugs. Maybe a good night's sleep is a better deal than we realize.

One more thing. An estimated 95% of people with sleep disorders are undiagnosed and untreated, according to *Power Sleep*. Maybe that has something to do with the observation that less than 1% of medical case histories make any mention of sleep. Fortunately, the American Medical Association has designated sleep a distinct medical specialty, encouraging public recognition and more research.

10

To Be or Not to Be

Is there no pity sitting in the clouds
That sees into the bottom of my grief?
—WILLIAM SHAKESPEARE

Despair is the price one pays for setting an impossible aim
—GRAHAM GREENE

There is but one truly serious philosophical problem and this is
suicide
—ALBERT CAMUS

...Suicides have a special language. Like carpenters they want
to know which tools. They never ask why build
—ANNE SEXTON

That is what chills your spine when you read an account of a suicide;
not the frail corpse hanging from the window bars but what
happened inside the heart immediately before
—SIMONE DE BEAUVIOR

"My Record Is Broken"

As I walked down the streets of Manhattan to the hospital, the city made a better visual impression than usual, thanks to spring. Bright bits of green had appeared on trees. Verdant grass returning to little squares, generously referred to as parks, and equally small patches of blue sky amongst the clouds broke the oppressive concrete appearance of the city. When I rounded the corner, the huge brush of a street-cleaning vehicle was sweeping briskly against the curb, removing the last dirt, litter, and vestiges of winter. Recent rains, though ineffective against the travel-worn sidewalks and stained streets, brightened the buildings. Energetic birds chirped melodically above the dissonance of automobiles, trucks, and buses.

My first patient of the day was a stark contrast to spring. As she walked into my office, I immediately felt her dark mood settle over the room. Martha Winslow had light gray hair. Brown-framed reading glasses hung on a strap around her neck. Dressed plainly but neatly, wearing little make-up, she looked kind and motherly, yet despondent. Even had she worn earrings, her face was too sad to have been adorned by them.

Mrs. Winslow volunteered the reason she came to the clinic: "I've been having some problems at home." Frown lines formed between her eyebrows. She seemed restless.

"What kind of problems?" I asked.

"Constant arguments with my husband. We've said things to each other I never imagined we'd say. We don't really mean to say them; I know it and so does he. I'm taking out my anger on him and he's unleashing his frustration on me."

"Why?"

"The usual reason—my attitude."

"I'm not following. What attitude?"

"It's about my daughter or former daughter—I don't know which to call her any more. I have to let go of her."

"Why? Has she moved away from home?"

"Grace died two years ago in a car crash." Mrs. Winslow put her right hand over her brow and bent her head down slightly.

I could see how close to the surface her pain still was. "I'm sorry. How did it happen?"

"A drunk driver hit her on Memorial Day. The other car crossed the median and collided with her head-on. She didn't have a chance."

"How sad."

"Yes, well, my husband has gone on with his life, but I can't let go. I still remember the phone call in the middle of the night like it happened yesterday. I had to identify my daughter in the morgue. No mother should ever have to do that." Her voice was barely audible.

"How old was she?"

"Only thirty-two."

"Did they catch the driver?"

"Yes." Mrs. Winslow nodded. "They arrested the woman who did it. She served time for involuntary manslaughter. But *she* gets out next month on parole and has her life ahead; *I* have no daughter." Mrs. Winslow began to sob softly into her hands. She opened her purse, found a tissue, and wiped her eyes and cheeks. "Grace was an actress, you know. She was going to audition for a part on a new TV series the following week."

"This must be very difficult for you to talk about." I leaned over and touched her hand.

"No. It's all right. I *need* to talk about it." She stopped to collect herself. "Ever since the accident I have felt so alone."

"Do you have other children?"

"No. Even if I did, I would still feel the pain. I am tired of feeling pain. Also, I've become a burden to my husband."

"Has he said that?"

"Not in so many terms yet. Someday he will. I can tell he feels that way. I'm a wet rag to him," she bemoaned, wringing her hands in her lap.

"What makes you think that?"

"I have a terrible problem giving up my daughter. I've been a mother to her for so long, I can't let go. My first therapist told me it was considered normal to grieve for six months, maybe a year, but going on for a few years is abnormal. They call it a morbid depression."

I listened attentively without speaking.

"Grace meant a lot to me. Some people have an avocation. They put in time and get good at it...it becomes a major part of their lives. I put myself into my daughter. She was the best part of my world. My husband and I wanted to have other children, but I couldn't." Mrs. Winslow heaved a deep sigh. "Grace was a perfect child, at least to me.

I remember one Friday, she didn't come home after school for two hours—she was only seven then. Imagine a whole two hours. I was frantic, thinking something terrible had happened to her. When she got home, she said she went to play with some girl-friends. I gave her such a lecture. I made her apologize and promise never to do that again. She didn't protest and said nothing in her defense.

Then over the weekend, on Mother's day, she produced a beautiful bouquet of daisies. They were tied together with a purple ribbon. She never told me—I found out later—she walked *two miles* to the florist's that Friday and used all the money she saved from birthday gifts and allowance to buy the flowers. That was one of the happiest and saddest days of my life. Since she died, every Mother's Day is an ordeal for me."

Mrs. Winslow fought back the tears. Grief contorted her face. After a brief but anguished pause she regained her composure.

"Grace was struggling to make it in her career. Everyone's trying to be an actress these days it seems; it was very competitive for her. She wouldn't accept help from my husband and me. She wanted us to save for our retirement because, unless she got her break, she probably wouldn't be able to help us out financially later. Grace was always thinking about us like that.

Then, suddenly, some drunk tore her out of my life." Mrs. Winslow's voice flashed rage momentarily then sank back into despair. "Now I have to go on." She paused. "I wanted to give my daughter so much, but I didn't get a chance. I didn't tell her enough how much she meant to me."

"I'm sure that she realized that, Mrs. Winslow."

"Don't wait to tell people what you want to tell them," she advised, ignoring my response. "You never know when you will run out of time."

"Do you have a picture of her?"

"Yes, of course." Excited that I thought to ask, Mrs. Winslow removed the silver locket hanging from her neck and opened it for me. "Grace had blond hair and lovely green eyes."

The picture was of a child not an adult. I wondered if Mrs. Winslow had already given me the reason why she chose to remember her daughter that way. "She was pretty."

"Yes," Mrs. Winslow replied wistfully. "I love my husband very much, don't get me wrong. He means everything to me. But a spouse is not the same as your own flesh and blood. I've never told anyone this," she confided, lowering her voice, "but I wouldn't mind—I mean it would be okay—if I died, if *somehow* I could see my daughter again and be with her."

I didn't like the sound of the remark. "You don't really mean that, do you?" I searched her eyes warily.

"I do. I want to be with her again." Mrs. Winslow stared off. "Do you believe in an afterlife?" she asked quietly a few moments later.

It was an unnerving tangent. "I don't know, I suppose I hope there is one."

"You must have watched many patients dying."

"Yes, I have." Too many, I thought.

"Did they talk to you about an afterlife?"

"Not usually. Most people kept their beliefs to themselves. Some didn't know they were dying or if they did, they didn't talk about it. I remember one demented woman asking me if I knew what happened to us when we die."

"What did you tell her?"

"I said I didn't know, but whatever it was, it would be okay. Nothing bad would happen to her. The answer seemed to calm her. She died shortly afterward. I hope I was right."

Mrs. Winslow looked pensive. "You'll have to excuse me. It's my morbid side coming out again. My therapist told me I need to go on another antidepressant."

"That would be a good idea since you've been struggling with this for so long. I can see your pain."

Just listening to Mrs. Winslow made me feel depressed. That was my rule of thumb: you could tell a person was depressed when talking to them depressed you. Depression was more contagious than the flu.

"I hate to take drugs."

"It may help you go forward. Your life may turn around."

"How can it? My record is broken. I don't want to be happy. It's not that I can't." She shook her head side-to-side. "I don't want to try."

I pushed the box of tissues toward her. "That's when you need medication."

Mrs. Winslow looked down again and seemed to stop listening. "I can still remember my husband when he was twenty-six years old and we were courting. I know it's terribly old-fashioned of me. He had curly black locks of hair. We were so young then. Just like you."

"I'm not young."

"Just think, you are younger today than you will ever be again."

"Now that's a very cheery thought." I was aiming for levity, but undershot my mark.

"I don't mean it that way. Take it as an invitation to feel young and act young...let your worries go. There's time enough for worries." She looked dreamy-eyed. Then the reverie ended. "Don't let me take up all of your time."

I asked Mrs. Winslow a number of other questions about her appetite, energy level, and sleeping pattern, looking for other signs of depression. When depressed patients admitted not only to thinking of hurting themselves, but had a specific plan, I considered them to be a suicide risk. Martha had suicidal ideation.

I was worried enough about her that I called over to the Psychiatry Triage Clinic and they agreed to see her. To make sure she did go I walked over with her. After she was evaluated and plans were made for treatment, I spoke with Albert Yazzie, the psychiatric worker.

"I probably shouldn't tell you this," he said, stroking his beard slowly and repetitively, "but as one professional to another, I will. When in doubt, it's better to err on the side of caution in these cases, otherwise you may experience what happened to me." The man's voice was calm, yet I felt its urgency. "Years ago I sent home a depressed man and he killed himself. I didn't think he was really suicidal."

Like the ancient mariner, he was retelling this story about the event that changed his life, a pathetic script he was forced to read from. His gray-green eyes revealed the incident had both enlightened and diminished him.

"It's a common problem. You can be deceived by someone clever. I remember that day well. My patient had been through the questions before with someone else. He knew if he admitted he was planning to do away with himself, he would have been hospitalized, so he told me he didn't want to hurt himself. I wish I'd seen through him...but I also know that you have to make decisions in real time, not in hindsight. It's made me even *more* careful."

"I don't like these life and death decisions. I never have," I confessed.

"They *are* difficult, but they're part of our jobs. What can you do?"

I wished they were not part of my job.

I saw Martha Winslow several more times over the following weeks and a bond developed between us. She seemed to be doing well on medication, but talked so much about her daughter that I thought I was getting to know her, too. Then Martha came by less often and was managed entirely by her therapist. Months passed before I heard word of her again. The news wasn't what I wanted to hear: she'd taken a *massive* overdose of drugs. When I learned that Martha was in the coronary care unit, I went to see her after work.

Being in the unit reminded me of my ICU days. The medicinal smell, the sterile look of the corridors, even the ceiling lighting brought back a flood of memories, uninvited, unwelcomed. I'd worked the evening shift many times and knew the routine. Seeing the nurses watch monitors, chart, and draw up medications put me back on the job.

I gazed beyond all the equipment and technology that would impress a non-medical person to the people behind the desks, the workstations, and their blue scrubs. I looked at their faces and into their eyes, watching their expressions, their movements, their interactions as they went about their tasks—custodians of all too frail and failing bodies and the breaking hearts of the families.

A nurse directed me to Martha Winslow's bedside. Martha was lying on her back with her eyes closed. She looked calm, all too calm. At least she was breathing on her own, I thought. I hoped that the woman's lack of movement indicated sleep, not coma.

A man with thick, black hair—hair that was too black—sat staring at her, looking like his mind was a million miles away. This must be Martha's husband, I realized. When he saw me, he stood up and mustered a smile. With bags under his eyes, his face had the expressionless appearance of someone in emotional shock. I introduced myself.

"I'm Charlie, Martha's husband," he replied softly. "My wife has told me about you."

"May I speak with you?" I motioned him away from the bedside, and he followed me out of the room. "I don't know what she can hear, so I don't want to talk in front of her. How is she?"

Mr. Winslow's face turned solemn. "They told me she's probably not going to make it. She could go at anytime."

My tight grip on my emotions all of a sudden slipped. Both sickened and saddened, I closed my eyes for a split second. "What have they found out?"

"Apparently she suffered a pretty major heart attack from the drugs she took. The doctors were surprised she even made it to the hospital. The heart muscle has been severely damaged and is not pumping effectively."

A strong sense of antipathy overtook me. All my efforts at getting her proper treatment were in vain; Martha was going to die anyway. Her depression hadn't released her mind from its chokehold. "What happened?"

He hung his head. "We had an argument this morning. It was our usual argument over our dead daughter. I blew up. I told her if she refused to try to go on with our own lives, I wasn't going to be able to live with her anymore."

Mr. Winslow leaned back against the wall, visibly tortured by his guilt. "You have to understand," he pleaded, "seeing the way she grieved all the time was draining the life out of me. It broke my heart. I not only lost my daughter, I lost my wife. Strange as it is to say, she was present physically, but her *soul* was gone.

It was becoming difficult for me to keep my job. My concentration faltered. My boss gave me yet another warning. I'm trying to hang on until I retire, which will be soon. We had such plans for our retirement, but Martha lost all interest. Her constant sadness alienated our friends. Even our extended family became estranged because fights erupted over the most stupid issues, things she *never* would have cared about before."

I listened quietly, knowing he needed to say all those things to begin the process of grieving. I watched as Charles Winslow agonized. Nervously he rubbed his hand on the back of his head and sighed.

"She was seeing a therapist and taking medications, as you know, and she was making strides, but not huge strides. Martha was a shadow of the woman I once knew. I was desperate. I hoped to shock her out of her depression." Mr. Winslow paced in front of me. "*I* am the one to blame. It was too much for her. She must have felt I was abandoning her. I caused her to overdose. I'm responsible for all of this."

He turned and looked at me plaintively. "Oh God, how am I going to live without her?" He bit his upper lip and his body quivered. Eyes flooded with tears, he stared off, absorbed in self-reproach. Then he appeared to remember me standing next to him. "If the paramedics hadn't resuscitated her, that would have been the last time I ever saw her. And the sight of her crying and the sound of my own harsh words would be all I have to remember for the rest of my life. At least, here, she has opened her eyes and I spoke to her briefly. She's not with it for very long. It must be the medications. I don't know the half of what's dripping in all her lines. Something's for the heart, something else is for the blood pressure."

My mind was translating his words into medical jargon. Martha Winslow was probably receiving antiarrhythmics and a dopamine drip, medications that would not sedate her. Needing a drip to support blood pressure wasn't a good sign. I touched Mr. Winslow's shoulder. "It's not your fault. It's no one's fault."

He tried to reply, then just nodded.

"Is she able to talk? Did she wake up at all tonight?"

He couldn't speak. "Yes," he said finally. "Not for long."

"May I go see her?"

"Please do."

I walked back into the room. Mr. Winslow sat on the edge of the bed next to his wife. "Martha," he said near her ear. "Can you hear me?" He placed his hand on hers.

After a pause, when I concluded he would get no response, she slowly opened her eyes. Seeming to recognize him, she attempted to reach out with her arm, but moved in slow motion.

"It's okay, Martha. Don't try to move."

Mrs. Winslow's features were soft in the dim lighting of the room. Serene and momentarily alert, out of place in the hospital bed, she had the look of someone in church at a contemplative moment, or the appearance of a person who, having lived a good life, in a flash now looked back and reflected on all that had been planned, all that had transpired, and all that mattered. In the uncertainty and angst of the moment, Martha was the only one who looked calm. Weakly motioning him to come closer, she moved her lips as if trying to say something. He drew close. When he put his head down near her lips, she tenderly kissed him.

"I am so sorry. Please, *please*, forgive me, Martha."

She smiled at him and gave him a look that only people who have loved each other for many years can give. Tears rolled down her cheeks. Slowly, she moistened her lips with her tongue. "A-l-w-a-y-s l-o-v-e y-o-u," she said, her voice faint but audible. Then her eyes closed and her muscles relaxed. Her face became expressionless and she stopped breathing. The heart monitor above sounded continuously. I saw that Martha was flatlining. Something had clearly left her body, some energy or force had ceased to empower her.

Before I could do anything, Mr. Winslow yelled, "*Oh, Martha!*" Seeing the only woman he ever loved lying still and unmoving before him, the raw power of love and guilt, strangely conjoined, threw him over the edge. Unaware of his surroundings, he flung himself over her, putting his arms around her lifeless form. He shook her body with his sobs of sorrow.

The medical team rushed in and I stepped out of the way and left the room. As I glanced back over my shoulder, I saw them trying frantically to do CPR and wheeling in the red crash cart. A nurse was escorting Mr. Winslow out of the room. He didn't want to leave, but he was too crushed to resist.

Charles Winslow sat in a chair down the hall like a piece of crumpled paper. I went over to console him, but he was inconsolable. My medical background prepared me for what had happened because I understood the futility of attempting to keep the dying heart of Martha Winslow going. I tried to make him understand. He looked at me vacantly without comprehension, beyond grief. His own words were ironic: now, literally, he *had* lost *both* women in his life.

I saw past this transient moment into a future time when Charles would also understand. In some sad and contorted reality, was he now not also free of the suffering caused by loving someone who no longer loves life? He had been a lifeguard who almost went under trying to save another person's life. Or had depression merely chosen a new victim? Determined that he would get aggressive, early treatment, I would keep in touch with him. Martha would have wanted it that way, too.

As Mrs. Winslow slipped away, I had the most unusual thoughts. I recalled how I shared in the woman's agony and implacable loneliness, her inner darkness and resolute yearning for a yonder world of distant memories and imperturbable tranquillity. The possibility of Martha somehow finding her daughter, however untestable and unknown, gave me satisfaction. I imagined the two of them meeting after their long separation and embracing tightly without speaking. What would they say? What would they do?

On the hithermost edge of this world, I bid Martha Winslow farewell forever.

SUICIDE

Anthony and Cleopatra committed suicide after their defeat by Octavian in a great sea battle near Actium in Greece. So did Earnest Hemingway, Adolph Hitler, and Vincent Van Gogh, men who otherwise could not have been more different. Whether the method is asphyxiation, drug overdose, hanging, jumping from heights, poisoning, self-inflicted wounds from firearms or knives, or other violent means, suicide is not confined to any one era or group of peoples. At the root of suicide is depression, but not all depressed patients become suicidal. Other than for the lemming—rodents noted for their fatal mass migrations into the sea—humans are alone in this behavior.

Suicide was the ninth leading cause of death in the U.S., accounting for more than 31,000 deaths in 1994. Considering that only an estimated 1% of suicide attempts succeed, the number of suicide attempters is astounding. Individuals with untreated depression have up to a 30-fold increased risk of suicide compared to people who are not depressed and commit 60 to 70% of all suicides.

The rate of suicide varies with a person's age, gender, geographical region, and racial or ethnic group, being much higher in the elderly, males, western states, Alaskan natives, Native Americans, and non-Hispanic whites. The geriatric population has the highest rate of suicide in the U.S. and the rate has continued to climb over this past decade. Suicide rates are lower among married persons than among people who are divorced, single, separated, or widowed.

Self-poisoning is a common method of suicide, usually with a single agent. Many individuals use prescribed medication to commit suicide. The concern is that a single prescription of antidepressants may be enough to commit suicide. Antidepressants, one of many drug classes used in suicide attempts, account for 10 to 20% of self-poisonings. They differ in their fatal toxicity index. Older tricyclic antidepressants and MAO inhibitors are more likely to result in death following an overdose, causing cardiotoxicity, convulsions, and hyperthermia.

Suicide attempters have also ingested analgesics, antipsychotics, cardiovascular drugs, sedative-hypnotics, stimulants, and street drugs. According to a study by the CDC, use of firearms is a leading method of suicide, accounting for more than half the suicides in every region except the Northeast.

Occasional reports of suicidal ideation taint most antidepressants, but the effect could be due either to the drug or the underlying depression. Paradoxically, patients being treated for depression are more likely to commit suicide when they begin to feel better. Presumably, only then do they possess the energy to carry it out. Rather than being falsely reassured, that critical phase is a time for increased vigilance and supervision.

DEPRESSION

English author David Herbert Lawrence observed, "I never saw a wild thing sorry for itself." Sadness is a unique and normal part of human life. How much time a person spends being sad depends on many factors often out of his or her control. Marcel Proust made psychological and philosophical sense when he said, "We are healed of a suffering only by experiencing it to the full." But when sadness preoccupies or incapacitates an individual, it becomes abnormal and part of a bigger issue: depression.

"Depression is a wimp of a word for a howling tempest in the brain," argues writer William Styron. It is a serious and formidable disorder of mood, prevalent in people of all ages. Depression destroys lives.

The National Institute of Mental Health referred to depression as "the common cold of mental illness." At least six percent of patients entering a primary care clinic, or 17% of the population, suffers from depression, and primary care providers are now more responsible than ever before for medical management of depression. An estimated 85% of depressed people show up in primary care clinics, but only 40% of them are recognized as being depressed. The annual direct and indirect cost of treating depression in the U.S. is 43 billion dollars.

No false reassurances: differentiating depression from physical illness can be challenging, particularly in older adults. They occur *together* 50% of the time in patients with cancer and 25 to 50% in heart disease. Physical signs like lack of energy, sleeping problems, and weight loss may be manifestations of depression or illness. Hypothyroidism and other reversible and treatable medical disorders should always be ruled out before concluding a patient has idiopathic depression.

"Atypical" depression is a syndrome of carbohydrate craving, excessive sleeping, and overeating. Instead, most people with "typical" depression don't eat and can't sleep.

Those who are depressed in late fall and winter but perky in summer—4 to 6% of the general population—constitute the "winter depression" category of seasonal affective disorder (SAD). The spring-onset pattern of "summer depression" is less common. Most episodes of SAD occur within unipolar major depressive disorders. Women, who are usually in their early twenties, outnumber men four to one. The problem is treatable. "Winter depression" responds to light therapy with therapeutic light boxes, monoamine oxidase inhibitors, or psychotherapy, whereas "summer depression" responds better to antidepressants.

Medical opinion is divided on the controversial chronic fatigue syndrome. Critics see it as a form of depression because more than half of those afflicted are depressed. Proponents focus instead on the association of fatigue and flu-like symptoms. The diagnosis should be considered although there is no specific treatment or cure.

Depression also frequently coexists with other psychiatric disorders such as alcohol and drug dependence, anxiety disorder, bulimia, obsessive-compulsive disorder, panic disorder, phobias, and posttraumatic stress.

Laboratory screening for depression includes complete blood count, blood chemistry panel, and thyroid studies. In the presence of an abnormal physical examination or supported by a suspicious history, other tests may be necessary.

GETTING OUT FROM UNDER THE CLOUD

The treatments for serious depression are psychotherapy, medication, a combination of both, or electroconvulsive shock (ECT). Selective serotonin reuptake inhibitors (SSRI's) and newer antidepressants, though more expensive, cause fewer side effects and are safer than older drugs, becoming first-line agents for many practitioners. SSRI's used in the U.S. are fluoxetine, fluvoxamine, paroxetine, and sertraline. Newer non-SSRI antidepressants include bupropion, mirtazapine, nefazodone, and venlafaxine.

Patients with a severe sleep disturbance may do better with a tricyclic antidepressant than with an SSRI, but fluoxetine is a good choice if they are sleeping too much. Antidepressants differ in their profile of side effects, such as sedation and sexual dysfunction. Several can be taken once daily. Usually, treatment should be continued for nine months after the depression has responded. In patients with ischemic heart disease, SSRI's may be safer than tricyclic antidepressants are.

Obstacles can get in the way. Several managed care organizations discourage the use of newer antidepressants because of their expense. Drug doses may be too low to be effective. Some people consider psychiatric disorders less serious than medical disorders. Because anxiety can be a symptom of depression, patients may be treated with the wrong medications. Patients should be warned that they may feel worse before they feel better. Mood may take a month to improve, although other symptoms like fatigue respond in days.

*   *   *

"I Can't Take the Pain Any Longer"

"You need to lose thirty to forty pounds, Mrs. Winters."

"I know. It's not easy for me. I've been struggling to do that for years." She patted her hips and smiled.

Edith Winters was a forty-seven-year-old patient I followed regularly for weight control and mild adult-onset diabetes. She was married to a high-ranking bank executive and had two, college-age children. At every opportunity, she showed me family photos. A fun loving woman, she laughed quickly, always had an interesting story to tell, and loved to travel with her husband. I looked forward to her visits.

"Your blood sugars are tipping over on the high side of one-hundred-forty to one-hundred-sixty. Losing weight would help that considerably."

She agreed. We worked together on trying to find a reasonable diet. The next step would be oral medication to control her blood glucose. Then, over a ten week period, I noticed that she missed several appointments with me. Previously, she'd been prompt and compliant. When I called her on the telephone, her voice sounded tired yet coherent. I was afraid that her blood sugar had sky-rocketed. I finally convinced her to come in to see me that day.

When she arrived in my office, to my amazement, she looked like a different person: weak, haggard, and old! She'd lost twenty pounds and her blood sugar was normal.

"You've lost so much weight. What happened?" I asked.

"I don't know," she said with a limp gesture of her arm. "I feel exhausted all the time."

"You're not on a crash diet, are you?"

"No, I don't feel much like eating. For once, I'm not trying to lose the weight." Her voice was faint.

"Have you been having diarrhea or any bleeding?"

"No."

"Do you have any pain?"

"Some, in my lower back and abdomen."

"Where?"

"I can't locate it very well."

After evaluating her, I ran some tests. The results seemed unbelievable. She had a primary cancerous mass on her right ovary that metastasized throughout her pelvis and into her bowel. Only nine months earlier her gynecological and PAP examinations were normal.

I referred her to Oncology Clinic. The prospect for treatment was poor. She opted against chemotherapy, choosing not to spend her remaining days vomiting and having diarrhea.

We continued our sessions together a few more times, but now she did little talking. Sometimes there was only silence and tears. Her pain medication controlled her discomfort in the beginning, but higher doses of pain killers became necessary. Eventually, she became too weak to keep her visits with me and the phone became our only connection.

One night her husband rushed her to the emergency room. She was admitted not for more treatment; she was admitted to die. The following day I went to her bedside, and she asked her family to leave the room. I didn't know what she was going to ask of me. In great pain and heavily sedated, she managed to talk with slurred words: "I can't take the pain any longer."

I held her hand. "I'm really sorry, Edith."

"If I can get myself home—" she said, pausing to gather her strength, "would you give me a strong drug that I could take to end the pain—forever?" she pleaded. Although her eyes looked glassy from the pain medication, I saw them struggling to read my face. She wasn't looking at my white coat or nametag; her eyes were fixed on me.

I didn't answer. Many thoughts ran through my mind. Euthanasia and assisted suicide were not practices I ever thought I'd condone or participate in. Even with all the publicity the issues received in the media, I hadn't decided what I would do if patients asked me to help them end their misery. I felt Edith's suffering, but asking me to take her life, even a terminal life, evoked some primal and abhorrent feelings within me.

"This cancer is eating me alive," she continued. "Can you help end my misery?"

I looked at Edith helplessly from the desolation of empathy. Only a glimmering of her old self remained in her eyes. Her voice was weak and she had the desperation of one who has lost all control over events. Now she had the look of belonging to her disease.

At that moment, her husband came into the room and she started to cry. I got up from the bed slowly feeling like I'd let her down. She must have read the answer in my face.

Edith Winters died soon after our bedside meeting.

ASSISTED SUICIDE

Mere mention of assisted suicide provokes strong opinions around the dinner table. Societal views are already polarized, with organizations such as the Hemlock Society and Choice in Dying (formerly the Euthanasia Society) advocating the "quality of life" over religious groups' advocacy of the "sanctity of life." The situation is volatile.

Since Jack Kevorkian, so-called "Dr. Death," kicked opened this door, attorneys have been battling over physician-assisted suicide in the courts. The *Quinlan* and *Conroy* cases affirmed the right-to-die years ago, but passage of Oregon's referendum to legalize physician-assisted suicide shocked many, including the neighboring state of Washington, which prohibits it even if the patient is terminally ill and in great pain. The public has shown a keen interest in the issue. *Final Exit*, a book containing instructions on how to commit suicide, was a national best-seller.

The debate over assisted suicide previously focused on doctors, but circumstances are changing. Patients are now appealing to nurse practitioners with prescriptive rights to participate. Their motivation may be severe depression, a painful chronic disease, or a fatal, agonizing illness with a slow death. With nurse practitioners so much more visible in today's health care market and many holding controlled substances prescriptive rights, we have become a new source of drugs to end life. We can prescribe narcotics independently of any physician involvement in fifteen states, and, in another nineteen states, we can write for controlled substances with some degree of physician involvement or delegation. Drugs for anxiety, depression, pain, or sleep are the same drugs used to kill patients.

Patients may be more inclined to ask nurse practitioners than to ask physicians for lethal prescriptions or advice on whether or not they should commit suicide. We are very much involved in this national debate. What should nurse practitioners say?

We must know our own ethical views regarding assisted suicide and euthanasia. We must also understand the laws. Many terms sound alike. As the laws on death change, the meaning of allowing a patient to die, assisted suicide, euthanasia, killing, and murder must be precisely defined because they have legal ramifications. The difference in the terms is not universally accepted.

Assisted suicide describes the act of helping an individual kill himself or herself. In contrast, euthanasia indicates that the helper does the killing. However, some courts consider it suicide rather than euthanasia if a person kills a terminally ill patient at his or her request. Killing, which means causing death, may be defined as euthanasia, murder, or suicide. Murder implies that a person is killed without his or her consent. Suicide is self-killing.

Measures to legalize assisted suicide have been or are being voted on in several states. In states legalizing assisted suicide, practitioners unwilling to participate will be required to transfer medical records to willing practitioners. Changes in the law may allow nurse practitioners to assist patients in euthanasia and suicide without legal punishment. Some national nurse associations condemn collaboration in assisted suicide. Nurse practitioners have the option of refusing to participate based on their own ethical objections.

ONE NOT TO MISS: OVARIAN CANCER

One alarm should sound loudly when caring for a woman with abdominal pain: ovarian cancer. It kills more women each year than homicides and suicides do. The tragedy is that 75% of ovarian cancers are not discovered until their advanced, hard-to-cure stage.

The symptoms are not impressive: abdominal pain, backache, fatigue, bloating, gas, constipation—everyday complaints. After all, the ovaries are only 1.5 inches long.

The cancer antigen CA125, transvaginal ultrasound, and color Doppler ultrasound are the best available tools to aid the diagnosis, but a strong index of suspicion is the first and foremost step. Especially suspect women with a positive family history for ovarian cancer, women with *BRCA* gene mutations for breast cancer, and women in their 70's. Up to 90% of familial cases of the breast-ovarian cancer syndrome have mutations of the *BRCA1* gene; the association with familial ovarian cancer is important but less strong.

*   *   *

"I Just Wants to Be Left Alone"

Alta Sweeney had the look of cancer. Sometimes you can tell when a patient walks into your office. The face of the Mississippi-born-and-bred, eighty-nine-year-old, tall, black woman was drawn and expressionless. Her clothes hung as if she had no shoulders. She weighed only about eighty-five pounds.

After evaluating her, I said, "We needed to do some tests to find out the cause of your weight loss."

I'll never forget the look conveyed by her large protuberant, lackluster eyes. "I just wants to be left alone, no one to bother me. I wants to die."

Later I found out it was her son who made the appointment for her because of the weight loss, and she saw me to humor him. She wanted me to do nothing.

"We need to see if you have something we can easily treat," I argued. "Maybe we can *help* you." As I spoke, my words sounded empty of conviction. Who was I kidding? I was grabbing at straws.

She looked at me like I didn't understand English.

A week later, I telephoned to see if she had the tests done. A woman with a thick Southern drawl answered.

"Are you Alta Sweeney?" I asked.

"I'm Alta's sister."

"How can I contact Alta?"

"She has pay-assed," the woman said. Her Mississippi accent was so pronounced that I didn't comprehend the significance of her words.

"What do you mean?"

"She dy-e-ed!"

Feeling more foolish than awkward, I asked her what happened. She explained that Alta died in her sleep a few nights earlier. The family declined an autopsy.

Alta Sweeney must have known all along that she had cancer. I was more concerned by Alta giving up than by her death itself. I tried to understand that for the longest time.

DEPRESSION IN THE TERMINALLY ILL

"Alta Sweeney" had the right to deny medical intervention and in doing so control the eventually of death on her terms. But did she seek no medical therapy for her disease because of depression?

According to researchers who assessed 200 patients with cancer to determine their level of clinical depression, a patient with cancer who wants to die may change his or her mind after receiving treatment for depression. Of the patients who wanted to die, 59% were diagnosed with clinical depression. In another study, six depressed, terminally ill patients who received comprehensive palliative care for 2 weeks changed their outlook about wanting to die. It's not a moot point.

Treating the mind for depression is just as critical as treating the body for a lethal disease. Depression is painful, but when recognized, can be treated to help ease the patient's already heavy burden. A positive outlook may also give the patient the best chances for surviving cancer.

SOCIETAL REACTIONS TO DEATH

We distance ourselves from death and try to shut out reality; it's human nature. Is death "a dirty little secret, a thing of shame," asks writer D. J. Enright, "the last taboo in an otherwise totally uninhibited world?" We view death as a failure of medicine and nursing, the enemy of society. It's not said aloud, but people think that if medicine and nursing were doing their jobs, no one should have to die.

As a health care provider, you pick up on that view and start to experience the death of your patient as a personal failure. So we try too hard to keep terminally ill patients alive. Isn't that what society wants?

That's not what the patient wants. You see it over and over again: dying patients push away their food, spit out medications, or refuse to cooperate with caregivers. Family members plead: "Please don't put her through that again" or "Can you just leave him in peace." It's difficult to stop offering patients things they don't need anymore. Sometimes the health care provider is the last one to accept the reality of death.

The findings of a 28 million dollar study, financed by the Robert Wood Johnson Foundation and published in 1995, were shocking. Nearly 80% of physicians misunderstood or ignored the requests of their terminally ill patients. About one-third of terminally ill patients did not want cardiopulmonary resuscitation (CPR), but half of them got it anyway. Against their will, many patients still die alone, in pain, and mechanically ventilated some 28 years since the living will movement began.

A nurse knows that for the terminally ill patient, a *good* death is a desirable outcome. Even though it tugs at your heart, you do all you can for your patient so that they accept their death with less fear and have a sense of closure with their loved ones. Accepting the reality of death doesn't mean that you're giving up on your patient or some sort of unfeeling person. Through refocusing care on compassion, love, and reassurance, we can look beyond ambivalence and confused emotions. It's about managing dying patients' pain, keeping them comfortable, gentle touching, holding of hands, the stroking of hair, and *listening* to what they want to say.

11

Private Parts

The three most important things a man has are, briefly,
his private parts, his money, and his religious opinions
                                                    —SAMUEL BUTLER

Civilization is the progress toward a society of privacy
                                                    —AYN RAND

Adolescence goes to at least the age of forty-nine
                                                    —ALAN BERMAN

Even the wisest men make fools of themselves about women, and
even the most foolish women are wise about men
                                                    —THEODOR REIK

Be not too hasty to trust or to admire the teachers of morality: they
discourse like angels, but they live like men
                                                    —SAMUEL JOHNSON

"I've Got an Itch Down There"

Spry, Irish-born Sarah Donnelly hadn't been seen by her primary physician for over a year. Hearing impaired, her face weathered and lined, she sat next to my desk and settled in. "I've got an itch down there," she screamed, pointing to her crotch. She felt she hadn't gotten a complete check-over, despite seeing various doctors. One doctor gave her some xylocaine local anesthetic for the itch. "I want to see my doctor."

"He's not in, but I'll examine you." I nearly had to shout at her to be heard. A hearing aid was now on my list of things to discuss with her physician.

Ms. Donnelly seemed very disappointed. "Oh, no. I want to see *him*."

"Why does it have to be him?"

"Because he's a handsome young man. I just *adore* him. I wanted to see him so bad that I put on a *new* pair of underpanties. I wouldn't have worn my new underwear if I knew I would see *you*."

"I appreciate your wearing new underwear," I said. "You should see some of the old underwear I have to look at."

She gave me a blank look.

"Your doctor didn't have time in his schedule this week to see you. He sent you here to be seen sooner. It's not a matter of coming in on another day to visit him. He sends all his patients to me."

Sarah Donnelly seemed to be pondering how she could overcome this cruel obstacle.

Her itch turned out to be nothing more than an attempt to get attention from the male doctor, as I suspected. But I was also suspicious about another hidden problem: her underpants were wet with urine.

"Do you dribble on yourself, Ms. Donnelly?"

She looked embarrassed. "Sometimes."

"Does it happen when you cough, laugh, or sneeze?"

"That's right."

Urinary incontinence revealed. I asked her more questions, we went over the possible causes, and I ordered an urinalysis to be sure she didn't have a urinary tract infection. When the urinalysis was negative, I referred her to a urologist.

"Is he a *male* doctor?" she yelled.

"Yes, and a handsome one at that."

Her eyes widened. Of course I wasn't sure, but I wanted her to show up for the appointment. That seemed to handle it.

The next day Thelma stopped in my office. "A patient named Sarah Donnelly wanted to be seen, but she left abruptly when she heard she'd be seeing you instead of her doctor."

"Oh, Sarah and her convenient crotch itch," I retorted.

"What?" Thelma asked.

"Never mind."

SEXUALITY AND AGING

Taking care of patients must encompass their sexual health. The subject can be difficult for patients and health care providers to discuss. Obtaining a sexual history requires sensitivity to cultural and generational values. It's best to seek permission to ask about sexual function.

The onset of menopause usually makes it easier to introduce the discussion with women, but men tend to be less comfortable. Many patients actually welcome an opportunity to discuss sexual matters with their health care provider. Although sexual desire and frequency may wane with age in some people, others remain sexually active into their 80's. Education about age-related changes can help them stay sexually healthy longer.

Couples sometimes develop sexual problems later in life because they are uninformed about the physiologic changes associated with aging. Out of confusion and frustration, they may stop having sex. For both men and women, arousal, plateau, orgasm, and resolution slow down. Older men require more penile stimulation, and attaining an erection takes longer. They may falsely conclude this is a sign of impending impotence; their partners may assume loss of interest.

In women, increased skin sensitivity may cause nipple stimulation to be irritating. Because more of the clitoris is exposed due to shrinkage of the labia, stimulation can be painful. Vaginal blood flow, lubrication, and size also decrease.

As many as 30% of postmenopausal women experience pain during intercourse (dyspareunia). Its causes are endometriosis, insufficient lubrication of the vagina, tumors, vaginismus, or vulvo-vaginitis. Inadequate lubrication is a consequence of incomplete sexual arousal and can be corrected with patient education and use of lubricants. When vaginal atrophy is the cause, conjugated estrogens or testosterone cream works well. Vulvovaginitis is due to infection or inflammation of the vulva and vagina. Vaginismus is voluntary or involuntary vaginal muscular contraction due to fear, pain, or sexual attitudes.

For post-menopausal women, estrogen replacement therapy can be instituted if there are no contraindications such as active gallbladder disease, estrogen-dependent cancer, thromboembolic disorders, or thrombophlebitis. A progestin must be added to the treatment to avoid uterine cancer except in the one-third of woman over 60 who have had a hysterectomy. Estrogen replacement therapy, a water-based vaginal lubricant, and masturbation may make the sexual experience more enjoyable.

Loss of libido afflicts both men and women. Depression, illness, medication side effects, and psychosocial issues, such as personal loss, are common causes. The sexual drive of women in their 40's to 50's may be improved with androgen therapy.

HIDDEN CONDITIONS

Social stigma, real or imagined, may prevent a patient from telling a health care provider about a medical condition. Urinary incontinence is one such "hidden condition" that affects 11 million women and 2 million men in the U.S. today and costs $16.4 billion. Other hidden conditions are depression, domestic violence, impotence, sexually transmitted diseases, and substance abuse.

Normally, the bladder wall muscle (detrusor) and sphincter muscle work together to allow the bladder to fill without leaking until it is emptied voluntarily. The teamwork sometimes breaks down. When urinary incontinence results, urine leaks involuntarily. It may occur at all times (total incontinence) or intermittently (stress, urge, or overflow incontinence).

Urinary incontinence usually strikes women 45 and older, but also 25% of those between the ages of 30 and 59. Women who are embarrassed by the condition may take more than a year to talk to their health care provider, according to a survey by the American Foundation for Urologic Disease. Stress incontinence, the most common type in older women, results from perineal muscle weakness often as an aftermath of childbirth. Coughing, exercising, lifting, or sneezing causes a loss of control. Without treatment, some women avoid certain social situations and experience discomfort.

Other types of urinary incontinence depend on whether the bladder is hyperreflexic (urge incontinence) or chronically distended (overflow incontinence). In old age, congestive heart failure, delirium, depression, drugs, hyperglycemia, and immobility are non-urological causes of urinary incontinence.

For mild stress incontinence, medications to increase urethral resistance or topical estrogen creams can be tried. Surgery is usually corrective. The treatment for urge incontinence is antispasmodic or anticholinergic drugs. Intermittent catheterization treats overflow incontinence.

*   *   *

"Forgive My Bluntness"

In the clinic hallway, Thelma leaned into me and whispered, "You're next patient is a real looker. Here's his chart. We haven't seen his likes around here before—believe me, I *would* remember." She arched her eyebrows for added dramatic flair and smiled a little too broadly.

"Contain yourself, woman. You act like they just released you from prison or something. Try not to flirt with our patients, it's bad for our image," I teased.

"See for yourself, Ms. Self-righteous."

I called James Videka from the waiting room. *Yep, he's cute all right—the body of Apollo himself. With his height, broad shoulders, and strong, sculpted, calendar model's face, he beams self-confidence.* It took less than two minutes in my office to discover how wrong my perception really was.

He extended his right hand; his handclasp was weak and moist. "Thanks for seeing me on short notice."

"How can I help you, Mr. Videka?"

"Forgive my bluntness. I have a problem getting a hard on, and if I do get one, I can't keep it up for long. This has been going on about three months. It's extremely embarrassing—you have no idea."

"Does it happen all the time?"

"Most of the time. When I'm with my fiancée, who looks better in a negligee than some of those magazine models, well, the wind goes out of my sail."

"Do you have early morning erections?"

"Not lately."

"Do you masturbate?"

"To be honest, I haven't felt the need to since I meet Crystal."

"Have you ever fathered a child?"

"From my previous marriage I have a child, but then I didn't have this problem either."

"Do you have any medical conditions like diabetes, sexually transmitted diseases, burning when you urinate, or pain or swelling of your scrotum?

"No."

"When did you get divorced?"

"About fourteen months ago, give or take a month. Why?"

"Sometimes emotional turmoil can affect sexual function. Have you been feeling depressed over it or other recent events?"

"Not anymore. We parted amicably and I see my little girl often. In fact, I'm very excited about getting married again. Crystal's great—very compassionate and the patience of a saint. I just don't want to start off the marriage on the wrong foot. Her patience won't last forever."

"When's the last time you had sexual intercourse and is she your only sexual partner?"

"She's been my only partner since our engagement four months ago, and the last time we had sex was a week ago, without success on my part."

I explained that I needed to do a complete physical and asked a female assistant to witness the genital and rectal examination. I found no abnormalities. The patient was in good physical health.

Mr. Videka was dressing behind the curtain, allowing it to act as a confessional. "You know, this is tough on a man's ego. Here I'm supposed to be this big macho stud—or so my friends say—and I can't even have sex with a woman, for cryin' out loud!"

The curtain opened quickly and caught me nodding to myself. I sympathized with the man's frustration. The cause of his impotence could be psychological. He was divorced and might well have anxiety over his new relationship, manifesting as performance anxiety. But the lack of early morning erections didn't favor that view. Something he said also bothered me.

"Mr. Videka, what did you mean when you said *not anymore* after I asked you about depression."

"Oh, right. About six months ago, I was down in the dumps for a while because I wasn't meeting women I really cared for. That's when I saw a shrink and he put me on this medication for depression. After about a month, I started to feel better."

"Are you still talking the medication?"

"Yes. I've been afraid to stop it because I don't want to feel that bad about myself again."

When he gave me the specifics about the drug, it dawned on me that his impotence easily could be drug-related or a mixture of physical and psychological causes. "I'd like to stop your medication."

He made a dubious face. "What if I get depressed again? My wedding is three months away."

"Well, if we don't take care of this problem, you might have another reason to be depressed. Besides, your divorce was a while ago and you say you're happy about remarrying. I suspect you won't need the antidepressant. If you do, we can put you on one that doesn't cause impotence."

I didn't hear from the patient again until over three months later when I found a postcard from Hawaii in my office mail:

Life is good again, and our marriage is off to a firm start. Thanks —James Videka

I knew we wouldn't be seeing the likes of Mr. Videka around our clinic anymore. Too bad—for Thelma.

IMPOTENCE

Priapus, the Greek god of procreation and guardian of gardens and vineyards, personified the erect phallus. The Romans set up crude images of Priapus in their gardens as scarecrows, representing him as a grotesque individual with a huge phallus. Young and old touched him for good luck. The term *priapism* now refers to an abnormally persistent and painful erection.

For males, the most common sexual problem is just the opposite: impotence. This consistent inability to get or sustain a firm enough erection for sexual intercourse affects 20 million men in the U.S., especially older men. The cause may be physical, accounting for up to 70% of cases, or psychological.

Physical causes are alcohol and certain prescription drugs, blocked or damaged blood vessels to the penis (arteriosclerosis, diabetes, groin trauma, hypertension, smoking), damage to the nervous system (brain tumor, diabetes, spinal injury, stroke), or reduced testosterone levels.

Evaluation of physical causes should exclude drug-related and hormonal etiologies. Penile doppler studies, which measure vascular pressure, help identify a vascular reason for the problem.

A new oral drug, sildenafil, enhances erectile response by increasing the penile mediator (cGMP) of nitric oxide (NO), the principal neurotransmitter in the penis. The drug works only when the patient is sexually aroused. One-third of impotent men do not respond to it and its use is contraindicated in those who take nitroglycerin for angina.

There are other methods. A vacuum cylinder creates negative pressure and draws blood into the penis, achieving an erection that may be maintained by applying a constricting band to the base of the penis to limit venous outflow. Self-injection into the penis with a vasoactive drug combination, such as alprostadil, papaverine, and phentolamine, produces an erection for 30 to 60 minutes. Penile implants are a surgical option for refractory impotence.

Psychological causes of impotence are anxiety, depression, guilt, marital problems, and performance anxiety. Signs of a psychological and not physical cause are early morning erections and successful masterbation. Simple solutions entail talking openly with your partner, relaxing, and seeking counseling.

*   *   *

"I Don't Want to Pee Anymore"

Janis Marks looked like she was confessing to grand larceny. "It burns when I pass my urine."

"How long have you been having burning?" I wondered why she

was so nervous.

"Since yesterday."

"Any blood with it?"

"It was a little pink this morning. That's why I came in." Self-consciously, she raised her collar to cover the hickey on her neck when she noticed me looking at it.

"Any fever or chills?"

"I don't think so."

"Have you felt any urgency to urinate?"

"Yes, but when I go hardly anything comes out."

"And do you go to the bathroom often?"

"Yes."

"Any other symptoms like nausea or pain in your back?"

"No. I feel okay otherwise."

"Have you ever had this before?"

"No."

"Are you having your menstrual period now?"

"No. It was two weeks ago."

"Have you had any change in habits recently? Bike riding, wearing tight jeans, a bout of diarrhea, a change in sexual habits or sex partners?"

She looked up at me. Her features were delicate and her blue-green eyes were clear. She had a dot-of-a mole on her left temple. "My boyfriend came home. He's in the Navy and I don't get to see him very much at all." She blushed. "I guess we had a lot of sex to make up for it."

"Are you using protection?"

"I make him wear condoms."

I nodded and told her I needed to examine her.

"There's more."

I looked up.

"He did a lot of oral sex this time." Her face was choked red with embarrassment. "Do you think that might have something to do with it?"

"Yeah, it might. Let's do your examination and check your urine first." I was able to tap the ribs over her flank without her showing signs of discomfort, so a kidney infection seemed unlikely. Her only physical abnormality was tenderness over the suprapubic area.

"Can you give me a urine specimen now?"

"I think so."

"Here's a cup. You can go into the bathroom over there."

She returned with the container one-quarter-full of pink urine, holding her crotch in discomfort. "It feels like everything's ripping open down there. I don't want to pee anymore. It's too painful."

"Your bladder goes into spasm after you urinate. It will subside in a few moments. Let me check this sample. I'll be right back."

I looked at the pink-tinged urine specimen under the microscope. It was full of white blood cells and bacteria, paradoxically a pretty mosaic visual pattern.

When I returned, Janis Marks was pacing with her hand on her lower abdomen, her face still pinched by pain.

"You have a urinary tract infection," I explained. "It's usually caused by bacteria getting into the bladder through your urethra."

I could tell this was not going to be a teaching moment because she was still hurting, so I cut it short. I handed her information to read later on the causes of urinary tract infections and proper hygiene after intercourse.

"Here is a sample antibiotic to get you started. This other medication is to decrease the burning sensation, but I'll warn you—it turns the urine orange."

"I don't care as long as it helps."

"I'll give you prescriptions to complete a three day course of antibiotics. That's all you'll need because it's your first infection. Then I'd like to see you back once. Push fluids, especially cranberry juice. As far as sex goes—"

"Don't worry. He's not coming *near* me until I'm better. This really hurts!"

"Well, pain does have a way of decreasing one's libido. It's best to give it a rest until you're off medications. And remember—push those liquids!"

URINARY TRACT INFECTIONS

Seven million persons in this country alone rush to their health care provider for urinary tract infections (UTI's). About 25 to 35 percent of women between the ages of 20 and 40 have isolated UTI's. In women, simple lower UTI's include acute infections of the bladder (cystitis) or urethra (urethritis). Kidney infections (pyelonephritis) involve the upper urinary tract. Recurrent infections are caused by reinfection, unresolved, or persistent infections.

Why are women so susceptible to UTI's? A major susceptibility is anatomic, because of the urethra's shortness and proximity to the anus and vagina. Changes in perineal flora, menses, and vaginal mucus or epithelial cells all further predispose.

Gram negative bacteria are the usual pathogens. *Escherichia coli* causes more than two-thirds of community acquired urinary infections. Other causative organisms are *Klebsiella*, proteus, *Enterococcus faecalis* (a fecal contaminant), and *Staphylococcus saprophyticus*. A simple urinalysis confirms the presence of pyuria and possibly bacteriuria. Dipstick urine testing alone will identify more than 95% of patients with positive urines.

Three-day treatment with trimethoprim/sulfamethoxazole may be more cost effective than the other commonly used alternatives such as amoxacillin, cephalexin, or nitrofurantoin. Failure to respond to initial treatment or relapse within a short time requires a urine culture with sensitivity testing. The presence of as few as 100 coliforms/mL in a clean-catch, midstream urine culture from a symptomatic woman is a positive culture.

Reinfection requires another course of antibiotics, and unresolved infection, which is usually caused by a resistant organism, requires a switch in antibiotics. Nitrofurantoin is a good choice for all but protei organisms. Reappearance of the same organism signals the need for further diagnostic studies and the possible presence of an underlying structural abnormality.

In men, UTI's are uncommon. The possibility of acute prostatitis, which presents as chills, fever, groin or testicular pain, and malaise, must be considered. Men with UTI's should be referred to a urologist.

Acute pyelonephritis causes chills, fever, flank pain, malaise, and nausea. Pyuria and white blood cell casts on urinalysis confirm the diagnosis. E. Coli concentrations in urine cultures (1,000 colony-forming units/mL) are usually less than those found in lower UTI's).

The management of acute pyelonephritis depends on the severity, ranging from a 14 day treatment with oral antibiotics as an outpatient to hospitalization for IV antibiotics (second or third generation cephalosporins or ampicillin plus gentamycin). In the later case, imaging studies should be obtained if fever persists on antibiotics. Patients with diabetes, neurogenic bladder, renal calculi, or who are pregnant are at risk for a renal abscess. Pregnant women are prone to UTI's and need to be treated quickly to avoid sepsis and fetal compromise.

*　　*　　*

"You Mean With Men?"

Yolanda Ruiz, a young, short, Hispanic girl, came in for a physical examination to return to college, where she was majoring in economics. Her flat belly peered out beneath her short, summer top. I'd seen her once before. On the previous visit, in discussing her sexual history, I asked if she was sexually active. She answered yes in a very shy manner. When I inquired if she had one partner or multiple partners, she said *several*. She made it clear that she really did not want to speak about sex.

I planned on this visit to do a gynecological examination and a Pap test and to go into more detail about her sexual history. Was she at risk for AIDS and other sexually transmitted diseases?

Ms. Ruiz replied to my question regarding sex partners with, "You mean men?"

"Yes, men." That was an odd response for a woman I assumed was heterosexual.

"Well, I'm not sexually active with them or at least I haven't gone all the way."

I was puzzled. "Are you sexually active with women?"

She seemed surprised that I had no idea about her sexual orientation. "Of course," she replied, quickly adding, "But I want to have children some day." The patient seemed to want to make it okay with me.

"It doesn't matter to me what your sexual preference is. You didn't tell me before."

Ms. Ruiz looked dumbfounded. "You never asked."

"I guess you're right about that," I admitted. "Have you ever had a Pap smear?"

"No. I didn't think I needed to."

"Why not?"

"I thought it's only for heterosexual women."

"No, it's for all women."

The stage was now set for a broader discussion about health care for lesbian women. After awhile she seemed to relax and we covered the main issues. I told her about Pap smears and we agreed to do one. Once I completed the physical, I filled out the examination form and returned it to Ms. Ruiz. When she left I realized if you don't ask the right opening question you won't get the right answer.

LESBIAN PATIENTS

About 2 to 10% of women of all ages in the U.S. are sexually active with other women. Lesbian patients often avoid medical practitioners because they fear a negative or hostile reception. Some forego routine health care as a result. Myths abound that lesbians cannot get cervical cancer or sexually transmitted diseases such as HIV infection. A further complication is that some women choose not to identify themselves as lesbian.

The best way to obtain an accurate history is to create an inclusive and sympathetic environment in which patients feel comfortable and safe. Ask questions in a non-judgmental way about sexual preference, including "partnered" relationships (in addition to single, married, widowed, or divorced) and "sexual contact" (instead of intercourse). The moment of disclosure should not be a conversation stopper. A full reproductive history must be obtained as in non-lesbian patients. Don't assume that a lesbian has never had sex with a man.

Lesbian and gay adolescents are two to three times more likely than heterosexual adolescents to attempt suicide and account for 30% of suicides among young people. Depression stems from rejection by family and friends, the stress of dealing with social stigma, and the difficulty of living a clandestine life for those who have not yet come out.

Sexual issues should be discussed candidly. Lesbian patients need to know about female-to-female transmission of sexually transmitted diseases, such as bacterial vaginitis, candidiasis, chlamydial and trichomonal infections, hepatitis, herpes simplex (types I and II), HIV, and syphilis. Such diseases spread by anal or vaginal penetration with devices or fingers, deep kissing, and oral-anal or oral-genital contact, and especially during menstruation. Statistics on HIV infection resulting from female-to-female sexual contact in the absence of sexual intercourse and IV drug use are lacking, but public health officials caution that unprotected female-to-female sex is not safe. It is also wise to acknowledge the sex partner and include her in discussions about these issues.

Lesbian women may have several risk factors for cervical cancer such as cigarette smoking, heterosexual intercourse at an early age, and multiple male partners. They need annual Pap smears. Lesbians are also at higher risk for breast cancer.

Although a lesbian partner's legal status varies from state to state, a woman may legally designate her partner as a health care proxy and grant durable health care power of attorney. Some lesbian patients raise issues of parenting, ranging from artificial insemination or natural childbirth to adoption or foster parenting. They may seek information or referrals. National organizations like the National Center for Lesbian Rights and the Gay and Lesbian Medical Association are useful resources for lesbian patients.

PAP SMEARS

Without exaggeration, the Papanicololaou (Pap) smear is one of the most effective screening tests ever devised and the biggest weapon against cervical cancer. Risk factors for cervical cancer are abnormal Pap smear, immunosuppression, lower socioeconomic status, multiple sex partners, sexually transmitted diseases, smoking, and young age at first intercourse. Chronic inflammation and the hormonal effects of oral contraceptives and pregnancy are possible cofactors.

Who needs a Pap smear? All women when they reach age 18 years or become sexually active—no excuses—should have an annual cancer screening by Pap smear and pelvic examination. The optimal time for a Pap smear is in the middle of the menstrual cycle. Although there is no consensus about how often to do a Pap smear in women older than 65, it matters most for those who have not have had adequate screening when they were younger.

Cervical cancer begins as a low-grade, well-differentiated, premalignant lesion and progresses over 1 to 7 years to high-grade undifferentiated disease. Human papillomavirus (HPV), which is found in 95% of cervical cancers, has a prevalence of 50-70% in sexually active adults. It is associated with various genital warts (condyloma acuminata).

Because cervical cancer arises at the junction of squamous and columnar cells in the cervix, a good Pap smear contains various cell types from this region. Otherwise it should be repeated. The technique is to rotate a plastic or wooden spatula in a full circle at the junction and then sample the endocervical canal in a full circle with a cytobrush. The two samples are spread thinly and separately on a glass slide and fixed before they can air-dry. The Pap smear's false negative rate is 5 to 45% due to errors in laboratory processing, misinterpretation of the slides, and poor technique of doing the procedure.

*   *   *

"My Lover Did It"

When I heard a knock on the door, I was trying to figure out what was in Freddie Bobbit's rectum. At that precise moment, double-gloved and behind the curtain, I had the index finger of my right hand as far up his rectum as I could and was reaching around inside.

Serai Alterman, one of the other clinic nurse practitioners, popped her head into the examining room. "Can I speak with you for a minute?"

"I can't talk, Serai. I'm a little busy right now with a patient." I spread the cheeks of his buttocks with my left hand to see if I could get my finger in farther.

"I'll drop by later when I get a chance," Serai said.

"Okay."

The door snapped shut.

Mr. Bobbitt jerked his head up. "Can *anyone* just waltz in here?" he asked with a grimace.

"Only clinic personnel—but don't worry, the curtain is pulled."

"It's always *rude* to drop in uninvited—even with people you know, let alone perfect strangers." His voice waxed peevish.

He lowered his head back down on the table.

I probed a bit more and felt something hard. Despite concentrating on what it might be, I couldn't discern it. When I tapped on the object with my fingernail, it felt almost metallic.

I pulled out my finger and cruised over to the cabinet for an anal speculum. Although I applied lubricant on the speculum, it was hardly necessary. Mr. Bobbit, who was overtly gay, had the characteristically loose anal muscle tone, and I had no difficulty inserting the speculum fully. Before I started the examination, I noticed that some of the tissue around the anus was torn. With mounting curiosity I bent over to look into his rectum through the spread anus. I couldn't believe my eyes.

After I relaxed the tension on the speculum, I went to the wall to flick off the overhead light. I cracked open the door of the examining room in order to find my way back. With a squeeze of the speculum, I pried open his anus and looked in, taking care not to get my hair near his buttocks and hoping that no gas leaked out of him while I had my face so close.

What the hell!

A faint light shone out of his anus! My wild suspicion was confirmed: *a flashlight!* He'd given no indication whatsoever.

"What did you stick up yourself?" I asked.

Mr. Bobbit groaned. "My lover did it as a joke. We were both drunk."

Making a point not to appear judgmental, I said, "Wipe yourself off and pull up your shorts. We have to talk." I turned on the lights.

Now I understood why he was disappointed to see me instead of his primary physician. I also knew why he insisted on being examined today. I discarded my gloves and washed my hands at the sink.

Freddie Bobbit sat down gingerly on the chair next to my desk. He was a lean, tall, white man in his thirties. I thought he would have been attractive under other circumstances.

"You told me you were constipated," I complained as I returned to my desk.

"Well, I didn't know what to say," he said timidly. "I was embarrassed."

"When did this happen?"

"Last night." I could tell he was chagrined and didn't want to dwell on it. Quick to understand his sensitivity, I didn't pursue the details.

I was amazed that the batteries hadn't worn out. This would make some battery commercial, I thought, in the off-color way that experienced practitioners do to add levity to a somewhat tense situation.

"How big is the flashlight?"

"It's a small one."

"One of those pocket lights?"

"No, bigger."

My eyes widened. "How big?"

"One of those glove-compartment ones, about an inch or two in diameter." He attempted to size it with his hand for me. "It was just supposed to be a joke."

Some joke.

There was inflammation in the bowel and the object was probably too large to pass out of the bowel safely on its own. I knew that if removal couldn't be accomplished with endoscopy, surgery would be necessary to cut through the abdomen and incise the bowel.

"I hope you're not going to need an operation to get that out."

"Operation! You mean surgery?" he asked, not anticipating this outcome.

"It's possible."

"And I'd have to be admitted to the hospital?"

I acknowledged with a brief nod.

"Oh, Robby's going to feel bad now," he said with boyish satisfaction.

"I can assure you abdominal surgery is nothing to be excited about. Let's hope they are able to put a scope into your rectum and extract the flashlight that way."

He looked disappointed.

"Why don't you get dressed."

I picked up the phone to the Rapid Assessment Unit in the ER. "I have a patient in my office who needs to be seen now."

"What's the problem?" a voice on the other end of the line asked.

"Oh, he's got a foreign body lodged in his rectum."

"Say what?"

"You heard me right." I let my eyes fall back to the chart.

"What is it?"

"A flashlight."

I heard a peel of laughter on the other end of the line. "A flashlight?"

"Yes." I looked over at Mr. Bobbit.

Again the person on the phone roared. "Now that's rich. You'll say *anything* to get us to see someone, won't you. Send him down."

I hung up. I had made someone's day. "I'm sending you to the ER, Mr. Bobbit. They will assess you and determine the best way of removing the flashlight."

"If my lover calls, don't tell him what happened. *I* want to tell him."

"I won't say a word," I promised and then sent him off to the ER.

I had to admit, Freddie Bobbit did get the morning off to an unusual start.

GAY PATIENTS

Many gay men face a unique set of health concerns besides those of the general adult male population. Infection with HIV heads a list that also contains bowel disorders, cancer, hepatitis, other sexually transmitted diseases, smoking, and substance abuse.

Flu-like symptoms may prompt a visit to the clinic for reassurance that the symptoms are not those of HIV infection. All gay men are not at equal risk for HIV disease. The health care provider should elicit a history of risk factors like blood transfusion, unsafe sexual practices, and substance abuse. The psychological impact of living at risk for AIDS should also be considered. HIV-discordant couples need special consideration because one partner may fear rejection and feel guilt or resentment. Providing terminal care can demand of one partner tremendous emotional, financial, and physical support.

Gay bowel syndrome presents as abdominal pain or tenderness, dehydration, diarrhea, or fever, and the stool may be positive for occult blood. Intestinal infections in gay men may be related to unprotected sexual contact or sharing of sexual devices. Gay men who have anal-receptive sex are at increased risk for colitis, enteritis, proctitis, and proctocolitis. The infections may be bacterial, protozoal, or viral in etiology. If an episode of diarrhea does not resolve in two to three days, stool diagnostic studies should be done. Gay men also may harbor anal fissures, foreign bodies, injury from trauma, or ulcers.

Although HIV infection is a top concern, sexually active gay men are at risk of contacting other sexually transmitted diseases including *Chlamydia*, herpes, gonorrhea, and syphilis. Unprotected sex with multiple partners also increases the risk for hepatitis B. Such individuals should be vaccinated prophylactically.

The risk of anal carcinoma is 25 to 50% higher in gay men who engage in anal-receptive intercourse due to exposure to human papilloma virus. The prevalence of prostate cancer also is disproportionately higher in this population.

*   *   *

"What Are You Going to Do With That Thing?"

Was this a reincarnation? James Whitney, the last patient of the day, came in with "leg pain." With his rotund body habitus and short neck, he could have been Winston Churchill. All that was missing was the beloved wife Clementine.

When Mr. Whitney saw my young, female, nurse practitioner student, he insisted that she leave the room. "This is a private matter."

In pursuing the story, it became clear that his leg wasn't the problem. He mumbled his responses to my questions and kept his head down.

"You need to tell me exactly where it hurts, Mr. Whitney."

"Down below."

"Down where?"

"Down low," he muttered.

"I'm sorry, I didn't hear that."

This went on for a bit. At last I told him if he wouldn't tell me, he should gown and show me, but he refused to put on a gown.

"Mr. Whitney, if you don't show me the problem, I can't help you with it. I take care of male patients all the time. I do genital and rectal examinations. It's all a part of my job."

His frustration escalated. He grew red in the face and looked like he was about to explode. Finally, he stood up and yelled, "Okay, okay, it's my BALLS! There! Are you happy now? Why don't you tell the whole clinic."

Mr. Whitney dropped his shorts indignantly and I stared at him in amazement. His scrotum was huge. It was swollen to at least ten times its normal size and looked very tense! He was carrying a virtual basketball in front of him. I didn't mean to stare and I hoped my mouth didn't drop open.

"Mr. Whitney, why on earth did you wait so long to come to the hospital?"

"It's humiliating, that's why. I was embarrassed. Do you think I like standing here like this before God and country?"

"I have an idea what caused that, but I need to examine you."

"Okay, just get it over with." He gritted his teeth and turned his head away like a boy awaiting a needle in the buttocks. The idea of a strange woman touching his private parts was almost intolerable to him.

Over at the counter, I snapped on some latex examining gloves, opened a drawer, and pulled out a flashlight.

"What are you gonna do with that thing?" he asked apprehensively.

"I'm going to shine it through your scrotum."

"Is this some kind of a game? I didn't come here to have somebody put a flashlight on my privates." He was about to yank up his shorts.

"No, no, Mr. Whitney," I pleaded. "I assure you it's no game. I think you have a hernia in your scrotum. That's why it's so large. If I'm right, when we shine the flashlight, the light should come through because the hernia is filled with fluid. That would be great news for you because the hernia could be repaired easily."

"Will it burn it?"

"*No*, of course not."

He thought it over. "Well, all right, if you put it that way."

Then I did the test. We both saw the light pass through, giving off a soft red glow. He had a hydrocele. "I need to put my finger on your scrotum to see which side the hernia's on."

"Okay, hurry up now." He closed his eyes tightly and grimaced.

Carefully, I moved aside his scrotum and put my finger up into the inguinal canal. The right side was closed; it was okay. When I did the left side, I felt a hole. I knew it lead into the abdomen.

"Mr. Whitney, you can pull up your shorts now."

He did so like a fireman off to a three alarm fire.

"Please sit down." I waited for him to be seated. "You need to have this hernia repaired. It's on your left side. There's an opening that's allowing fluid from your abdomen to fill your scrotum. Your scrotum will keep getting bigger if you don't have the operation. Eventually, a segment of bowel may also protrude into the scrotum."

Whitney looked worried. "I don't know about that."

"Why not?"

"I don't want anyone cutting around my"—He made a wavy motion over his groin.

"No, they won't cut the penis, if that's what you mean. This is a totally different operation. You won't have to worry about that."

"They're not going to castrate me, are they?" he asked, knitting his eyebrows in genuine concern.

"No, no, Mr. Whitney. What kind of a place do you think this is?"

"Well, I've heard stories of things that can go wrong. A man came in for an appendectomy and they accidentally did a sex change operation on him."

I looked up at him. He was serious. Instantly, all my professionalism evaporated and I broke out laughing. I covered my mouth with my hand to suppress further giggles, but the harder I tried to stop, the more I laughed. The singular absurdity was irresistible. He had burlesqued the problem. Caught up in the contagion, Mr. Whitney joined in.

After several moments, when the laughter had run its course, I said, "That was a good one, my friend. Now you stop worrying about all that and I'll fill out the paperwork to send you to urology clinic. Urologists are the doctors who do the operation. They will tell you all about it." Catching his reluctance, I added, "And promise me that you will show up there. Your wife would want you to do this."

"Sure, my wife wants me to do a lot of things I don't do."

I gave him the evil eye. I could tell he was still waffling. "It's only going to get worse, Mr. Whitney. They can fix it easily."

Preoccupied with the decision, he rubbed the fingers of one hand over his cheek repetitively like he was molding clay. "Okay," he conceded gruffly. "Okay."

After I completed my charts, locked my desk, and got ready to leave, I thought back to James Whitney's comments, imagining him after a sex change operation... a Winston Churchill in drag. I chuckled. He was certainly a character.

SCROTAL MASSES

A mass in the scrotum can be many things. The painful masses are acute orchitis, epididymitis, strangulated hernia, and testicular torsion. A painless lump may be benign—caused by a hydrocele, spermatocele, or varicocele—or perhaps cancerous.

Palpate the testes to be sure they are both present and normal in size. If a testicle cannot be palpated, examine the inguinal canals and lower abdomen. Shed light on the subject: transilluminate all testicular masses and swellings. Light will not transmit through a solid tumor.

Epididymitis is the most common cause of painful swelling of the testes in adults. Fever, pyuria, urethral discharge, and urinary symptoms are present, and the epididymis is sensitive to examination. Because a bacterial urinary tract infection is the usual cause, a Gram's stain and culture should be done. Treat with bed rest, local ice therapy, non-steroidal anti-inflammatory drugs, and scrotal elevation. In young adults, a sexually transmitted disease should be considered.

The term hernia simply indicates intrusion of one inner body part into a space where it doesn't belong. Hernias in the groin may be inguinal (usually men) or femoral (women). The hernia may contain abdominal fluid or a loop of protruding bowel. The danger comes from entrapment of the bowel in the hernia where its blood supply may become strangulated (incarcerated hernia). Patients with large hernias should not fly in nonpressurized aircraft due to danger of strangulated bowel. For simple hernias, trusses or other belts afford symptomatic relief. Surgical repair is curative.

A hydrocele is a collection of fluid between the two layers of the tunica vaginalis. Transillumination of the scrotum helps differentiate hydrocele from testicular tumors, varicocele, or other scrotal masses. About 10% of testicular tumors, which are most common in young men and usually germinal in origin, may have an associated reactive hydrocele. Because most testicular cancers metastasize, early detection and treatment may be life-saving.

Just as women do monthly breast examinations, men need to examine their testes every month.

PROVIDER GENDER ISSUES

It's a significant issue: *men* who don't want to be examined by a woman and *women* who don't want to be examined by a man—or anyone at all. Sometimes the fear can be so great that it prevents a person from seeking medical care until it is too late. If provider gender issues are important to patients, they should be given the option to change providers. In large practices, the request can be accommodated easily even if it means rescheduling the patient for another day.

At other times, gender-related issues are a *reason* for patients to come to the clinic—a disguised reason. Practitioners should ask a third party from their medical practice to step in as a witness to breast, genital, and rectal examinations when the gender of the health care provider and the patient is different, regardless of who is the male and who is the female.

*　　*　　*

"What Do You Think I Should Do?"

A young woman on the phone asked to talk to a female health care provider. Thelma patched her through to me. I discovered her name was Jamie Kwon. She hemmed and hawed. "I have heavy and painful periods."

"How old are you, Ms. Kwon?"

"I'm thirty-five years old—and it's Mrs. Kwon."

"Excuse me. How long have you been having this problem?'

"About a year, but it's gotten worse the past couple of months."

"Do you spot between your periods?"

"Yes. It almost feels like I'm about to start my period, but I don't. Now I'm spotting in-between periods also. I can't go anywhere without bringing along a pad. It's like having a continuous menstrual period. This problem is a sexual turnoff for both my husband and me. I was at a friend's house—a baby shower. I started cramping and when I stood, there was a great big, bloody spot on the off-white, linen upholstery. I had blood on my silk skirt, and blood trickled down my legs. I was horrified. I can't live like this anymore."

"Have you ever been treated for uterine fibroids, endometriosis, or a sexually transmitted disease?"

"No." She also denied missing any recent periods, which made pregnancy unlikely, and used barrier contraception, not an IUD or oral contraceptives.

"When was the last time you saw your gynecologist?"

"We just moved here a year ago and I haven't gotten one. I kept putting it off. What do you think I should do?"

"I can see you and do a Pap and pelvic examination."

"If you don't mind, I'd prefer to see a gynecologist."

"Sure, I'll give you the phone number to the gynecology clinic here. Tell them your problem and ask for an appointment soon. Don't put it off or accept an appointment months from now."

"Do you think it's serious?"

"I can't say for sure over the phone. That's why you need to get it checked out."

ABNORMAL MENSTRUAL PERIODS

Abnormal menstrual bleeding may be painful or painless. In painful bleeding (dysmenorrhea), the pain—cramping, undulating, pelvic in location, and radiating to the back or thighs—stems from uterine anoxia, contractions, and vasoconstriction. Although it is usually idiopathic (primary), dysmenorrhea can be caused by cervical or uterine structural problems, endometriosis, an IUD, or pelvic inflammatory disease.

Nonsteroidal anti-inflammatory drugs should be started at the onset of bleeding. In severe cases, oral contraceptives suppress ovulation and prevent dysmenorrhea. Only about 5.5 per 1,000 women require a hysterectomy.

Dysfunctional uterine bleeding (DUB) is the most common cause of painless abnormal bleeding. DUB occurs at the extremes of reproductive life: 50% of the cases after age 45 and 20% in adolescence. It is usually an effect of unopposed estrogen stimulating the uterine endometrial lining. Exogenous estrogen, multiparity, obesity, and polycystic ovaries are contributory factors.

*   *   *

"I've Been Having Terrible Pain"

A woman shuffled down the hall, trailed by a peculiar odor that caused everyone to turn and look. She was a dark Hispanic in her early twenties, slightly overweight, with black hair and orange-tinted highlights. I knew I was in for some sort of a gynecological problem.

When I stepped into the examining room, the patient was already gowned, naked below the waste. The wave of odor made me want to vomit.

"Call me if you need me," the assistant said as she scurried out.

I tried to mouth breath. "Hello, Ms. Delgado?"

She nodded, studying me with fright in her brown eyes.

"Tell me what's wrong." I noticed her underwear on the chair were foul smelling, saturated with a green, slimy, puss-like discharge.

"I've been having terrible pain in my stomach." She pointed to the area over her pubic bone. Her English was passable with a little extra concentration on my part. "It really hurts. I have this bad smell. I don't know what's wrong."

"How long have you had it?"

"About a week."

A week!

A surprising number of my female patients were woefully ignorant of the female physiology yet alone its pathology. Some had disdain for it; others denied it. They tolerated problems that no one else would.

"Do you have fevers?" I asked.

"A little."

"Nausea, vomiting, or back pain?"

"I got sick to my stomach a few times." She let her eyes wander over the strange surroundings.

After asking her other questions, I explained that I'd have to do a pelvic examination. She consented. When she spread her legs in the stirrups, the stench was so repugnant, I jumped up, excused myself, and fled the room. I returned with my assistant, armed with face masks, into which we'd placed a few drops of tincture of peppermint.

When I reinserted the speculum into the patient's vagina, copious amounts of discharge gushed out. I barely had enough time to pull myself and my stool out of the way to avoid being splattered. My assistant gasped and ran out of the room with her hand over her mask. This was a most distasteful part of my job. The woman's disease assaulted the senses. I felt physically ill. Yet she lay there moaning in need of my help.

Once I swabbed her vaginal vault, I could see the cervix, which was inflamed and bleeding. I did cultures for sexually transmitted diseases. After removing the speculum, I proceeded to the bimanual examination.

"It might be a little tender inside." I inserted the first two fingers of my double gloved hand into her vagina so I could feel her cervix while my left hand rested on her abdomen over her uterus. As I pressed on her uterus from above, more fluid drained into her vagina against my hand. When I wiggled my fingers, she let out a scream and reached for the ceiling.

"Aye-e-e-e, aye-e-e-e-e-e-e. *Mucho dolor.*"

Here was a positive test for pelvic inflammatory disease: the *chandelier sign*. She could not tolerate me palpating her other pelvic organs either. I had her sit up. "Ms. Delgado, you have an infection of your female organs called PID."

"How did I get this?"

"It's sexually transmitted from a partner with an infection. Does your partner have an infection?"

Angelina Delgado hung her head. "I have many partners... I'm a prostitute. I was afraid to tell you in the beginning because I thought I wouldn't get any care."

Bearing up under pain that would have immobilized many lesser-willed people, this unfortunate woman suffered more from shame than from her illness.

"I'm glad you did tell me. We're here to help you. You will need to be admitted because this infection has gotten way out of hand. In the hospital you'll be treated with intravenous antibiotics. I'll give you something for pain right now. After a while, you'll start to feel better."

Her story was all too common. Fortunately, most genital infections were not that rampant. No one should wait so long to seek medical help.

Pelvic Inflammatory Disease

Sex has been described as "the gateway to life" and as "one of the great life-mysteries." Others characterize it as Pandora's box. Sexually transmitted diseases (STD's) affect 12 million persons a year. The human costs of STD's are fear of discovery, the probability of infecting others, and risks of serious complications. The total financial burden is estimated at $17 billion annually. Some people secretly find a certain poetic justice in the selection of those who catch STD's; they have not seen the human suffering caused by STD's.

Internal female reproductive organs keep company in the pelvis, the "basin of the abdomen," with the urinary bladder, the rectum, and the sigmoid flexure of the colon. Upper genital tract infections in women, usually referred to as pelvic inflammatory disease (PID), may be life-threatening. Young, nulliparous women who are sexually active with multiple sex partners are at highest risk. Douching, non-white race, and smoking increase the risk of PID, while barrier or oral contraceptives decrease it.

Appendicitis, a bleeding or ruptured ovarian cyst, ectopic pregnancy, enteritis, pelvic abscess, and septic abortion can mimic PID. Recent intercourse, history of PID or sexually transmitted disease, menstrual period, or use of an IUD favors the diagnosis of PID. A serum pregnancy test rules out ectopic pregnancy. Direct visualization by culdocentesis and laparoscopy is indicated in complicated cases.

The causative organisms include *Neisseria gonorrhoeae, Chlamydia trachomatis*, anaerobes, enteric gram-negative rods, and streptococci. In 1993, the CDC recommended routine annual screening for *Chlamydia* in all sexually active females who did not use barrier contraception or who had new or multiple sex partners during the preceding months. There are 4 million new cases of *Chlamydia* in the U.S. each year at a cost of 2 billion dollars.

The medical treatment of PID is intravenous antibiotics, analgesics, and supportive measures. Preferred IV antibiotics are cefoxitin or cefotetan plus doxycycline. Surgical intervention may be necessary to treat abscesses, resulting in loss of the ovaries and tubes (salpingo-oophorectomy), uterus (hysterectomy), or both. Despite treatment, 25% of women with PID develop chronic sequellae such as dyspareunia, ectopic pregnancy, infertility, pelvic pain, or recurrent infection.

VAGINITIS

Vaginal discharge and vulvar itching are the most common reasons for a woman to seek gynecological care. Although many women fear that a sexually transmitted disease (STD) is the cause, not all vaginal discharges are caused by infections. Atrophic vaginitis, local irritants, and physiologic leukorrhea are non-infectious causes.

The vagina in adult women is normally acidic (pH 3.8 to 4.2) because it is colonized by non-pathogenic bacteria (Lactobacillus) that produce hydrogen peroxide. A rise in pH (less acidic) is one factor that may indicate infection. The normal, protective lactobacilli decrease in number as other flora overgrow the vagina.

Females of all ages fall prey to vaginal infections. The infections remain local (vaginitis) or, depending on the underlying organism and adequacy of treatment, spread to infect pelvic reproductive organs. Etiologies include STD's and treatments that alter vaginal flora (antibiotics, excess douching, or immunity-compromising disorders like AIDS and diabetes). The type of causative organism depends on the patient's age. Bacterial vaginosis, candidiasis, and trichomoniasis account for more than 90% of vaginal infections.

Bacterial infection, the usual source of vaginal discharge, causes up to one-half of all vaginitis. Organisms include *E. Coli*, group B streptococcus, *Staphylococcus aureus*, and other agents. Bacterial overgrowth from the gastrointestinal tract may incite bacterial vaginitis in postmenopausal women. In pregnant women, failure to treat adequately precipitates premature birth and infection of the infant.

In the "whiff test," adding a few drops of 15% potassium hydroxide solution to vaginal secretions releases an unpleasant, "fishy" odor. Finding more than 20% "clue cells," vaginal epithelial cells stippled by adherent coccobacilli, on a wet mount is another diagnostic criterion. Intravaginal preparations cause fewer problems than oral medications do in non-pregnant women, but they don't reduce the morbidity associated with pregnancy. Clindamycin and metronidazole are the drugs of choice.

Candidiasis presents as a thick, curdled, white discharge in a red, excoriated vulva and hyperemic vagina. The pH is normal, not increased as in other types of vaginitis. Hyphae and budding yeast, seen under the microscope, confirm the diagnosis. *Candida albicans* is the usual fungus, but other varieties are becoming more prevalent. Most organisms causing acute infections respond to treatment with clotrimazole and miconazole, and recurrent infections may be treated with fluconazole.

Trichomonas vaginalis, a sexually-transmitted protozoan, creates a foul, frothy discharge and punctate cervical hemorrhages. The motile organisms, which can be seen on wet mount, respond to treatment with a single dose of metronidazole. The sex partner must also be treated.

12

Telltale Heart

*Louder! louder! louder! louder! .... here, here!—it is the beating of
his hideous heart!*
—EDGAR ALLEN POE

*Symptoms, then, are in reality nothing but the cry from suffering
organs*
—JEAN-MARTIN CHARCOT

*In each human heart are a tiger, a pig, an ass, and a nightingale.
Diversity of character is due to their unequal activity*
—AMBROSE GWINETT BIERCE

"I Freaked Out"

"Ahhh-chooo."

"Bless you."

Laura Flanack winced as she wiped her red-rimmed nostrils with the clinic's harsh, standard issue tissues. "Thanks," she replied in muffled, nasal tones.

Reminded of my own box of softer tissues from a recent cold, I opened a desk drawer and gave her several tissues.

She made an effort to smile, but her mouth quickly dropped open again to breathe. Her whole face, despite make-up, seemed puffy and drooping with illness. She looked closer to fifty than to her real age of forty-one.

"Let me venture a guess as to why you're here," I said as I settled into my chair. "Head cold or allergies?"

"It's probably a cold. I'm leaking quite a bit from my nose the past three to four days. I generally feel achy and so-o-o-o tired."

Her history seemed to fit a viral upper respiratory illness, but I wanted to be sure she didn't have allergies. "Have your eyes been itchy, excessively red and watery lately?" I asked.

The reaction to my routine question was unanticipated. Her face went into an agonized contortion. Tears suffused her eyes, then spilled over, trickling down her cheeks and onto her hands. Her red nose was now a running faucet.

"I don't usually get such a response to that question." I offered her more tissues.

"I'm sorry, I'm not handling this well."

"What's troubling you? It's obviously not the cold."

"My sister just committed suicide two days ago. She shot herself." Tears sprang up again, washing away the last trace of her make-up. "I knew she broke up with her boyfriend, but Christine didn't seem *that* depressed." Laura Flanack wiped her eyes with more tissues.

"My sincere condolences. Do you have someone to counsel you and your family through this difficult time?"

"We've been talking with our minister, which kinda helps. I must be really stressed-out. I lie awake at night feeling my heart beating fast. Even before my sister's death I felt uptight and irritable. Must be chronic PMS or something."

She reached for the tissue box. It was empty. This was the first time anyone asked me for a second box.

We talked for a while and then I examined her. Her physical examination also was consistent with a viral upper respiratory illness. Although her heart was rapid—about one-hundred beats per minute even after fifteen minutes of sitting—it was regular.

I noted she was taking pseudoephedrine daily over the past several days as a decongestant. When I asked her about caffeine intake, she confessed to drinking six to eight cups of coffee. Both pseudoephedrine and caffeine could raise the heart rate. I advised her to cut back on caffeine and decongestant use and told her to call me if the symptoms persisted after her cold had passed.

Mrs. Flanack returned in less than two weeks, complaining of fatigue and emotional lability. When I walked into the examining room, she was so startled she jumped out of the chair. Her exaggerated reaction frightened me.

"I'm falling apart at the seams. Either I'm crying or fighting with everyone I know, and I've given up on sleep these days. This past week I noticed that my left ankle is swollen and the swelling's going up my leg. Two years ago I had some blood tests done that showed I was anemic. I freaked out. I thought I might have some kind of cancer, so I never returned. Medical tests *terrify* me." She said all this without taking a breath.

I waited for a break; it came with tears and sobbing. Overwrought with emotion, she abruptly referred to her sister's death. Given recent events, her cavalcade of emotions could be appropriate, but I was starting to get the nagging feeling that something else was going on. I couldn't identify the problem; nonetheless, my sensors were on yellow-alert.

While she struggled to regain her composure, I reviewed her last lab tests. She had a persistent, marked, microcytic anemia. I questioned her as to possible causes, including cancer, but she denied weight loss, excessive menstrual blood loss, or rectal bleeding. The questionnaire about depression she filled out scored her as severely depressed. Mrs. Flanack denied having suicidal thoughts.

I examined her shins because she'd mentioned swelling. When I pressed in my thumb, it left a dent. So, pretibial edema, I thought. Her heart rate remained regular but elevated at one-hundred, which would be acceptable if she were a child. The remainder of her physical examination was normal.

I discussed her case with Dr. Janet Ressor, who puzzled over it a moment. She advised me to obtain a chest x-ray to make sure her heart size was normal, give the patient cards to test for occult blood in the stool, start her on an iron supplement, repeat a complete blood count in two weeks, and prescribe an antidepressant.

The chest x-ray turned out to be normal, making a cardiac cause of the elevated heart rate unlikely. We agreed that the rapid heart rate might be in response to her prolonged anemic state and should decrease as her anemia improved. I continued to mull over that heart rate. Why was it so high?

One night about a week later, I was watching a sitcom rerun on television in a mindless daze when I had an epiphany. It had nothing whatever to do with the show but everything to do with my patient. Suddenly it all came together. The prospect intrigued me, but I couldn't do anything about it until the next day.

The following morning I searched for her records in the alphabetized office files. F, Fl, Fla—there it is—Flanack. I pulled her chart and riffled through the pages. Sure enough, a thyroid test had *not* been drawn.

Excited and hopeful, I called Mrs. Flanack, who agreed to get the blood test done that day. I reassured her it was not for cancer, but to find out if her thyroid was overactive. Her voice registered concern. I wasn't sure if she was going to start crying.

"Would *this* be the reason that my heart beats so fast and I'm so terribly nervous and jumpy?" she asked.

"It certainly could be. It would account for all of your symptoms including your anemia, anxiety, depression, and heart palpitations."

"And what happens if it *is* a thyroid problem?" Her voice revealed another twist of tension.

"Then we'll treat you and correct it. Don't worry. As soon as I get the result, I'll call you."

The report came back the next day: hyperthyroidism. Immediately, I conferred with an endocrinologist who recommended a few more studies, like antithyroid antibodies and a thyroid scan, to determine the cause. Was this her body's immune system attacking the thyroid or a tumor of the thyroid gland?

Mrs. Flanack agreed to do the further tests with trepidation only after much encouragement on my part. She also consented to an appointment with the endocrinologist for the following week. I started her on the heart medication propranolol to help slow down her heart rate. It would protect her from the danger of a *thyroid storm*—a term I came to respect as an accurate portrayal of the provoked thyroid's fury unleashed upon the unsuspecting body. Without this protection, she could die.

We waited. Fortunately the thyroid scan showed no tumor or nodule, but the thyroid was clearly enlarged. The case for Grave's disease, an autoimmune disorder, was mounting. She would need chemical or radioactive treatments to shrink her thyroid or reduce its output of hormones. The endocrinologist was now in charge.

A few months later I saw a woman who called herself Laura Flanack, but she was not the same person. She entered the room on a waft of perfume, smartly attired in an ankle-length shift, toting some shopping bags. With her light brown hair pulled up in a high ponytail, her animated, pale green eyes, and the little mole on her right cheek, she looked attractive, if not youthful.

"How are you doing?" I inquired.

"I feel like a new woman." Her smile didn't wane. "I'm calmer and stronger. No more racing heart. The other doctor said my heart rate was seventy-six! Of course, I still miss my sister a lot, but I'm able to deal with it now."

"That's the best news I could hear. I'm glad for you."

She rustled a bag and, like a magician, extracted a large box of tissues. "These are the softest tissues I could find. They're moisturized, perfumed, reinforced—whatever. I thought you could save them for the next patient who comes into your office as strung out as I was."

I laughed. "Okay. Thanks."

"And those clinic tissues"—she wrinkled her nose and quickly shook her head a few times— "they've *got* to go."

After she left, I recalled how her illness had evolved. As grateful as I was to have made the diagnosis, I berated myself for not having thought of it sooner. Easily I might have referred her to a psychiatrist if I focused on the depression instead of the heart rate. What if she had run into trouble? Could the head cold have taxed the thyroid gland and made her symptoms worse? If so, she was lucky to have caught the cold.

As I considered the possibilities, self-reproach changed to amazement that a single hormonal imbalance could throw a person into such disarray, and correcting it, just as dramatically, put the pieces back together again. The coincidence of her sister's suicide, the pseudoephedrine decongestant, and the excessive caffeine intake, together with long-standing anemia, had masked the obvious. Her body had finally given up one of its secrets.

Edgar Allen Poe would have been pleased. The telltale heart had saved her.

THE RAGING THYROID

How can a butterfly-shaped gland weighing only 15 to 20 grams—worn like a bow tie under our Adam's apple—have such profound effects on body weight, bowel habits, energy level, heart rate, menstrual periods, mental outlook, metabolism, muscle strength, skin texture, and voice quality? The story of the thyroid gland: too much or too little of a good thing can be life-threatening.

Here's the chain of command. The brain's hypothalamus orders the pituitary or "master gland" to secrete thyroid-stimulating hormone (thyrotropin, TSH), which directs the thyroid gland to form thyroid hormones. Thyroxine (T4) is the most abundant thyroid hormone, but tri-iodothyroxine (T3) is the most active. A serum TSH is a sensitive test for primary hyper- and hypothyroidism.

What does that mean in human terms? Patients with hyperthyroidism or "thyrotoxicosis" exhibit fatigue, heat intolerance, irritability, loose stools, menstrual irregularity, nervousness, staring, tachycardia, tremor, warm and moist skin, weakness, and weight loss. The most common form is Grave's disease, an autoimmune disorder, eight times more prevalent in women, who are usually 20 to 40 years old at its onset. Often it follows a very stressful or upsetting life event. Bulging eyes (Grave's exopthalmos) and edematous shins (pretibial myxedema) are not obligate features. Stimulatory plasma antibodies to TSH receptors circulate in 80% of such patients.

"Thyroid storm," the most severe but rare form of thyrotoxicosis, is a medical emergency. A toxic thyroid nodule also causes thyrotoxicosis. Some other forms of thyroid disease begin as hyperthyroidism, but "burn out" into a hypothyroid state.

Beware of imitations. An elevated T4 alone is not synonymous with hyperthyroidism because many acute illnesses (AIDS, hepatitis), high estrogen levels (estrogen replacement, oral contraceptives, pregnancy), and various drugs can cause it.

Hyperthyroidism may be misdiagnosed as anxiety or mania; the reverse is also true. About 30% of patients with acute psychiatric disorders have elevated levels of T4 without thyrotoxicosis. Unlike in real hyperthyroidism, TSH is not suppressed. With treatment of the underlying psychiatric condition, the T4 level eventually returns to normal.

The treatment of thyrotoxicosis depends on its etiology and severity, but must be prompt. Propranolol and newer beta-adrenergic blockers afford symptomatic relief of the anxiety, diaphoresis, tachycardia, and tremor until the hyperthyroidism resolves. Thiourea drugs reduce thyroid hormone production, but must be taken chronically. Radioactive iodine, which is used to treat about 70% of adults with hyperthyroidism, and thyroid surgery are permanent and curative. Overshooting causes hypothyroidism and requires daily maintenance thyroid hormone.

MEDICAL SOURCES OF PSYCHIATRIC SYMPTOMS

Medical diseases and their treatments mimic most "psychiatric disorders." They produce behavioral, cognitive, or emotional disturbances, such as anxiety, dementia, depression, and psychosis. Patients with medically-induced psychiatric symptoms are sometimes first referred to a psychiatrist before the correct diagnosis is made.

Hyperthyroidism is only one representative condition from an extensive list of disorders. The main categories are cardiovascular disorders, connective tissue and immunological disorders, degenerative disorders, drug withdrawal, endocrine disorders, infections, intoxication, medications, metabolic disturbances, neoplasms, nutritional deficiencies, respiratory disorders, seizure disorders, and trauma. Some notable examples include psychosis induced by corticosteroids, phencyclidine (PCP), or the hypercalcemia of multiple myeloma; depression caused by hypothyroidism, amphetamine abuse, clonidine, or sedatives; dementia caused by cerebrovascular and degenerative neurological diseases; and anxiety from caffeinism or cocaine abuse.

*   *   *

"*I Promise I'll Go to the ER*"

Thelma stopped by my office looking frazzled. "Are you on hold?" she whispered. "I need to talk with you about a problem with scheduling."

I glanced up, still entranced by the *Jupiter Symphony* playing on the phone. As beautiful as Mozart's music was, Thelma had uttered the magic words that commanded my full attention. Reluctantly I hung up. "O.K., I'm putting myself on alert. What's up?"

"Dr. Conley's wife just went into labor. We canceled his patients today without a hitch, except this one woman demands to be seen. All the other docs are double-booked and are asking if you could see her. Her only complaint is chest congestion. She thinks she's catching a cold." Thelma gave a crooked grin, implying, how bad could it be.

I thought it over. "Okay, Thelma, I'll see her."

Mahalie Mercer was a regally handsome woman in her late sixties. Her sprayed, silver hair, worn in a French twist, and soft-spoken manner suggested a wonderful gentility. She was the picture of the late Princess Grace of Monaco. Her face reminded me of ivory with just a touch of pink to the cheeks and a few wrinkles gently carved by nature. I wanted to take a snapshot of her as a role model on how to age well.

While listening to the symptoms of what sounded like a viral upper respiratory tract infection, I discerned her shortness of breath. She gasped between every fourth or fifth word. Because her lips were painted pink as were her nails, it was impossible to gauge their true color. I wondered if they were mildly cyanotic.

Mrs. Mercer seated herself on the examination table. "I hope you can give me something for this awful chest cold." Her voice was distinguished and agreeable.

I began my examination as usual, working down from the head to the chest. I expected to find congestion in her bronchial airways or lungs, but they were clear. The surprise came when I laid my stethoscope over her heart. It filled my ears with bongo drum-like sounds, jamming together in different rhythms.

I glanced at Mrs. Mercer to make certain she was not about to pass out. As I auscultated her heart, I felt her pulse. Her pulse counted out to one-hundred-and-ten, but her apical heart rate was much faster—so fast and irregular that I could not keep up with it. This woman was in atrial fibrillation!

"Well, are you going to give me something for this cold? You spent more time on my heart than on my lungs," she accused.

"Mrs. Mercer, I'm going to get a electrocardiogram on you. Your heart is racing and it's irregular."

She appeared to think I'd gone quite mad. However, the tracing confirmed atrial fibrillation with a rapid ventricular response of one-hundred-sixty. Now I realized why she felt short of breath. Fortunately I didn't hear any signs of impending heart failure—yet. After reviewing her ECG with Dr. Janet Ressor, I broke the news to Mrs. Mercer that she needed to be evaluated in the ER.

"Oh, my dear, I *can't* go to the ER. I'm expecting the electrician today to fix some bad wires in my house. I've waited three weeks for him to come out. I simply cannot go *anywhere* but home after this."

"Your heart is the reason you're short of breath, not a cold."

"Can I at least go home and make some arrangements first? I promise I'll go straight to the ER afterward." She took on the appearance of an aged Girl Scout about to hold up two fingers and make the pledge of allegiance.

"You may use the phone at the receptionist desk to make any arrangements. We're talking about your heart here. It's in a dangerous rhythm even as we speak and can slip into a lethal pattern without any warning. My attending physician and I both feel that you need to be seen urgently in the ER. You'll probably be admitted to the hospital."

With a resigned nod she acquiesced. I helped her into a wheelchair and escorted her to Thelma's desk. Mrs. Mercer called a neighbor to take care of her two poodles and canceled the electrician. She was clearly upset with me. In this profession, it's the messenger who gets shot.

"Guess I'll also miss my usual afternoon glass of Merlot, my favorite wine, you know."

A hidden sleuth within me woke up with a jolt. What was that she said? The information sparked a series of thoughts. New Year's Eve was three days ago.

"How was your New Year's Eve?" I asked innocently.

"Oh, it was wonderful! We went out to dinner. Speaking of wine, my son ordered two bottles of 1992 Merlot—it's not a wine with a great deal of staying power, so you can't wait too long to drink it. I couldn't believe it, but we finished them both. I felt a little giddy, but it was a most enjoyable evening ...." She continued on, but I stopped listening after the part about the bottles of wine.

"How many glasses did you have?" I interjected.

"Hmmm, it's hard to remember. Maybe three. But who's counting? I should mention my daughter ordered me a dry martini. I think she did that in memory of my husband, who use to make one for the two of us before dinner. It would relax us at the end of the day. We always kept it to just one, mind you." She raised the pointer finger of her right hand for visual emphasis. "It did taste exquisite." Her eyes now partially hooded, and with a faint smile, Mrs. Mercer was spiritually transported for a moment.

Thelma's phone rang suddenly and broke her reverie. It was the ER requesting a report about my patient.

I was in a reverie of my own: the "holiday heart." Drinking alcohol or withdrawal from it could precipitate irregular heart rhythms in susceptible people. Most people drink more on holidays, hence the name, but even small amounts can trigger it. As I wheeled Mrs. Mercer to the ER, I made a mental note to mention that the holiday heart may be pertinent. The patient's love of wine wasn't noted in her chart.

I showed a copy of the ECG tracing to the triage nurse. At times, pictures say so much more than words do. It took less than fifteen seconds for her to call stat for the attending ER physician then jump up and wheel the patient to a monitored bed cubicle. Triage nurses are worth their weight in silver and gold.

At the end of the day, I found out Mrs. Mercer was admitted to a step-down cardiac unit. Her nurse informed me she was put on an antiarrhythmic IV drip and converted to a pulse of eighty-two within hours of admission. They also added an anticoagulant as a precaution to avert a possible stroke caused by blood clots from the heart—a potentially fatal consequence of A-fib.

The nurse laughed lightly and said, "This patient keeps asking if we serve Merlot, like we're a restaurant or something."

I had to smile. Two weeks later, I was waiting outside Dr. Conley's office to discuss a case, when his door opened and Mrs. Mercer stepped out. I surprised her. After exchanging pleasantries, I asked how she was feeling.

"Well, you should know I got my frayed wires repaired eventually." She started walking down the hall.

Not wanting to miss a beat, I inquired, "Your heart or the electrical wires at home?"

She turned around in mid stride. "Both—and I might add—the electrician cost less and didn't take so long to do the job."

She was right. On the other hand, what would the electrician have charged to rewire the city? *That* was the complexity of the heart.

KEEPING PACE

2,000 beats per minute: the racing heart of the ruby-throated humming bird, less than 3 inches long and weighing 7 one-hundredths of an ounce, empowers its annual 500 mile, non-stop flight across the Gulf of Mexico.

10 beats per minute: the sluggish heart of the hibernating brown bear, pumps just enough blood to sustain the 10 foot long, 1700 pound body through winter. A whale's heart beats only 9 times a minute.

Healthy human heart rates fall in between these extremes:150 beats per minute in the fetus, 72 in healthy adults, 60 in the aged, and 40 to 50 in the conditioned athlete. Usually, resting heart rates above 100 (tachycardia) and below 50 (bradycardia) in average adults are abnormal.

Heart rates may exceed these parameters under several physiologic or environmental situations while keeping a regular rhythm. Alcohol consumption and alcohol withdrawal, anemia, drugs, emotion, exercise, fever, pain, shock, and thyrotoxicosis drive the normal heart to extremes (sinus tachycardia). Fever alone accelerates the heart rate by 10 beats per minute for every degree of increased body temperature. Heart abnormalities, such as cardiac failure, do the same. Another major cause of tachycardia is tachyarrhythmias.

KEEPING THE BEAT

Music, electricity, and heart rhythm. To pump efficiently—fill with blood and empty—the heart must contract with a steady, regular rhythm. Heart muscle cells are inherently contractile. Placed in electrolyte solution, the detached heart of a frog or rat will beat for hours. But the contractions must be regulated.

"Pacer cells" in the heart's atrial wall (sinus or sinoatrial node) keep the beat; they pace the heart. An electrical network connects the chambers of the heart to coordinate their activities. Nerve impulses from the right atrium travel the slender bundle of His to the atrioventricular (AV) node and its branches to each ventricle.

When this system fails, there's chaos. The atria beat at their own rate of 400 to 600 beats per minute, driving the ventricles at a lesser but dangerously high pace; ectopic rhythms from atria or ventricles emerge and take over, producing unusual, coupled rhythms; or the ventricles fibrillate uselessly on their way to cardiac standstill.

Arrhythmias are irregularities in heart rhythm which secondarily alter heart rate. They result from abnormalities of impulse formation or automaticity, impulse conduction, re-entry, or triggered activity. Some may be fatal; others are physiologic, linked to the phase of breathing (sinus arrhythmias). When arrhythmias impair blood flow to the brain or heart, dizziness, syncope or near syncope, even sudden cardiac death may result.

Tachyarrhythmias may be supraventricular or ventricular. How they are tolerated depends on the health of the heart. When there's underlying heart disease, tachyarrhythmia leads to congestive failure or myocardial infarction. Ventricular tachycardia, which is likely to deteriorate into ventricular fibrillation, isn't tolerated for more than 30 seconds. It can degenerate into to lethal ventricular fibrillation.

Those at risk for life-threatening arrhythmias must be monitored in the hospital or as outpatients. Portable devices (event recorders or transmitters) can be worn for prolonged periods of time to record rhythm tracings. Other monitoring techniques include exercise testing, signal-averaged ECG's, studies of heart conduction (intracardiac electrophysiologic studies), and tests of autonomic nervous system function (tilt-table testing).

Antiarrhythmic drugs are tricky: they can induce or block arrhythmias and have side effects. There are four main classes. *Class I* drugs (a to c) block membrane sodium channels. *Class II* drugs (beta-blockers) slow AV conduction. *Class III* agents (amiodarone, sotalol, bretylium) prolong action potential. *Class IV* drugs block slow calcium channels. *Class V* drugs are heterogeneous.

Supraventricular tachycardia responds to Class Ia, II, III, IV, and V drugs; Ic drugs are for refractory cases only. Ventricular tachycardia responds to Class I and Class III drugs.

ATRIAL FIBRILLATION

Atrial quivering (fibrillation), the commonest chronic arrhythmia, strikes about 20 per 1,000 persons. It is acute or chronic, occurs in people with normal or abnormal hearts, and may be either an asymptomatic, incidental finding or precipitate cardiac decompensation. Atrial fibrillation is the only common arrhythmia in which rhythm is very irregular and ventricular rate is rapid (80-180 beats per minute). Not all ventricular beats produce a peripheral pulse.

In patients with normal hearts, atrial fibrillation is triggered by alcohol (mild consumption, intoxication, or withdrawal—the so-called "holiday heart" syndrome), chest surgery or trauma, lung disease, medications (beta-adrenergic agonists, theophylline), pericarditis, and thyrotoxicosis.

With heart disease (atrial septal defect, mitral valve prolapse, dilated or hypertrophic cardiomyopathy, valvular disease), rapid atrial fibrillation can lead to heart failure or pulmonary edema. The risk of a fatal outcome doubles.

Prepare for the worst, even if a patient appears stable. The priority is to control ventricular rate. Other goals are to restore sinus rhythm and identify any underlying heart disease. The tools are chemical conversion or electrical conversion. Beta-blockers, calcium channel blockers, or digoxin control heart rate and can be given intravenously if there is hemodynamic decompensation. Because digoxin has a slower onset of action, it should not be given alone.

If chemical conversion is unsuccessful, electrical cardioversion may be necessary. Electrical cardioversion (a jolt of electricity through paddles applied to the chest of a sedated patient) is extremely painful and is unsuccessful in 20 to 50% of patients with atrial fibrillation, so it should be reserved for the sickest, unstable patients. Avoid it in the presence of digoxin toxicity.

Beyond 48 hours after onset, cardioversion carries a risk of embolization. The formation of clots is unpredictable and may occur in 20% of patients who have had atrial fibrillation for less than 72 hours. Transesophageal echocardiography can detect the clots.

After atrial rate is controlled, most patients with acute atrial fibrillation need to be converted to sinus rhythm. If arrhythmia has been present for more than 48 hours, first anticoagulate them for 3 to 4 weeks. Pharmacologic conversion should be tried prior to electrical cardioversion. Alternative options are a class I or short-acting class III antiarrhythmic. After electrical cardioversion, atrial function in the "stunned" atrium returns only gradually. Warfarin anticoagulation is just as important 4 to 6 weeks after cardioversion as before cardioversion.

How do things turn out? About 80% of patients with new onset atrial fibrillation revert to normal sinus rhythm during hospitalization. Only 25% of patients who are converted from atrial fibrillation maintain sinus rhythm beyond one year. Chronic anti-arrhythmic therapy boosts the number to 50%, but carries significant risks. Patients with structural heart disease are more likely to require chronic treatment with antiarrhythmics.

Chronic atrial fibrillation is a major risk factor for stroke. The risk ranges from 2 to 20%. Advanced age, diabetes, heart disease, and hypertension increase the risk. Patients at high risk for stroke need to be treated with warfarin; others should be treated with aspirin or other antithrombotic agents.

13

Stalked from Within

Mental health problems do not affect three or four out of every five persons, but one out of one
—WILLIAM MENNINGER

The pain of the mind is worse than the pain of the body
—SYRUS

Sanity is very rare: every man almost, and every woman, has a dash of madness
—RALPH WALDO EMERSON

A man who is 'of sound mind' is one who keeps the inner madman under lock and key
—PAUL AMBROISE VALÉRY

If you talk to God, you are praying. If God talks to you, you have schizophrenia
—THOMAS SZASZ

"There Are Martians on the Telephone"

"You're not going to believe what I just heard!" Susan Crawley exclaimed as she rushed into my office at 10:15 A.M. Her look of animation and confidential manner piqued my curiosity. "Remember that psychotic patient that you and I ping-ponged back and forth this past month—the one who keeps coming to walk-in clinic?"

My mental list of such patients included more than one name, but I thought I knew who Susan meant. "He's a big, bald, black man with a round, chubby face? He always wears a plaid shirt with corduroy pants and his eyeglass frames are held together by scotch tape in the center?"

Susan nodded.

"John something."

"John Lance," Susan quickly replied. "Well, I just saw him and I *still* can't stop laughing."

I knew Susan realized that mental illness is no laughing matter. I guessed it must have been something John Lance said or did. Things that psychotic patients say take even the most experienced clinician off guard. Sometimes humorous, sometimes tragic, the words of the seriously mentally disturbed can even be prophetic. "What was so funny?"

"John had a bee in his bonnet from the moment he walked into my office."

"Why?"

"He kept insisting that he was listening to people from Mars on the telephone."

"Hallucinations?"

"Well, he *is* schizophrenic. It made sense."

I recalled that John Lance had disturbed and disordered thoughts. He also exhibited the typical indifference about appearance. His clothes were worn and soiled and he didn't bathe. He had a tendency to discontinue his antipsychotic medications. "Did he stop taking his meds again?"

"He claims not." Susan waited to see if I had anymore ideas. When I offered none she went on. "So I gave him the usual psych nurse response. I told him that I was sure he really thought he was talking to people from Mars, but if there were people on Mars, they wouldn't be talking on an ordinary telephone. I asked him how long had he been hearing those voices. He denied he was hearing voices and insisted they were real Martians.

As I spoke to him, he was getting angrier with me and I was starting to get worried about what he might do next. I said that if he was going to act upset, I would have to go and call some people who would come over and calm him down. When's the last time either of us did psych nursing? What are you supposed to do?" She threw her arms up to frame a question.

"What did he say then?"

"He wanted to prove it to me."

"Okay, so what did you do?" I wanted the punch line, but Susan enjoyed spinning a yarn.

"I figured this guy is really psychotic, right, so what could it hurt to pacify him. This is the good part."

"Yeah, yeah," I said impatiently.

"He told me to call this number on the telephone and to listen carefully. He said I would hear aliens talking."

I laughed. "And did you?"

"You bet I did," said Susan as she broke into a cascade of giggles, "right there in front of him. And to top it off—he was right."

I looked at her puzzled.

"I dialed the number and it kept on ringing until an answering machine clicked on and delivered a high pitched voice announcement." She paused to build the suspense. She knew it was driving me crazy.

"So what did it say?" I finally exclaimed.

"It said *You have just reached Mars. We're out of this world. Leave a message or call back later.*" Susan howled.

"You're kidding. What was going on?"

"I know, can you believe it? Someone has this crazy answering machine and just when I told Mr. Lance he was imagining things. I tried to reassure him it was just a gag message on an answering machine, but I know he walked out of the office still believing there are Martians on Ma Bell."

A smile spread over my face. "That's too much, Susan. Where do you come up with these stories?"

"Somebody has to take care of the patients." She shrugged. "Well you know what they say about psychiatrists, don't you?"

"Go ahead. I'm game. What?"

"A neurotic is the man who builds a castle in the air, a psychotic is the man who lives in it, and a psychiatrist is the man who collects the rent."

"Who said that?"

"I don't know."

"Don't you have work to do?"

She grinned. "Okay, I get the hint."

After Susan left my office, I found myself recalling my conversations with Mr. Lance. He was usually a gentle man who spoke softly. When he became agitated, his speech had the force of a locomotive. If I questioned the rationality of the voices in his head, he made sweeping hand gestures to convince me.

I truly felt sorry for him. He was a tormented soul. The visits at our clinic offered Mr. Lance a dose of reality. I always made sure he was taking his medications and keeping his appointments with his therapist. I felt that we were throwing him a life vest as he treaded on the murky, undulating sea of incessant paranoia, but he swam the other direction into engulfing darkness.

Then I got to thinking about the dark humor of health care providers. We usually prefer to joke amongst ourselves about matters that are otherwise too difficult to handle. I guess it provides an innocent release. When nursing and medical students first hear it, they're shocked. I can remember as a student thinking that people who joke about patients are jerks. After you have been in the business a while, you start doing it to keep your sanity.

MENTAL ILLNESS

Young and old danced uncontrollably in the streets and fields, screaming and foaming at the mouth. Such was the situation around 1374 A.D. in Aix-la-Chapelle, a city in West Germany near the Belgian and Dutch borders. In retrospect, the cause was probably hallucinogenic ergots, a fungus contaminating the rye they used to make bread. Like other people with mental illness, especially hallucinations, who did not fare well in early societies, they were persecuted as heretics or witches.

In the middle ages, next to nothing was known about the origins of mental illness. Borrowing from the Greeks, physiologists believed that the distinguishing mental and physical characteristics of a human being resulted from dominance of one of the four "humors":

black bile, blood, choler, and phlegm. With nothing more substantive to go on, the dark ages of mental illness far outlasted those of European history.

Now, in what we hope the future will consider a "renaissance" of attitudes and approaches, we know that mental illness is caused by brain dysfunction. Modern neuroimaging studies have found brain correlates for some psychiatric disorders. Evidence of brain chemical alterations, especially of neurotransmitters and other chemical messengers, has guided and validated the use of psychoactive medications. Genetic abnormalities identified in some individuals at increased risk are promising. For most psychiatric disorders, however, the basic chemical, genetic, or structural abnormalities are unknown.

Mental illness takes many forms: disorders of behavior, cognition, emotion, and perception. The health care provider must recognize and handle them all because they often first present to primary care settings under the guise of medical complaints. The thickness of the *Diagnostic and Statistical Manual of Mental Disorders* (DSM-IV), which catalogs all of the 410 psychiatric diagnoses, makes it easy to appreciate how mental health costs run about $19 billion a year.

Given that so many people have occasional or intermittent symptoms of mental illness, the problem is where to draw the line in deciding who to diagnose as abnormal and treat. Some experts argue that we are living at a time when it's easier to medicate individuals than to address the broader societal ills that cause them to become symptomatic. Drugs are also a quick fix compared to time-consuming introspection and counseling. Antidepressants and anxiolytics are prescribed so liberally, they might well attain the status of "soma" in *Brave New World*.

While these issues are germane to the neuroses, patients with psychotic disorders undeniably need prompt and effective drug intervention. Many new drugs with fewer side effects are now available. Many more are being engineered or are already in clinical trials.

SCHIZOPHRENIA

The word *schizophrenia* often conjures the desperate and sorry state of affairs depicted in *One Flew Over a Cuckoo's Nest*, complete with forced institutionalization and cruel frontal lobotomies, or the distraught Vincent van Gogh cutting off his earlobe and presenting it to his horrified roommate, Paul Gauguin, after one particularly heated argument. As dated as these images are, they do convey a very realistic picture of the pain and suffering experienced by schizophrenics to this day.

Schizophrenia is one of the three most common mental health problems seen in primary care settings. Referred to as "malignant," it is the most chronic and disabling of the major mental illnesses. Schizophrenia torments one percent of the population or about two million Americans, and more than 300,000 persons with it are hospitalized each year. The inability to control one's own thoughts and the intrusion of directive "voices" makes schizophrenia a frightening and lonely experience.

Being out of touch with reality (psychotic), delusions, disordered thought, hallucinations, and inappropriate affect are key features of schizophrenia. Symptoms of schizophrenia are classified as "positive" (features not found in normal people, such as hallucinations) or "negative" (loss of normal functions).

There is no single cause of schizophrenia. Both genetic and environmental factors contribute. Children of a schizophrenic parent have a ten times higher risk of developing schizophrenia than other children have, but no causal gene or biochemical defect has been identified. Schizophrenia may not even be a single disorder. The first psychotic symptoms occur in the teens to twenties in men and a decade later in women. Because not all psychotic symptoms result from schizophrenia, the search for other reversible conditions should be thorough.

Schizophrenic patients have difficulty establishing and maintaining relationships with others. Because schizophrenia presents during the years when other people are establishing a career or learning a trade, schizophrenics lack social and work skills, too. Their occupational, psychological, and social problems are best handled by psychosocial approaches, such as rehabilitation, individual psychotherapy, family therapy, group therapy, and self-help groups. Short-term residential care, partial hospitalization, outpatient treatment, and halfway houses provide useful adjuncts to treatment with antipsychotic medication.

The outcome of schizophrenia is variable. Although half recover at least partially, only 25% recover fully, and another 25% require long-term care. With a lifetime suicide prevalence of 10% compared to 1% in the general population, suicide is their leading cause of death.

Schizophrenia can be treated, not cured. Antipsychotic medications (neuroleptics) abate psychotic symptoms and improve function. The drugs are more effective against the positive than against the negative symptoms of schizophrenia: agitation, confusion, delusions, distortions, hallucinations. Antipsychotic medications help the patient differentiate between psychotic symptoms and the real world. With continued use, about 40% of recovered schizophrenics relapse within two years after hospitalization, compared to the 80% relapse rate when the medication is discontinued by those who deny they need medication.

The acute side effects of antipsychotic drugs include blurred vision, dry mouth, drowsiness, muscle spasms, and restlessness. The most serious long-term side effect is tardive dyskinesia, an involuntary movement disorder affecting the lips, mouth, tongue, and sometimes the limbs. Use of the lowest effective dosage prevents unwanted sedation. Newer atypical antipsychotic drugs are less likely to cause the movement disorder possibly because they block serotonin more than they block dopamine receptors. They also reduce rehospitalization in compliant patients by one-third.

*   *   *

"The X-Rays Burnt Me"

When I introduced myself as a nurse practitioner to my next patient Roxanne Delacruz, she complained bitterly.

"Why do I have to see a nurse practitioner? I thought I would be seeing a physician. Where's the doctor?"

Ms. Delacruz was a short, stocky, very plain-looking, twenty-five-year-old Hispanic with long, black hair and wire-rimmed glasses. The small moles on her face looked like they'd been splattered by the whimsical fling of an artist's paint-filled brush.

"Your doctor asked me to evaluate you. He could not see you right now because he's already seeing scheduled patients and you don't have an appointment."

"That pisses me off." Ms. Delacruz's face was contorted by instantaneous rage.

Some people prefer not to see a nurse practitioner, but the reaction is not usually so strong.

"Tell me what's wrong and maybe I can help you out?" I said neutrally.

She sat for a moment without speaking, as if cooling off. Reluctantly, she told me her story. "I've had a burning tongue after having x-rays at a chiropractor's office yesterday."

Oh, great, this is going to be just terrific. Is anything really what it seems?

"What x-rays were done?"

"He x-rayed my entire spine. It was a *sloppy* job."

"Why were x-rays done?"

"Because I told him I had pains."

"What pains?"

"My tongue has been burning since the x-rays were taken, all right? It goes down my throat as if I have been washing my mouth out with a strong mouthwash. It never subsides. My tongue feels swollen and my speech is different. *Can't you tell?*" The patient glared obliquely at me.

When it came time to examine Ms. Delacruz, I inspected her mouth carefully. She had copious postnasal drainage in her posterior pharynx. It looked like a case of sinusitis. "I want one of the physicians I work with to take a look at you."

The walk-in clinic attending coverage for me that day was Dr. Eva Romerez, a black/Hispanic woman in her late thirties. She wore her white coat open, pockets stuffed with manuals and booklets. I asked her to examine the patient with me. She agreed with my examination and discussed the diagnosis of sinusitis with the patient.

Roxanne Delacruz became enraged. "You're wrong and stupid. It's *not* sinusitis. The x-rays burnt me."

"Uh-huh, uh-huh, well okay," Dr. Romerez replied. "Well, we want to help you. The nurse will tell you what to do." Skillfully she moved toward the door. Her tone was one of insincerity and false solicitude.

The patient looked at me as if to say who is this strange person you brought in with you.

When Dr. Romerez left the room I said, "It really looks like you have a sinus problem. I can prescribe an antibiotic and decongestant for you. You should feel better soon."

"I don't have a sinus infection."

"Perhaps you'll want to see your own personal physician tomorrow. Maybe he'll want you evaluated by a throat specialist in ENT clinic."

"This is real piss poor care," the patient yelled with a brusque movement of her arms. "You're an asshole and dumb bitch! I'm not making an appointment to see *anyone*."

I eyed her warily. "Well, that's up to you. We recommend you do."

"I'm not going to." Her rage was molten. She had spittle in the corners of her mouth. "And how are you going to write this up? Are you going to include the part about the x-rays being done? That's the cause of this, you know. The *x-rays* burned me. *You* don't want to admit it."

"Why would I not write what you told me?" Illogical as it was, she seemed certain I was going to falsify the history. The flavor of her comments was one of paranoia.

"I don't know. You're just being an *asshole*."

I realized I'd been clenching my teeth. As the rampage continued, I let out a silent, long, deep, inner sigh—one of chronic exasperation and annoyance. Was I running a psychiatric clinic here? Had someone changed the sign on the outside of the clinic? I wasn't going to get into it with this patient. I gradually persuaded her to leave the room.

On her way out, the patient reviled me in a loud voice to the secretary and the other patients. "They have NURSE PRACTITIONERS back there. They don't know what the hell they're doing! Get your asses out of here. *Don't let them fuck with you!*" Her seditious comments trailed off.

Thelma came back to my room. "Child, you are blessed with the best cases. Here's the chart for a patient referred from the rapid assessment unit in the ER." Thelma started to leave the room. "Oh, and please tell your patients *not* to swear at my desk on the way out," she said with a sardonic smile.

"I just bring out the best in them, Thelma. What can I say."

PERSONALITY DISORDERS

"If your dislike of a patient ... is severe, the patient either has a serious personality disorder or he or she may be acting out an aspect you despise or disown." This aphorism is rule number 28 of *A Little Book of Nurse's Rules*.

Personality disorders come in multiple varieties. The main types are antisocial, avoidant, borderline, compulsive, dependent, histrionic, narcissistic, paranoid, passive-aggressive, schizoid, and schizotypal.

The most severe personality disorders—antisocial and borderline—which bring the individual into greatest conflict with society and result in legal problems, have a guarded prognosis. Borderline personalities are aggressive, impulsive, and unstable, lacking in self-control and self-fulfillment, and prone to abuse drugs and attempt suicide.

Behavioral treatment techniques are aversive conditioning and operant conditioning. Social and therapeutic environments, which utilize peer pressure to modify behavior, include day hospitals, halfway houses, and self-help communities. Group therapy is useful when social interaction is severely impaired and patients act-out. Under stress or decompensation, personality disorders mimic other psychiatric disorders, such as anxiety, depression, and psychosis. Then the patients require medication.

*   *   *

"I Want to Kill Her"

This time the ER sent *me* a patient. Cecilia Rolanda, a woman in her twenties, sat facing away from me most of the time and never looked me straight in the eyes during the interview. She was accompanied by her mother.

"Why are you here, Cecilia?" I picked up my pen to start writing.

"My mother made me come here," she replied, looking contemptuous.

"I want her to be examined and have some blood tests done," the mother said. "She's not acting right. I *know* she's got something wrong in her blood."

I was getting a very bad feeling about the two of them. Was I up for a walk on the wild side? "What's been going on, Cecilia?"

"You're not going to touch me," she insisted. "I don't want to be touched." The young patient was not about to give me a history.

I turned to her mother. "Tell me what you mean by not acting right?" The question seemed moot.

"She has been depressed for three or four years. This past year she changed jobs every few months. She's argumentative at work, hostile toward others, and has a short temper, which tends to get her in trouble."

As the medical history continued, I gleaned that Cecilia's relationship with her mother was poor, and she was also estranged from her father, who called only to bother her. She was hospitalized in a psychiatric ward after throwing scalding water on a coworker because he "pissed her off."

"Mrs. Rolanda, I'm going to ask you to step outside for a little bit while I talk to your daughter and examine her. Then I will come and get you in the waiting room and we'll all talk some more."

Mrs. Rolanda left reluctantly, viewing me with suspicion. Her daughter seemed to relax more after her mother left.

"Cecilia, do you drink?"

"Yes."

"How much?"

"I drink one or two fifths of Scotch if I am depressed or angry at someone who pissed me off. I'm not supposed to take my anger out on people because I get in trouble, so I drink to get drunk 'til I pass out."

The list of problems was growing. Substance abuse was now an issue. I was becoming more alarmed. "Are you having other problems?"

Cecilia paused momentarily. "My stomach bothers me. I feel nauseated, but it's nothing compared to the time when I overdosed myself on aspirin and wine." The exuberance of her responses contradicted the content of her words.

"When was that?"

"That happened a couple of years ago. Someone dumped me off at an ER."

"Do you have thoughts about hurting yourself?"

"No."

"Do you want to hurt others?"

"Yes." She was not at all reticent or remorseful.

"Why?"

"It makes me feel good." The corner of Cecilia's mouth curled up unnaturally.

I felt uneasy on hearing her answer. "And do you want to hurt someone today?" I asked gingerly.

She hesitated long enough to make me wonder if she'd heard the question. "No, not right now."

I was relieved. "Do you ever feel bad after you hurt someone?"

"Sometimes. A few years ago, my cat knocked some paint onto the floor, so I grabbed the cat by the tail and threw it against the wall." She snickered. "The cat survived, but walks funny now."

I thought about my own cat at home. The very idea of what Cecilia did repulsed me. I reminded myself that she was a patient seeking my help.

"Once I was standing in line at school when I was little and another kid kept bothering me. I turned around and belted him in the face. I made his nose bleed," she said without emotion. "Another time, a little black kid was making fun of me and got me upset, so I jammed him with a desk against the wall and ended up cracking three of his ribs and sending him to the hospital."

I stopped writing and looked up. "Why did you do that?"

"'Cause he made me get mad. I told him he shouldn't make me mad. After that, my mother had to walk me to school and back everyday for a year so the black kids wouldn't beat up on me."

Still thinking about the unconscionable acts I just heard, I watched Cecilia revel in her dark deeds. My unease was mushrooming.

"I told a little white girl not to tease me," she continued, "but she teased me about my name. She said my last name sounded like a first name. So I grabbed a clump of her hair and pulled it out. That made her stop," Cecilia said with a cruel smile.

I was aghast. "Are you seeing a psychiatrist?"

"No."

"Are you getting counseling?"

"Yes."

"Where?"

She told me where casually and I made a note of it. "Why do I have to go through all this?"

"Because I need this information for your chart."

"Do you know I almost joined the Navy?" Cecilia unexpectedly confided, as if I were her best friend. "I wanted to escape reality by joining the Navy until I found out they might send me to some ungodly place for years. So I got myself out before I was sworn in."

I thought I'd heard quite enough, but as a matter of standard practice I asked, "Is there anything you wish to discuss in your mother's absence?"

Cecilia gave the question careful consideration. "I want to kill her," she whispered.

I looked up from my notes. "You're just saying that, aren't you?"

"No. I'm *serious*," Cecilia insisted. The wild look in her eye convinced me of her intent.

"Have you actually made plans for how you're going to kill her?"

"Yes." Cecilia smiled.

"How?"

"When she's sleeping."

"But how?"

"With knives. We have long sharp kitchen knives. My mother's afraid of knives. It will be perfect." Cecilia continued to be preoccupied with the idea.

"Why would you want to kill her?" I recoiled at the thought.

"Cause she ruined my life, that's why." Cecilia became very angry. The muscles in her face and neck tightened. "I hate her."

This was no idle threat. She had a plan with specifics. "Have you discussed that with your therapist?"

"No."

"You really should."

Cecilia just stared at me.

I completed her history taking and cajoled her through the physical examination. After we finished, I excused myself to discuss the case with Dr. Eva Romerez, who'd seen my other patient.

"Eva, this patient told me confidentially that she wants to kill her mother. She's an adult not a minor. I'm not sure what my obligations are to the mother."

"Do you think she's serious?"

"Yes."

"And she's already seeing a therapist?"

"Yes."

"A lot of good it's doing, right?"

"Right."

Dr. Romerez deliberated. "Well, let's go talk to the daughter."

When she and I walked into the room, the patient looked calm. "Cecilia, I'm Dr. Romerez. I understand that you're not too happy about your mother."

Cecilia Rolanda's facial expression was blank. "What do you mean?"

"I heard you have plans to kill her."

"I never said that."

"Didn't you say that you wanted to kill her in her sleep?"

Cecilia broke out into a spine-tingling laugh. "Where did you come up with that? *I* never said that. My mother and I get along fine. She's my friend." Cecilia stared at me from behind a self-satisfied countenance and burst into another round of laughter.

Dr. Romerez looked over at me, obviously not amused, and motioned for us to leave the room. "What's going on?"

I shook my head incredulously. "That's what she told me. I don't understand it. She's lying to one of us."

Dr. Romerez didn't know what to make of it either. Nonplused at this encounter, she said, "Call her therapist today and relay the information."

I brought the mother back into my office. "What is to be done for her?" she demanded to know. "What blood tests are you going to order, and are you concerned about her cholesterol? I think her cholesterol may be making her act this way."

I sighed as I reassured the patient's mother that I ordered blood to be drawn for routine tests, including cholesterol. "The results of Cecilia's physical examination were normal. Blood pressure, heart rate, and the like were all fine. Cecilia's behavior is not likely due to problems in her blood." I looking directly at Cecilia and said, "She needs to continue to work *intensively* with her counselor."

The mother did not take the news well. Her daughter was indifferent. As the two left my office, I didn't know who should rightfully be called the patient. The daughter's prognosis for a productive life was dismal. I also understood that had I referred the Rolanda's to the psychiatry clinic, the clinic only would have sent them back to their local counselor or therapist.

I did call Cecilia's therapist and discussed her behavior. The therapist was not surprised by what I told her and reassured me that Cecilia was a pathologic liar. She planned to see the patient in the next few days.

With her comments fresh in mind, I was left with the macabre thought of Cecilia Rolanda standing in the darkness, brandishing a long, razor-sharp blade above her sleeping mother's throat.

SUBSTANCE ABUSE AND PSYCHIATRIC DISORDERS

The risk of substance abuse disorder is higher in those with a psychiatric disorder. Compared to the 16.7% of the population who have substance abuse disorder, the risk is 3.4 times higher in patients with bipolar depression, 2.8 times higher in schizophrenia, and about 1.5 times for anxiety disorders or major depression.

Such patients often frustrate health care providers by being difficult, non-compliant, and resistant to making needed changes. When they present to primary care settings, they have multiple somatic complaints, overuse services, and fail to respond to treatment.

Substance abuse is underdiagnosed in psychiatric patients. The clinical interview, toxicology screening, and use of screening questionnaires help to make the proper assessment. When used chronically, barbiturates, benzodiazepines, marijuana, and PCP can be detected for 14 days, whereas amphetamines, cocaine, opiates, and propoxyphene are detectable for only a few days.

The main interventions are counseling, patient education, and medications. Community self-help groups like Alcoholics Anonymous (AA), Controlled Substances Anonymous (CSA), Narcotics Anonymous (NA), and "Double Trouble" may benefit patients who can tolerate group involvement.

*   *   *

"If You Put Something In, Something Has to Come Out"

The sight of Agnes Bullocks walking into my room triggered the memory of Alta Sweeney, the woman with end-stage cancer. Ms. Bullocks was a walking skeleton.

Oh, no, another terminal patient. How sad.

The bird-like, short, middle-aged woman positioned herself in the chair. "I feel weak and don't have much energy." Her breath was sour, like that of someone starving.

"How long have you been this thin?" My mind was organizing the blood tests and procedures I would need to order to evaluate her weight loss. The appearance of her face, skin drawn over the bones, was disquieting.

"I'm not thin. I wish I were." She was very matter-of-fact.

I was dumbfounded. "You don't think you're too thin?"

"No. I feel fat."

"Why is that?"

"I don't know. I've always been too heavy."

That was my wake-up call, loud and clear. "Have you been trying to lose weight?"

"No, not really."

"What do you mean, not really?"

"Well, if you put something in, something has to come out," Ms. Bullocks explained.

There was a moment of silence. "Say that again."

"If you put something in your mouth, it has to come out of your bowels."

"That's normal."

"I don't want that," she snapped. "It's dirty."

So much for cancer. That was the positive side. But an eating disorder posed as pernicious a threat. I needed more information. "Why are you concerned about your bowels?"

"Bad things grow in me. I need to be cleaned out."

"Do you use laxatives?"

"Why, yes, doesn't everybody?" Ms. Bullocks appeared somewhat surprised by the question.

"How often?" The trail was becoming hotter.

"Everyday, sometimes several times a day."

Yes, the pattern of a laxative abuser. "So, you're having diarrhea all the time?"

"That's why I don't eat until I really have to."

"Tell me about your bowel habits."

"I clean off the germs around my rectum several times a day," she said with deliberate precision. "I change my underwear frequently so they don't get contaminated with the germs."

After obtaining a full history, I told Ms. Bullocks that I needed to do a complete examination. She consented, but refused a rectal examination, insisting that I would introduce germs into her anus and the germs might be of a strain that her body couldn't fight off. Curiously, she did allow me to do the routine vaginal exam and Pap smear. What was so special about the anus to this patient, I wondered.

I passed the case by Dr. Romerez, who, apparently remembering her experience with my previous patient, decided not to see Ms. Bullocks with me. She did agree with my plan.

I focused on two tasks. I needed to obtain a complete blood panel. Chronic laxative use may have altered the blood chemistry; low potassium could be lethal to the heart. I sent the blood off stat. The harder task was to get her a psychiatry appointment.

I went to the empty conference room to use the phone. "I have a patient who needs to be seen soon."

"We have no openings. Sorry."

"Look, this woman is a walking cadaver from an eating dis-order—God only knows how low her potassium is—and you *can't* see her? This is clearly psychiatric."

"We are overbooked." The voice had grown stern.

"My attending, Dr. Romerez, wants her seen today."

"I don't care *who* wants her seen. There are no available acute ap-pointments. We're swamped. If your patient is that ill, she should go to the ER."

I couldn't believe it. I called the Rapid Assessment Unit of the ER, hoping to be able to force a psychiatry consult from the ER. They didn't want her either because she had no medical problem. Agnes Bullocks was to be a pawn of war.

Although I spent more time on the phone trying to call the psy-chiatry on-call consultant, I couldn't convince anyone that this was an emergency. Who would give me back-up? I wished that Dr. Con-ley, Dr. Ressor, or Dr. Santini were on clinic duty. What could I do?

Thelma came into the conference room. "So, there you are. I've been looking all over for you. The lab called with the results of your stat blood tests. They want to talk with you. Please call them back right away."

"Thanks, Thelma." Quickly I dialed the lab and reached the tech. "Is there something wrong?"

"Yes, the potassium on Agnes Bullocks was only 2.1 and some of the other electrolytes like chloride and bicarbonate are abnormal, too." I copied down the numbers with amazement.

"Thanks! Thanks a lot!"

I felt strangely relieved on receiving the news. Ms. Bullocks now had a medical problem and a serious one at that. Her potassium was critically low. At least my patient would be taken seriously. I called the ER. "I have a patient with a potassium of 2.1 and a metabolic acidosis."

"Send her right down."

I quickly got Agnes Bullocks ready and shuttled her over in a wheelchair. I returned feeling fatigued. The clinic closed at five P.M., but I stayed until twenty-after-six completing my charts. Without the distracting buzz and interruptions of the clinic, I could get caught up at the end of the day.

EATING DISORDERS

A P.O.W.? A terminal cancer patient? A victim of involuntary starvation? No. A person with an eating disorder. When the brain does not regulate eating behavior, things go terribly wrong. Eating disorders, which are often unrecognized, cause death about 15% of the time from cardiac arrhythmias, gastric hemorrhage, and suicide. This potentially lethal aberration has been known since the 9th century, when the followers of St. Jerome starved themselves, but was recognized as a discrete medical entity only in this century.

The obsession is with thinness: skin and bones. The big two—anorexia nervosa and bulimia—are now the stuff of documentaries, commercial movies, and tabloids, raised to public attention largely by affected celebrities. They afflict women far more often than they afflict men. Anorexia nervosa racks about 1% of the population.

The anorexic patient, morbidly afraid to gain weight and feeling powerless while striving toward culturally aesthetic thinness and perfectionism, becomes emaciated. Secrecy is the rule. Anorexia so distorts body image that the mirror may lie, reflecting back an image of obesity rather than of cachexia. The prepubertal pattern of hormone production found in anorexia nervosa leads to amenorrhea. Medical disorders that cause weight loss, like cancer, diabetes, hyperthyroidism, and malnutrition, must be excluded.

A "chipmunk face" is a clue to bulimia. Patients with bulimia—maybe 5% of the population—binge and then purge by inducing vomiting. Purging causes the parotid glands to swell and puff out the cheeks. Diet pills, diuretics, exercise, fasting, and laxatives are all tools of the bulimic. The patient's dentist may make the diagnosis by noticing erosion of dental enamel from vomiting. Other disorders that provoke vomiting may be confused with bulimia: brain tumors, gastrointestinal reflux, infections, and migraine headaches.

The eating pattern is one of alternating restrained and unrestrained food intake. Once bulimic patients eat a forbidden food, like candy, chips, or sodas, they binge. Excessive eating triggers a return to food deprivation. Can you imagine what it must feel like to induce yourself to vomit 10 times a week—the average number of times for bulimics—for weeks, months, or years?

What happens if you binge at least twice a week for 6 months, but don't purge? Such a person is a binge-eater. Binge-eaters can ingest 2,000 to 3,000 calories, a whole day's caloric intake, at one sitting! How much do they weigh? Only 20% over ideal body weight suffices to make the diagnosis. So what's different about binge-eating and obesity? Binge-eaters exhibit extreme lack of control, frustration, self-anger, and shame.

A multifaceted approach to the treatment of eating disorders works best: structured food intake, psychotherapy, and drug treatment. Psychotherapy probes issues of chaotic eating, conditioned responses, fear of expressing feelings of anger and sadness, hunger, impulse control, and inadequate caloric intake. Serotonin, a brain chemical that regulates eating behavior, is low in people with eating disorders. Antidepressant drugs, especially ones that sustain the activity of serotonin and norepinephrine, are useful.

The story does not end here; it goes on with a twist. "Agnes Bullocks" probably had something more than a simple eating disorder. Psychological disorders can produce the same symptoms. The spectrum includes affective disorders (unipolar and bipolar), anxiety disorders, obsessive-compulsive disorder, personality disorders (borderline, histrionic, narcissistic), and schizophrenia. Stimulant abuse (cocaine and amphetamines) leads to weight loss, too. As many as half of people with an eating disorder also carry another psychiatric diagnosis.

14

The Gatekeeper

There is only one cardinal rule: One must always listen to the patient
—OLIVER SACKS

When we are well, we all have good advice for those who are ill
—TERENCE

I recommend frequent doses of that rare commodity—common sense
—VINCENT ASKEY

When a lot of remedies are suggested for a disease, that means it can't be cured
—ANTON PAVLOVICH CHEKHOV

The major concern of the nurse is to know the person with the disease as a person
—ROSALIE HAMMERSCHMIDT

"He's Confused"

"Are there any patients to be seen, Thelma?"

"No, but you have lots of phone messages to catch up on."

"Okay, hand them over."

"A few are patients of the doctors, but the doctors want you to call." Thelma looked at me as she handed me the stack. "You know how this place works," she said with a wink. "But this last call does seem more urgent."

I picked up the beige desk phone in my room and began returning calls. This part of my job made me feel like a telephone operator. Some of the patients wanted results of their blood tests from earlier that week. Others had questions about their illness that they didn't think to ask in the office. Sometimes there were new problems.

"Hello, Mrs. Jordan. I'm a nurse practitioner at the clinic. What can I do for you?"

A woman with a sweet but wavering voice answered. "The problem's with my husband."

I heard a voice in the background—shrill and peculiar: "Help! Help me! Help!"

"Shut up, Pauli. I'm on the phone," she shouted.

I was rattled by the rough exchange. "What's going on? Is that your husband?"

"Good heavens, no. That's our parrot."

Under other circumstances, mistaking a woman's parrot for her husband would have been laughable. But the tone of her voice indicated this was no laughing matter.

"My husband is a diabetic. He takes insulin every day. Today he's confused. He doesn't know where he is or who I am." Her words were knitted together by anxiety.

I felt embarrassed, but recovered quickly. "How old is he?"

"He's seventy-five."

"Is this a new problem?"

"Yes."

"Did he get his insulin today?"

"Yes he did."

"Has he been sick at all?"

"I think maybe he's running a little fever. He hasn't felt much like eating."

"Can he drink liquids?"

"Yes."

The choices weren't good. Either he was having a hypoglycemic reaction from his insulin and bottomed out his blood sugar, or he was harboring an infection, as diabetics are prone to do, and his confusion was from that—or both.

"Mrs. Jordan, I want you to give him some orange juice or other sweet fruit juice now. Then call 911. Don't wait, okay?"

"Okay. Thank you."

"Thank you! Thank you!" Pauli had to have the last word.

TELEPHONE TRIAGE

A massive electronic network across the country connects people like nerve cells in an organism. As Elie Abel said, "No blare of trumpets announces a modern crisis.... in these matter of fact times, a telephone call will do." The telephone is the entry point for many people into the health care system, whether from the honeycombed isolation of inner-city, high-rise projects or the rugged expanses of rural America. The professional sitting on the other end of the line must determine the level of risk, the appropriate referral, and the most reasonable time-frame for dealing with the problem. There are no visual cues; only the voice and the pauses between words.

Nurse practitioners perform telephone triage. They are "gatekeepers" in the unique way they treat patients with acute, self-limiting problems and stable, chronic illnesses. The training and experience of the nurse practitioner are crucial to knowing when to see patients or appropriately and cost-effectively refer them to physician specialists. Many problems can be managed over the phone. Telephone triage gives added meaning to Dr. Richard Smith's advice: "If you listen to the patient, he or she will tell you the diagnosis."

Unfortunately, critically ill patients or their spouses may be placed on hold when they call the clinic due to the volume of callers. Most offices and hospitals with an automated answering system now instruct patients with emergencies to hang up and call 911 immediately. Patients should rush to the ER rather than try to schedule a clinic visit when they are seriously ill.

CONFUSION

Confusion in persons over the age of 65 is usually a symptom of delirium or dementia. In as many as 25% of demented individuals, delirium and dementia coexist. Delirium acutely and abruptly alters consciousness as well as cognition, whereas dementia is a slowly progressive disorder of cognition. The mental status of a patient with delirium fluctuates throughout the day, sometimes moment to moment, and attention span is short. Physiological and psychomotor changes may be marked. Delirium is more often reversible or treatable than dementia is.

Causes of delirium include infections, medications, and metabolic disorders, such as diabetes. The medications most likely to induce delirium are anticholinergic agents, antihistamines, benzodiazepines, cardiovascular drugs, hypoglycemics, narcotic and nonnarcotic analgesics, and psychotropic drugs. Almost any new drug in a delirious patient must be viewed as the possible reason for delirium.

*   *   *

"They Are Little White Pills"

The next caller on my list was Ralph Alphonso. "Oh, yes, thank you so much for calling back," he said. "My wife takes pills for her heart and cholesterol and she's running out. She has only a few more left. They are little white pills."

If you only knew how many kinds of small white pills there are.

"Okay. Do you have the bottle there?"

"No, but my wife laid them out on the counter." He began rattling off descriptions of all the medications before I could stop him. "This here one's football-shaped and kinda pink. There's two little white ones: one has a crack down the middle, the other's smooth. Then there's this one little one—I guess it's peach colored." He finally stopped.

"I really need the names of the medications."

"I thought you're supposed to know the names of the drugs based on the appearance of the pills."

I chuckled. "When was your wife last seen in the clinic?"

"Well, it's been awhile. She missed a few clinic appointments."

"I'm going to have her chart pulled. If she hasn't been seen recently enough in the clinic, I can't refill her prescription. Her heart condition may have changed, she may have other problems, or the medications she takes may not agree with each other."

"But she *needs* her medicine," the man argued, sounding more protective than persuasive.

"Mr. Alphonso, I want to help you. I'll phone in a small refill to the pharmacy once I confirm the drug and dosage in her chart. That will be enough to last until she can get an appointment. You must phone in to make her an appointment today, because patients who take these kinds of heart medications need to be examined regularly. We really want to make sure she is safe. No one will give you any more refills after this."

"Okay."

Ralph Alphonso was one of many callers who expected nothing less than clairvoyance. How could people with serious conditions think they should get refills indefinitely without being seen again? It would be too dangerous that way.

DRUG INTERACTIONS AND ADVERSE REACTIONS

Drug incompatibilities and adverse drug events cost $136 billion a year, according to *The Essential Guide to Prescriptive Drugs*. Although adverse drug events are a potential problem for people of all ages, the aged, who account for 35% of prescription drug expenditures, are at highest risk.

About 75% of independently living, older individuals take more than one prescription drug and also regularly use non-prescription drugs. Roughly half may take three or more drugs (polypharmacy). They are more likely to have side effects from polypharmacy than younger patients are due to age-related changes in the body's response to drugs and drug disposition, such as reduced drug metabolism and excretion. As the number of medications grows, so do the possibilities and unpredictability of adverse interactions. One medical problem of the aged patient may deteriorate due to treatment of another, such as osteoporosis worsened by steroid treatment of COPD.

To reduce the risk of adverse interactions, avoid polypharmacy or simplify the drug regimen. Stopping a drug that induces liver enzymes may raise blood levels of other drugs, so both dosages should be reduced. If multiple drugs are necessary, use the least toxic drugs at the lowest effective doses. Nonpharmacologic approaches may replace drug treatment or allow drug dosages to be reduced. Intermittent re-evaluation of a patient's need for medication will signal when a drug is no longer necessary or safe.

Educate patients about possible adverse drug interactions. Make sure patients do not to swap medications or fragment their care by seeing multiple health care providers who prescribe different but equivalent medications. Point out that a patient's use of alcohol, caffeine, and cigarette smoking influences drug efficacy and safety. A careful history will identify bad habits that cause disease and create a need for medications, such as excessive caffeinism and anxiety, or smoking and peptic ulcer disease.

Certain drugs don't mix: antacids and quinolone antibiotics, alcohol and chronic warfarin. Some drugs are no-nos for particular diseases: ibuprofen in chronic renal disease or hypertension, beta-blockers in asthma, cisapride in urinary incontinence. In aged patients, increase safety by making the following substitutions: risperidone for haloperidol in aggression-dementia, SSRI's for tricyclic antidepressants in depression, salsalate for indomethacin in chronic pain, and donepezil for tacrine in dementia.

Pharmacists usually function as a check-and-balance system for prescribing health care providers, but patient education about drugs and diseases provides extra security.

*   *   *

"It's a Yellow Powder"

"Hi, this is Aida Guzman. I have a question for you."

"Sure, how can I help you?" I asked.

"I want to know if I can take something with my medication."

"What is it?"

"I've been taking arthritis medication."

"Which one?"

"I don't know."

"Do you have the medication bottle?"

"Yes. I'll go get it."

I heard the clunk of the receiver and her fading footfalls as she ran to get the bottle. My mind filled the time—*she must have gone into another room*—by imagining a shiny, checkered linoleum floor. Perhaps I was merely probing my own distant past.

When she came back, she was a little out of breath. I had her spell the name of the medication for me.

"Okay," I said. "Now what's the other medication you have the question about?"

There was silence at the other end of the line. I started thinking about what else she might be on.

"Well, it's sorta medication."

"What do you mean?"

"It's a yellow powder."

"What?"

"You know—a powder. I'm supposed to put it in my tea or mix it with something."

"Where did you get the powder from?"

The woman hesitated. "It's from a healer that my people go to."

"Do you know what's in the powder?"

"No."

"Does it say anything on the jar?"

"No. She told me it's supposed to be good for arthritis. I once had cancer and she gave me some bad-tasting blue water to drink for a month. Now the cancer's gone. My doctor say's it's a miracle. So I believe her when she tells me anything."

I was astounded that the patient didn't know what the powder was yet she would take it into her body. I told her I couldn't advise her on the powder because I didn't know what it was. It was not a useful answer, but was an honest one. As far as the blue water—I would need a lot more convincing about that.

Aida Guzman was not an exception. Many of our culturally diverse patients sought alternative medical opinions. Along with seeing their own clinic health care provider, they consulted a local, respected, folk healer. This person usually charged five or ten dollars for their time and gave out remedies ranging from spiritual counseling to benign herbs. I felt that they took advantage of those who already were living on a tight budget, but the patients thought otherwise.

A cardinal rule of my practice is that my own personal beliefs and values shouldn't interfere with the patient's care as long as alternative methods cause no harm and the patient believes their well-being has improved. I prefer that my patients tell me who else they're seeing and what alternative remedies they are taking. It's better to work with your patient and have an open, trusting relationship than have one with secrets.

ALTERNATIVE THERAPIES

Many Americans don't need convincing. More and more people are relying on alternative therapies for medical problems today, ranging from easing the mind to fighting the flu. It's estimated that one-third of all Americans, most of whom are educated, upper-income whites between 25 and 50 years old, use "unconventional" medical treatments. In 1990, more Americans sought out providers of unconventional therapy than they sought primary care providers. This is clearly something the public wants.

What's so unconventional? These therapies include acupuncture, biofeedback, chelation therapy, chiropractic manipulation, guided imagery, herbal remedies, homeopathic treatments, massage therapy, megavitamin treatments, naturopathy, relaxation techniques, therapeutic touch, and others. The National Institutes of Health, at the instruction of Congress, now funds studies of alternative therapies.

The return to herbal medicine is fueled by how profitable plants have been to modern medicine. Digitalis, a heart medication from foxglove, is one of the best known, plant-derived drugs. Aspirin once was extracted from the bark of the willow tree. Atropine, curare, ephedrine, morphine, physostigmine, reserpine, and many other drugs were obtained from plants. Even common household foods and spices, like blueberries, broccoli, cayenne, cranberries, garlic, green tea, grapes, licorice, soy, and tomatoes, hold medicinal value says James Duke, author of *The Green Pharmacy*.

Four billion persons, 80% of the world's population, use herbal medicine in primary health care according to the WHO. Benefits of herbal remedies are highly touted in the lay press. The resurgence of herbal therapies is due to a renewed interest in naturalism and the health care system's changing focus on preventative care. The result is a booming, largely unregulated market for herbal preparations. It's big business—about $20 billion big—analysts say.

Plants upstaging pharmaceuticals? Saint-John's-root is the most popular antidepressant in Germany. Many people pop Enchinacae to boost the immune system and prevent infection. In the U.S., only nine herbs are approved by the FDA for selected indications. The German Commission E reviewed information on the more than 1,400 herbal drugs, but most have not been evaluated in humans. The WHO has listed more than 20,000 plants as being used for therapeutic purposes.

Herbal medicine sounds wonderful. The answer, it turns out, is not simple. Support for herbal remedies is largely anecdotal. Herbs must be considered as drugs with all the potential risks and side effects of drugs. They can be harmful or fatal. Hepatitis has been reported after ingestion of asafetida, chaparral leaf, Chinese herbs, gentian, germander blossoms, hops, mistletoe, senna fruit extracts, skullcap, and valerian. Kola nut and Ma huang, which contain caffeine and ephedrine, can cause death, heart attack and arrhythmias, psychosis, seizures, and stroke.

Are natural phen-fens safe? Watch out. Since the phen-fen drug combination was yanked off the market by the FDA for fatal heart problems, many people have clamored for natural alternatives. Unfortunately, Ephedra, the active ingredient in many such preparations, has also caused deaths.

The following are guidelines for herbal use. Do not to take herbs during pregnancy, while attempting to become pregnant, or while nursing. Babies or young children should not be given herbs. Herbs should not be consumed daily or in large doses. Avoid preparations that fail to list all ingredients and quantities or that contain comfrey.

As Eric Hodges said, "A miracle drug is a drug that will do what the label says it will do."

*   *   *

"Is This Something New You Gave Me?"

"I just had my prescription filled. The name of the medicine on the new bottle is different than on my old bottle. You might remember me from the clinic today. My name is Ray Palmer."

"Mr. Palmer, what does it say on the new bottle?"

"Okay, I have it here. I can't pronounce it so I'll spell it: *C-l-o-n-*

a-z-e-p-a-m. Is this something new you gave me?"

I was appalled. His hypertension was well controlled on clonidine and a diuretic. Clonazepam was an anticonvulsant. "Did you take any yet?"

"No."

"Good. You've gotten the wrong medication. I'll call your pharmacist and get it cleared up."

"Okay. I'm real careful about that sort of thing. My brother-in-law got a medicine supposedly for migraine headaches and he got a hard-on. It lasted for a day. He was in quite a bit of pain. I don't want that to happen to me." He laughed.

I didn't expected him to say that; at least he wasn't upset over the mix-up. When I hung up the receiver, I wondered if I had written the wrong prescription. Those two drugs are frequently mixed up by prescribers and pharmacists. I pulled his clinic chart and found a photocopy of his prescription. It said *clonidine.* I breathed a sigh of relief.

The pharmacist I contacted pulled up the script. "No, it's clonidine on the prescription. What did the patient get?"

"He says he got *clonazepam.*"

"Oh shoot, that's our fault. Damn. Did he start taking it?"

"He says no."

"Have him come back and I'll redo the prescription. Thanks for calling, Doc."

Whoops! To err is human; to admit it makes a good pharmacist in my eyes.

LOOK- AND SOUND-ALIKES

Over 1000 drug names look or sound alike. The spelling of Clonopin™ was changed to Klonopin™ as a result of confusion with clonidine. Zantac™ and Xanax™ or zithromycin and cipromycin also sound similar. "Sound-alikes" cause problems with telephoned prescriptions. Some are catastrophic.

To help prevent errors, examine your prescription carefully. Check the drug name and disorder and read the written instructions. Compare the labels with the written name of the drug from your doctor. More than one-half of patients take prescription drugs incorrectly. A little time spent double-checking can prevent a serious error.

*   *   *

"I Want to Play Touch Football"

"It's my back. It wakes me up at night. I have pain when I do certain movements, sit, or stand too long." Erin Bromberg, a man in his late twenties, worked as a junior executive in a downtown office building.

I questioned him about additional symptoms, like bowel or bladder problems, arm or leg weakness, or loss of sensation, but he said he felt fine otherwise. When I first started to examine him, there were a lot of possibilities. As I went along, the field narrowed. "Does this hurt?" I asked, lifting his leg into the air while he lay flat on his back on the examining table?

"Ah, slightly. Not much."

I lowered that leg and tested the other one.

"No, it just pulls in the back of my knee some."

That was a negative straight-leg-raising test. Patients with acute disk pain could not tolerate such a maneuver. He was able to walk on his toes. Even pressing on his spine while he stood leaning forward or to either side did not bother him. I took the time to do a careful deep tendon reflex examination, but I could find nothing neurologically wrong with him. He did have moderate muscle tenderness and spasm over the lower back.

"Are you sure you didn't do anything that could have triggered this?"

"Not that I recall."

"Think back over the past two weeks. Any heavy lifting, falling, or working in unusual positions?"

He thought it over. "Well, a couple of weeks ago, I helped move some boxes in the storage room at work, but I felt okay. It wasn't a big deal."

"How about the weekends? What kind of physical activity do you do?"

"I pal around with my buddies."

"Doing what?"

"Well, we like to play football."

"And does that give you any problems?"

"I am pretty sore after that."

"Do you think it could be the football activities."

"Well, I suppose it could be, but—*nah*. I've been doing this for years."

Here was a guy with a sedentary job approaching thirty. He had the build of an ex-jock. Now he was having trouble admitting that football could be the offender.

"This weekend I want to play touch football. I'm too young to start cutting back. I used to have washboard abs and pump iron. At least I still have weekend football. Do you have any pain pills?"

"I would suggest you take ibuprofen. The obvious thing is that you shouldn't play this weekend. You've got muscle pain and spasm. That means you've got some strain injury and inflammation. Re-injury will make it worse. Some people end up with a chronic problem because they did not go easier at the beginning. Let pain be your guide. You may find some back strengthening exercises useful."

He laughed. "Well, thank you very much for checking me over."

"I can tell by the look on your face that you're going to play football again this weekend."

"Of course, I'm gonna. I'll just take more ibuprofen."

So goes another weekend warrior.

LOW BACK PAIN

The primary source of physical discomfort among Americans is back pain. We must fight for a healthy back. One enormous obstacle is sitting. How can something so natural be so bad for your back? Prolonged sitting places 40% more pressure or load on the vertebral disks than standing does. Static posture is unavoidable even if you're not one of the 50 million office workers or so called "desk jockeys" in the U.S. We sit to drive automobiles, chat on the phone, check our e-mail, eat, pay bills, watch TV—to name a few activities. Most adults sit in front to the television more than two hours a day.

A simple backache stems from "mechanical" irritation of muscles or tendons in the lumbosacral region, buttocks, or thighs. According to a survey by the National Center for Health Statistics, musculoskeletal disorders account for more clinic visits than any other problem. Backache usually affects otherwise healthy people between the ages of 20 and 55 years. The risk factors for back pain becoming chronic are adversarial medicolegal proceedings, depressive symptoms, heavy smoking, low job satisfaction, personal problems, poor physical fitness and health, poor trunk muscle strength and endurance, and psychological stress.

The solution? Ninety percent of back pain subsides on its own within a month, usually aided only with over-the-counter pain medications or lifestyle changes. For chronic, uncomplicated back pain, the current recommendation is staying active as much as possible (rather than bed rest), back exercises, and ice-pack self-treatments.

In more difficult cases, acupuncture, electrical stimulation, massage, physical therapy, short-term manipulation, or ultrasound treatment are options. In selected patients only, there may be a role for local steroid injections into trigger points. Drug therapies include non-narcotic analegesics, muscle relaxants, and antidepressants. Only 1 to 2% of adults with low-back pain should be considered surgical candidates.

Back pain also results from injury to nerve roots or spinal cord disorders. Nerve root inflammation, usually from lumbosacral spine disk disease, produces pain and numbness over an area controlled by one nerve root. Half of such patients recover in 6 weeks with conservative management, otherwise they need to be referred for further evaluation. When a serious spinal cord condition is present, especially at the base of the spine (cauda equina syndrome), patients may have leg weakness and absence of reflexes in the legs, loss of anal sphincter tone, "saddle" anesthesia (anus, genitals, perineum), and urinary incontinence. Treatment of the underlying problem is essential. About 2.9 back surgeries are done each year per 1,000 persons in the U.S.

We're picking on the back. Other areas get their share of aches and pains. Having a finger get stuck in "trigger finger" position is common in rheumatoid arthritis, but can happen to anyone. Carpal tunnel syndrome and tenosynovitis are common wrist problems due to repetitive tendon irritation. "Tennis elbow" and "golfer's elbow" are forms of epicondylitis. The two most common causes of an acutely painful shoulder are bicipital tendinitis and deltoid bursitis. A "frozen shoulder" is a sign of adhesive capsulitis, a deeper malady than rotator cuff inflammation. Bursitis attacks heels, hips, and knees as well. A variety of joint injuries produce the "giving way," "locking," "pop," or "tear" that should prompt a referral.

*   *   *

"My Toe Is Throbbing"

Mark Blandon, a fifty-year-old man, was dressed impeccably. His white shirt looked starched, his yellow power-tie was fastened with a gold pin, and his business suit was well tailored. Only one thing did not fit the picture: he had taken off his left shoe and sock. At work on his laptop, he spread his papers over the examining table. The freckles on his scalp were visible through his thinning, gray-streaked, red hair, which he wore combed from ear to ear in a futile effort to cover his baldness.

The patient didn't acknowledge my arrival. As I tried to take a history, he kept working and answered my questions only after episodic keystrokes and brief delays.

"Excuse me, Mr. Blandon, could you put away your computer while I talk to you?"

"Oh, sure, sorry. I've got a deadline to meet. I hate wasting time." He smiled a half-second smile.

Wasting time?

"So what brings you here today?"

"I've had gout before in my foot. It seems to have flared up again. Just when I need to be on my feet and on the go, my damn foot is acting up. It's probably my fault—I've been entertaining clients quite a bit. And that includes rich foods, desserts, and alcohol. Can you give me something for the pain so I can get going? I have a meeting in an hour." A brief glance at his watch revved him up more. "I know it's gout, I don't need an x-ray. It's the ball of my left foot. I can't put it into my leather shoe without extreme pain. It should be obvious to you I can't wear a tennis shoe with a business outfit."

The foot, which was red, excessively warm, swollen, and exquisitely tender to touch, *did* match the description of gout. I put him on a high dose of a non-steroidal anti-inflammatory drug. He packed it up and left precipitously—a mini-twister.

A week later, I got a call from Detroit. It was Mark Blandon.

"My toe is throbbing and killing me again. Can you call in a prescription for me? I'm holed up in my hotel room and can't get around to see a doctor. I'm going to be here over the weekend."

"Did you bring your medicine with you?"

"No, I stopped it because I was doing better."

Why am I not surprised?

"I can't call it in out of state, but I'll get one of the doctors here who can."

"Great. Get on that right away," he said in his command voice.

We arranged for Mr. Blandon to get his medication. But this was a new experience for me. I had never been in the military before.

THE ATTACK OF GOUT

When Anton Van Leeuwenhoek invented the microscope in the late 17th century, one of the first things he inspected was crystals from a gouty joint. Gout, a metabolic disease, once called a "disease of kings," has been with us a very long time. In the 17th century, English physician Thomas Sydenham said of it: "Gout, unlike any other disease, kills more rich men than poor, more wise men than simple."

Deposits of urates (tophus) cause a reactive, recurrent arthritis, usually of the first toe (metatarsophalangeal joint), but sometimes of the ankle, foot, knee, or shoulder (polyarthropathy). Overproduction or undersecretion of uric acid is the cause of the hyperuricemia. Over time, urate deposits in bone, cartilage, joints, and subcutaneous tissues leads to deformities (destructive arthropathy). Gout sometimes runs in families. Nearly 90% of patients with primary gout, which is common in Pacific islanders, are men over 30 years of age.

Attacks are sudden. The pain usually begins at night. Symptoms of the attack respond dramatically to non-steroidal anti-inflammatory drugs or colchicine, analgesics, bed rest, and corticosteroids if necessary. After the acute episode subsides, the skin over the affected joint desquamates and itches. Simultaneous treatment of the hyperuricemia and the gouty arthritis is a common mistake, which can aggravate the attack.

The time to treat the hyperuricemia is during the asymptomatic periods between attacks, when it will reduce the frequency and severity of attacks by minimizing urate deposition. Potentially reversible secondary causes of gout are certain medications (low-dose aspirin, nicotinic acid, thiazide, and loop diuretics), frequent alcohol consumption, high purine diet, and obesity. Patients with a single episode of gout who lose weight and stop drinking alcohol may not require medications for gout. If drug treatment is necessary, uricosuric drugs, which act on normal kidneys to help lose urates to the urine, or allopurinol may be used.

When a large joint is acutely painful and has an effusion, it should be aspirated. The joint fluid provides clues to the diagnosis. Normal joint fluid is very clear, viscous, and low in white blood cells (less than 1000/μl). In gout and other inflammatory diseases, the fluid is turbid and white blood cell counts climb to 30,000 to 60,000. The urate crystals of gout under a polarizing microscope look brilliant against the dark field. In the presence of joint infection, the synovial fluid turns very turbid or purulent, white blood cell cells soar to 100,000 to 200,000, and the Gram's stain reveals organisms.

While aspirating a knee is straightforward for most experienced health care providers, aspiration of other joints should probably be referred to a rheumatologic or orthopedic specialist.

15

Overheating the Engine

Time and fevers burn away
—WYSTAN HUGH AUDEN

Fever itself is Nature's instrument
—THOMAS SYDENHAM

Show him death, and he'll be content with fever
—PERSIAN PROVERB

*I reckon being ill as one of the great pleasures of life,
provided one is not too ill and is not obliged to work until one is
better*
—SAMUEL BUTLER

*I enjoy convalescence.
It is the part that makes the illness worth while*
—GEORGE BERNARD SHAW

"Last Night It Was One-Hundred-and-Three"

I picked up the phone to hear a woman coughing. It was a coarse, deep, moist-sounding cough that lasted for about fifteen seconds. In the background, a baby cried vigorously, pausing briefly before hitting the big crescendo.

The woman took a deep breath and identified herself as Keiko Nakasugi. "I don't feel too good. I caught a head cold from my baby a couple weeks ago. That went away, but I can't seem to shake this cough."

"Do you have a fever?"

"Yeah. Last night it was one-hundred-and three."

"Are you taking anything for it?"

"Ibuprofen. The temperature doesn't go down much and I have chills. I seem to get real hot then chills."

"Any other symptoms?"

"My back aches a lot the past couple days. And when I lie down, it's harder to breath. The cough keeps me awake at night. My husband's sleeping on the couch because of it. I have a sore throat from coughing so much now. My ribs hurt and I get a bad headache every time I have a coughing spell. My muscles hurt so bad, I brace myself with sofa pillows when I start coughing."

"Do you bring up anything when you cough?"

"This dark brown-green stuff. It tastes terrible and makes me gag it's so thick."

"Do you have an appetite?"

"No. I feel nauseous, but I'm not vomiting."

"Are you taking any cough medicines?"

"Yes, but nothing's helping. I've gone through two bottles of cough syrup."

"Well, you may have pneumonia and you should be seen. We probably have to do a chest x-ray. You should come to the clinic today."

"I need to bring my baby in with me because I don't have a babysitter."

"That's okay."

She said good-bye and hung up. A few moments later, the phone rang again. "I forgot to tell you, I'm breast-feeding. Does that make a difference?"

"Yes, you can't breast feed while you're on medication. But you still need to be treated."

A week later, Keiko Nakasugi contacted me again. She explained that she'd been evaluated by her own physician who treated her with an antibiotic for pneumonia. Even while alternating acetaminophen and ibuprofen every two hours, she had a fever of one-hundred-and-one to one-hundred-and-two for three days and slept most of the time.

"The fever finally broke. What I'm calling about is being so washed out. I don't feel like doing anything. Do you know how hard it is to take care of a baby and a husband when all you want to do is lay down and sleep? My mother, who lives in town, had to come over to help with the baby. Thank God for her. I can't get through the day without a two or three hour nap. My husband complains I don't make conversation. I'm told I stare off until someone calls to me or touches me. Am I depressed or something?"

"Do you have headaches?"

"Only when I get to coughing a lot."

"Do you have a stiff neck?"

"No. I can move my head all around."

That makes meningitis unlikely, I reasoned. "Are you drinking lots of fluids?"

"Yeah."

"Are you peeing clear?"

"Well, it's yellow."

"Okay, you need more fluids. You may be a little dehydrated. Are you eating three meals a day?"

"Yes. My husband went shopping and got me some stuff I can fix for myself during the day."

"Good. It sounds like you have post-viral syndrome. I think your illness was probably viral pneumonia because your temperature stayed up for a couple of days even on antibiotics. Let's be sure you're on an antibiotic for mycoplasma pneumonia because mycoplasma can do this and should be treated longer than the usual pneumonia. If things get worse or the fever returns come back to see us. I suspect you will improve a small amount each day. It may take a few weeks to bounce back to normal. Get the rest you feel you need."

THE SPECTER OF PNEUMONIA

When you consider that as many as 50 million bacteria can reside in an inhaled droplet of liquid, how respiratory infections spread so rapidly in a community is frightfully clear. Prior to the antibiotic era, hospitals opened their windows to reduce droplet transmission of infectious diseases.

Pneumonia, a persistent, major health problem, is an infection of the lower respiratory tract. Evidence of pneumonia has been found in Egyptian mummies. Hippocrates diagnosed pneumonia long before the modern stethoscope had been invented. Charlemagne, conqueror of the largest empire of his day, died of it; so did the American novelist, Thomas Wolfe. The aging Sir William Osler, English physician and educator, was riding on a train when the dipping of the train car made him aware of fluid in his chest. He diagnosed his own fatal pneumonia, calling it prophetically "the old man's friend" and the "captain of death."

Today society spends four billion dollars yearly on hospitalization for pneumonia alone. Approximately 15% of the 4 million Americans who contract community-acquired pneumonia (CAP) each year are hospitalized.

What are the warning signs? Coughing that brings up blood, even specks, or persists for weeks, fever over 101° F, shortness of breath, and wheezing warn of a serious infection. Acute bronchitis, an infection of the bronchial tree that produces swelling and mucus, can be confused with pneumonia. In both bronchitis and pneumonia, the cough produces purulent or clear sputum and may last several weeks. Coughing alone is rather nonspecific because it can be triggered by allergies, asthma, sinusitis, or upper respiratory tract infections. While the same organisms may be involved in either infection, viruses cause up to 95% of the cases of acute bronchitis. Both infections trigger bronchospasm.

How does pneumonia take root? Microorganisms invade the lung from the blood or the airways by aspiration or inhalation. Identifying the specific infectious agent is difficult, so newer terminology that differentiates between CAP and hospital-acquired pneumonia (HAP) has supplanted older terms that attempted to classify by microorganism. The usual pathogens are *Streptococcus pneumoniae* (pneumococcus), *Haemophilus influenza, Mycoplasma pneumoniae, Chla-*

mydia pneumoniae, and respiratory viruses. Miscellaneous organisms include aerobic gram-negative bacilli, endemic fungi, *Legionella*, *Moraxella catarrhalis*, *Mycobacterium tuberculosis*, and *Staphylococcus aureus*.

While a chest x-ray is part of the initial evaluation of a patient with pneumonia, sputum studies should be reserved for suspicion of fungi, *Legionella*, mycobacteria, and *Pneumocystis carinii*. An arterial blood gas analysis, blood cultures, and complete blood count are helpful adjuncts to clinical decisions about treatment and hospital admission in seriously ill patients. In the presence of symptomatic pleural effusion, especially when a bacterial cause is suspected, it's time for thoracentesis, with cell counts, chemistries, cultures, and gram stains.

How aggressive should therapy be? The treatment of CAP is based on patient age, evidence of severe infection (altered mental status, dehydration, high fever or low body temperature, hypoxemia, tachypnea, and other factors), and presence of comorbid diseases. According to the 1998 recommendations of the Infectious Diseases Society of America for CAP in *otherwise healthy* outpatients younger than 60 years of age, treatment for 10 to 14 days with a macrolide antibiotic or with or doxycycline is adequate. In older patients with comorbidity or *hospitalized* patients, a second- or third-generation cephalosporin, sulfa combination drug, or a beta-lactam combined with a beta-lactamase inhibitor is preferable. The patient usually improves before the chest x-ray does.

Here's good news. Preventative vaccines for pneumonia have had a beneficial impact and could be used much more often than they are. Many of the 40,000 persons in the U.S. who still die each year from pneumococcal infections could be saved by vaccination. The Advisory Committee on Immunization Practices recommends the pneumococcal polysaccharide (23-valent) vaccine for everyone 65 years of age and others with various risk factors. They should be revaccinated every five years. Although vaccines are available only against pneumococcus and influenza, the development of vaccines for other organisms is an active area of research.

VACCINATION

An Inquiry into the Causes and Effects of the Variola Vaccine, a Disease Discovered in Some of the Western Counties of England, Particularly Gloucestershire, and Known by the Name of Cowpox.

The year was 1798. Edward Jenner had written the treatise that would lead to the world's first compulsory vaccination program in 1835. Despite its long-winded title, the work explained clearly how to use harmless cowpox to immunize against the deadly and disfiguring smallpox. The devastating disease that Fernando Cortez's men inadvertently introduced to the native population of Mexico and later re-emerged with greater virulence in Europe could now be prevented. The term *vaccination* was coined from the Latin *vaccinia*, meaning cowpox.

Thomas Jefferson took great interest in the first vaccinations performed in the U.S. in 1799. He was so pleased with the results of Professor Benjamin Waterhouse's "experiments" that he had 18 members of his household vaccinated. Most royalty and dignitaries in Europe had taken the precautionary step of having smallpox vaccines tested on commoners before allowing their own families to be inoculated, according to the medical historian Frederick F. Cartwright.

Vaccines continue to protect us from many microbial infections, mostly viruses, whether through active immunization with live attenuated viruses or passive immunization with inactivated whole or split viruses. No one needs to contract diphtheria, measles, mumps, polio, rubella, or tetanus. For patients at risk due to chronic diseases or a compromised immune system, vaccination against hepatitis, influenza, and pneumococcus are now commonplace.

The Advisory Committee on Immunization Practices strongly recommends that all health care workers be vaccinated against hepatitis B, influenza, measles, mumps, rubella, and varicella, unless they have documented immunity. Under certain circumstances, but not routinely, immunization against diphtheria, hepatitis A, meningococcus, pneumococcus, smallpox, tetanus, tuberculosis, or typhoid also may be indicated. These recommendations apply to emergency personnel and those who work in health departments, hospitals, laboratories, nursing homes, private physicians' offices, and schools.

Sadly, even as the search for new vaccines against cancer and AIDS marches on, the public pendulum has swung away from compulsory childhood vaccination. A new generation once again faces the possible re-emergence of the dreadful diseases vaccinations protected us from. This is a modern tragedy.

TOPPING THE THERMOMETER

Fevers. They proceed in three stages. As the body temperature rises, the patient feels cold, has chills and headache, and may shiver violently. The skin's cold and pale. Then the skin becomes flushed and hot; the temperature plateaus. As body temperature falls, the patient perspires profusely and may urinate.

How high can they skyrocket? During infections, certain white blood cells (monocyte-macrophages) produce chemicals (pyrogenic cytokines) that act on the hypothalamus to increase body temperature. Due to the convulsions, irreversible brain damage, and lethal consequences that would result, the brain doesn't usually permit human body temperature exceed 107° Fahrenheit (41.1° centigrade) except during heat stroke and malignant hyperthermia (a muscle disease). Anyone who has had a fever of 103° F can imagine how 4 more degrees would feel!

The highest recorded fever: 115.7° F. The patient had heatstroke and wasn't discharged from the hospital until 24 days later.

*   *   *

"I Can't Eat Nothin'"

The telephone rang again. This time it was a young man who called himself Tyron Wells. "How are you doing?" I asked.

"I wouldn't be calling if I was feeling well."

Oh boy, here we go.

"Tell me what the problem is."

"I can't leave the apartment. I've got the runs. It's been this way for three days. Yesterday I was vomikin', but that stopped. Now every time I drink somethin', I run to the toilet five minutes later. Yesterday, I messed my pants 'cause I didn't make it in time. I'm weak and dizzy. I can't eat nothin'. Lordy, I'm in trouble."

"Do you have any medicine for diarrhea at home?"

"No. That's why I'm callin'."

"Do you have a fever?"

"I don't know. I feel hot, but we ain't got no ter-mom-o-ter."

"Do you have any blood in your stool?"

"In my what?"

"In your poop?"

"I don't look at that stuff. It smell bad, too."

In the background I heard: "Get off the phone, Tyron. I need to call my boyfriend."

"Do you have any other symptoms, Tyron?" I asked.

"I feels sick to my stomach."

My fact-finding mission hadn't gone smoothly, but I was getting the picture. "It sounds like you have gastroenteritis."

"*Gastro-extra-itis*? What's that?"

"No. *Gastro* means stomach and *enteritis* means bowels. It's a virus that affects your stomach and your bowels. You have to give them a rest."

"Is it the flu?"

"No."

"So how do I get rid of it?"

"Take it easy until it passes and drink clear liquids."

"What are they?"

"If you can see through it, you can drink it—water, weak tea, apple juice, that sort of liquid. Keep them at room temperature because any extremes of temperature will stimulate your bowels. Drink until you pee clear."

"When can I eat again?"

"Wait forty-eight hours, then try some light food. You can have applesauce, bananas, rice or noodles, dry toast or crackers. If you do okay on that for a day, then try some soup. *No* salads, *no* vegetables, *no* fruits, and *no* milk."

"How 'bout pizza?"

"Are you kidding?"

GASTROENTERITIS

The culprit goes by many aliases: stomach virus, the grippe, the runs, Montezuma's revenge. Invisible, it strikes unexpectedly, willing to ruin a weekend or vacation, spread through a whole school, or publicly embarrass a President, showing no mercy toward the weak and vulnerable. It can be devious, hanging around a lot longer than it should, but there's no escaping it's real identity.

Viruses are responsible for an estimated 30 to 40% of infectious diarrhea in the U.S. They attack both the upper and lower gastrointestinal tract (gastroenteritis) or lower tract alone (enterocolitis). Enteric adenoviruses and astroviruses are common viral diarrheal pathogens in adults. Rotaviruses spread from infected children to adults, and the Norwalk agent makes the rounds among institutionalized patients.

Most cases of acute viral gastroenteritis are self-limited and require only supportive measures. Common reasons for prolonged illness or complications are advanced age, compromising medical conditions, dehydration due to inability to take clear liquids, failure to restrict the diet, or severe infection.

Other bad guys: bacteria (*Campylobacter jejuni, Yersinia*) and various protozoa (*Giardia, Entamoeba*). Without specific exposures or suspicions, these diagnostic considerations do not come into play unless symptoms last longer than 3 to 4 days, the diarrhea is bloody, or fever persists.

In food poisoning, which may cause vomiting or diarrhea, a person ingests toxins already produced by bacteria growing in the food (clostridia, staphylococci) or is infected by the organisms themselves (*E. coli, Salmonella*, shigellae, vibrios). Botulism (from clostridia), one of the most dramatic and serious of the food poisonings, results in paralysis.

Infections can't take all the blame. Non-infectious causes of vomiting and diarrhea include drug side effects, emotional stress, food intolerance, and poisoning by nitrites, mushrooms, or shellfish.

*   *   *

"I Want an Antibiotic"

"Oh-h-h-h-h."

What a dreadful voice. The woman on the other end of the phone sounded like she had a clothespin on her nose.

"I feel like a truck ran over my body."

I learned that the caller was Camilla Lucovski, a middle-aged woman who was in good health until she came down with a fever, muscle aches, fatigue, nasal congestion, and a cough a few days ago.

"Do you have a fever now?"

"I had one for three days, but it passed. I'm still sneezing and have a sore throat and cough."

"Did you have a flu shot this year?"

"No, I didn't get a chance to."

"You may have the flu. It's the right time of year. Plenty of people are calling in with the same symptoms."

"I want an antibiotic."

"Why?"

"My doctor *always* gives me one when I have the flu."

A precedent had been set; it's hard to argue against precedent. "Were you in good health before you caught the flu?"

"Yes."

"Then you probably don't need one. If you did, I'd be happy to give it to you. But we have to be a little careful here."

"Why?"

"Antibiotics aren't appropriate for treating viral illnesses. The flu is caused by a *virus*. Antibiotics don't kill viruses. The flu runs its course over a few weeks with or without antibiotics. If you take antibiotics when you really don't have to, they may not work when you absolutely need them. They can also give you diarrhea, yeast infections, and allergic reactions."

"I never had any of that stuff before. If I don't get an antibiotic, I'm not going to get better." Her voice implied pouting.

"Sure you will," I cajoled. "It's going to require time. The flu is certain to pass no matter what you take. You have to make sure you drink enough fluids, eat, rest, and get some extra sleep."

"Well, I don't know." She was mollified only a little.

"Mrs. Lucovski, if your fever comes back, you're doing worse, or new symptoms develop, give me a call. You may have to come in to

be seen if that happens. I'll be glad to check you over."
"Well, all right."

THE ANTIBIOTIC CRISIS

The ancient Egyptians treated infections with moldy bread, anticipating the serendipitous discovery of penicillin mold by Alexander Fleming at St. Mary's Hospital in London by a few millennia. But the understanding and proliferation of antibiotics was a phenomenon of the twentieth century that has produced a multi-billion dollar industry. Surgeons in the Civil War and WWI would have given anything for a few of our outdated, first-generation antibiotics when they were forced to pile amputated limbs outside tents for lack of antimicrobials. When first introduced in the 1940's, antibiotics were haled as miracle drugs. Inadvertently we have diminished the miracle.

Antibiotics or not? Infectious disease experts reported that in 1992, more people were treated with the powerful antibiotic zithromycin than voted for George Bush! Bronchitis, head cold sinusitis, and other upper respiratory infections (URI's) account for one-third of all antibiotics prescribed. If more than 90% of are caused by viruses, why are antibiotics prescribed for 50 to 70% of patients with these conditions who seek medical attention?

One part of the answer has to due with human nature. Sick patients who visit their health care providers expect or demand a prescription for antibiotics. A common belief is: "If you don't get an antibiotic prescription at the doctor's office, he or she is not a good doctor." Many health care providers admit that antibiotics are probably not necessary, but cave in anyway. Another factor in antibiotic resistance is the crowded conditions of the inner city.

The consequence? Dangerous antibiotic resistance is now a worldwide crisis. While only about 1% of *S. pneumoniae* organisms were penicillin-resistant in 1980, as many as 25 to 30% are now; some are resistant to macrolides. *S. aureus* and enterococcus resistant to vancomycin have emerged in the 1990's.

When are antibiotics necessary and when is it better to watch and wait? Patients with community-acquired pneumonia and those with acute exacerbations of chronic bronchitis warrant an antibiotic. Otherwise healthy patients with acute bronchitis and patients with a sore throat without tonsillar exudate or adenopathy probably do not need an antibiotic. How "toxic" a patient appears, how long the symptoms have persisted without significant improvement, and the patient's overall state of health are all mitigating factors.

When antibiotics are required, a narrow-spectrum drug suffices if the most likely pathogen has been identified. If not, a broad-spectrum agent is preferable. Patients with family members in the same household who have taken antibiotics recently or work in a child day-care facility or long-term care center for the elderly may harbor resistant organisms. If compliance is apt to be a problem, choose an antibiotic that can be taken once or twice a day for the shortest period of time. Possible side effects and cost-saving factors need to be weighed individually.

THE FLU

I have a little bird and its name was Enza,
I opened the window and in-flew-Enza!
—ANONYMOUS

So cheerful little girls sang as they played in 1918 while influenza dispassionately annihilated 20 million individuals, including 1% of NYC's population. As common as influenza is today, it is not something to take lightly. Caused by an orthomyxovirus, it usually occurs as an epidemic. Influenza (the flu) was so named because the evil "influence" of the stars supposedly caused the disease.

Viruses have altered history as decisively as armies. They destroyed emperors, kings and queens, impacting on politics and the development of nations. Influenza may have transformed the outcome of WWI. In the summer of 1918, the German assault on France came to a grinding halt due to the influenza A outbreak, giving the Allies precious time to reorganize. Influenza caused more deaths than the war itself. In 1918 the virus circled the globe in 4 months. Today such an outbreak would travel infinitely faster and exact a higher toll of the world's 5.9 billion denizens—a sign of the times.

Influenza spreads by the respiratory route through tiny droplet nuclei. A simple sneeze expels droplets at up to 103 miles per hour; that covers a lot of territory in a hurry. Infected persons are miserable with chills, fever, headache, malaise, muscle aches, nasal stuffiness, non-productive cough, sore throat, and substernal soreness. Patients with influenza feel much worse than those with the common cold, which is spawned by different viruses. Both are common viral upper respiratory tract infections in adults.

The "flu shot," usually dispensed in the autumn, confers partial immunity for a few to several months, slashing the mortality and morbidity of influenza infections. Because the prevalence of influenza A, B, and C strains changes, the vaccine's antigenic configuration must also be changed yearly. Health care workers, nursing home residents, anyone over age 65, and those with lung or other debilitating diseases should be vaccinated. It takes two weeks to build up immunity after vaccination. Influenza vaccination is reimbursable by Medicare.

Once a person has contracted the flu, treatment is symptomatic. You've heard the advice before: analgesics, bed rest, and cough preparations. Oral or aerosolized antiviral drugs are reserved for severe cases or debilitated patients. Antibiotics, which are greatly over-prescribed for viral illnesses, should be saved for the treatment of bacterial complications, which can be otherwise fatal or result in chronic lung disease. Because influenza destroys the respiratory epithelium, bacterial infections of the ears (otitis media), bronchi (bronchitis), lungs (pneumonia), and sinuses (sinusitis) sometimes occur. Most healthy people recover completely.

*   *   *

"My Smokes Have Lost Their Taste"

How often do you get a call from a person complaining his cigarette's have lost their taste? That was Dino Papadinos' problem. I puzzled over that. Whatever the cause, I was starting to wish this could happen to all my heavy smokers. Then it hit me: this was not a good thing.

"What do you mean, Mr. Papadinos?"

"Well, they taste like cardboard or something, I don't know. I don't even feel like smoking them anymore."

"How long have you been a smoker?"

"Oh, about twenty years I'd say, maybe more."

"How many packs a day?"

"One to two." His gritty, smoking-deepened voice attested to the veracity of his statements.

"Tell me what else is going on?"

"Well, I haven't been feeling well. I'm tired. Then I wake up I don't have the energy to get going. I've been dragging myself to work, but I'll tell you, it's getting harder to do. Finally, today, I couldn't go in. That's why I'm calling now."

"Any fever?"

"I haven't checked. I feel warm to myself."

"Did you have any nausea or vomiting recently? Any cold or flu-like symptoms?"

"I did have a cold or something over the past couple of weeks."

"Do the whites of your eyes look yellow?"

"Well, it's funny you should ask. My wife's been saying my eyes look different."

"Yellow?"

"Just a minute." He shouted into the background, "Do my eyes look yellow to you?"

I heard a woman's voice growing louder. "Who are you talking to?" she asked.

"I called the clinic. Come on, she's waiting."

"I can't see," the woman said to him. "Look into the light here...ah... yeah, they're yellowish."

"Mr. Papadinos, are you a hemophiliac or have you received any blood products?"

"No."

"Have you ever been diagnosed with AIDS or HIV infection or do you have any reason to think you might be at risk?"

"No, nothing like that, but I've been traveling."

"Out of the country?"

"Yeah, eating out and all that."

"Do you eat shell fish much?"

"Well, yeah, I have been lately. Why?"

"You'd better come to clinic so I can check you over and run some tests. I think you may have hepatitis."

"Is it serious?"

"It can be. You need to get it checked out. We'll talk about it more then."

"When are my cigarettes going to taste okay again?"

Never, I wish. It's an idle thought and, of course, quite illogical:

Maybe someone is trying to tell you something.

HEPATITIS

When the Titan Prometheus stood chained to a rock in punishment for stealing the fire of Olympus for mortals, an eagle, red with blood, feasted in fury on his liver. So mighty Zeus got his revenge. True to the amazing capacity of the liver to regenerate, but false in the extent and speed of recovery, Prometheus' liver grew back for the next day's excruciating ordeal. We are told that Hercules slew the eagle and released Prometheus from his bonds—the undisputed value of having the right friends.

While eagle bites are low on the list of liver injuries in today's world, there is no shortage of other causes of serious liver injury. Hepatitis, a highly infectious inflammation of the liver, is foremost. The letters A to G are signatures of the many viruses that cause hepatitis in about 500,000 persons each year. Blood levels of liver enzymes rise with injury to liver cells, and the body produces antibodies to the virus, providing a means of making the diagnosis through blood tests. Although it's not possible to know the early history of hepatitis, outbreaks of jaundice were reported by the ancient Greeks in the 5th century B.C. and by the ancient Chinese.

Hepatitis A and B cause similar symptoms and signs: fever, loss of appetite (anorexia), malaise, nausea, pain in the right upper abdomen, vomiting, and aversion to smoking. Dark urine, light-colored stools, and jaundice (scleral icterus) are specific signs. Hepatitis A, which is usually spread by the fecal-oral route in contaminated food or water, is contagious for 2 to 6 weeks during the incubation period and can cause epidemics, but it is not likely to be chronic, fatal, or fulminant. Hepatitis B spreads by sexual contact or infected blood and blood products, has an incubation period of 6 weeks to 6 months, a high recovery rate, and 1 to 2% risk of becoming chronic and fulminant.

The prevalence of chronic hepatitis C is about 4 million compared to 1 million for hepatitis B, according to the CDC. Hepatitis C virus infection often is indolent and clinically silent until it has become chronic. Jaundice is unusual, and patients may have no early symptoms or vague symptoms such as arthralgia, fatigue, and myalgia. The predominant route of transmission is parenteral, not sexual, from accidental needle stick, blood transfusion, ear piercing with unsterile equipment, and street drug injection. About 60 to 80% of patients progress to chronic infection, with twice-normal levels of liver enzymes (ALT), and 20% develop cirrhosis. The prognosis is worse in those who consume large quantities of alcohol. Hepatitis C is the nation's leading reason for liver transplantation and the second leading cause of cirrhosis.

Hepatitis D, caused by the delta agent, is endemic in Mediterranean countries. Hepatitis E is an enterically transmitted virus that occurs in epidemics in Asia, Mexico, and North America. Hepatitis G has been recently identified, but diagnostic tests are not yet available.

In immunocompromised hosts, such as patients with AIDS, consider other causes of hepatitis, such as cytomegalovirus infection, herpes simplex, infectious mononucleosis, and spirochetal diseases. Not all hepatitis is infectious. Autoimmune hepatitis, drug exposure, shock liver, and, rarely, metastatic cancer of the liver may produce a similar picture. Patients with chronic hepatitis should be referred to a gastroenterologist for further studies such as a liver biopsy and possible antiviral therapy using interferon α-2b and ribavirin.

*   *   *

"It Used to Take Three Days"

Greg Newsome swallowed hard. He was a freckled, seventeen-year-old who wore several friendship wrist bracelets. A clump of thick, blond hair crowned his otherwise shaved head. Around his neck hung a leather cord with a pendant and some kind of symbol, and a wisp of a beard struggled for existence under his chin. "I've got a lump in my throat," he complained.

"Anything else?"

"I had a fever."

"How high?"

He shrugged.

"It was one-hundred-and-one degrees," his mother said. "He just got it over the past couple days, but he keeps complaining about his throat."

We talked about other possible symptoms, but he had none and was in good general health. The time for talking was over.

"Open wide," I said wielding a dry wooden tongue blade and pocket light.

Like scared animals crouched in a cave, his tonsils hid in the shadows of his beefy red throat covered with yellow-white discharge. They were quite swollen. "I have to swab the back of your throat. We'll know if you have strep in five minutes."

The mother was impressed. "It used to take three days."

"I hate when people stick things in my throat," Greg protested, unimpressed by the technological advances. "It makes me gag." He shuddered.

As I put the swab into his mouth, I exclaimed, "Oh, here's a surprise."

"Sorry, I forgot to tell you. I've had it so long I forget about it. I'll bet you think it hurts."

"No. I've seen people in the ER take a couple of stitches in their tongue without much problem."

"Oh, cool."

I shouldn't have been surprised by his pierced tongue. I'd seen my share of body piercing. My mind flashed back to a woman with a gold ring through her labia and a small butterfly tattoo on her inner upper thigh to keep it company. Stainless steel and gold "barbells" and studs through the tongue, finger-sized rings through the hood of the clitoris, labia, lateral eyebrow, naval, nipple, nostril, penis—what part of the body can't be pierced? I guess it's been a long time since ear-piercing was radical. But, for some reason, piercing the tongue seemed the strangest of all.

"All right, back to business. Open up again."

Greg Newsome made a horrible face as I thoroughly swabbed his throat. The odor from his mouth was foul and sulfurous like he hadn't swallowed in days. Ironically, while complaining of *me* gagging *him*, *he* was now gagging *me*. Except for some palpable cervical lymph nodes and a few chest rhonchi, the rest of his physical examination was normal.

With swab in hand, I marched off to do the strep rapid diagnostic test. Five minutes later I returned. "You don't have strep throat and I know it was a good swab. Can you vouch for that, Greg?"

"That's for sure."

I was left with one small irony: how one with such an aversion to throat swabbing found tongue piercing and stitching perfectly acceptable. I supposed I lacked the makings of a body piercee.

The Common Cold

Entombed but not dead—not alive in the usual sense either—viruses have laid dormant for centuries under conditions that no other organism could survive. Aptly called "a piece of bad news wrapped in a protein" by Nobel Prize laureate Dr. Peter Medawar, viruses (Latin for *poison*) are nothing more than a fragment of nucleic acid—either DNA or RNA—inside a protein coat. Because they're only 20 to 300 nanometers wide (just millionths of a millimeter), they can't even be seen under an ordinary light microscope. Whatever else they need to live and proliferate they coerce their unsuspecting host to make for them by using the surprisingly few genes they possess. How diabolical. Most viral diseases discomfort rather than kill the host. How convenient.

Case in point: viral rhinitis, the common cold—man's sidekick. It's the most common contagious disease in the world. The average person catches 2.5 colds per year, the primary cause of absenteeism in U.S. schools and industry, accounting for 150 million missed days. Colds make us feel that we're at the edge of death's door. School children know the drill: headache, nasal stuffiness, scratchy throat, sneezing, watery, runny nose. As common as respiratory tract infections are, they still constitute more than 10% of all office visits to primary care providers. According to the National Center for Health Statistics, cough was the third most common reason for visits to health care providers in the U.S.; sore throat was the sixth.

Consumers spend $1 billion each year on cold remedies. Cold tablets, gargles, inhalers, liquids, nasal sprays, syrups, and throat lozenges in seductively colorful packaging stuff shelves in pharmacies, supermarkets, and other stores and promise us a good night's sleep or a moment of easy breathing. We would all probably be willing to spend more if they worked better, but this is one area in which modern technology has let us down.

Why don't we develop immunity to colds early in life? After all, we catch so many colds in childhood. The explanation is the more than 100 different varieties or serotypes; we couldn't possibly have contracted them all. Unfortunately catching one does not protect us from others.

When is a sore throat something other than a simple cold? Beware of look-alikes: allergies, strep throat, and viral infections, such as mononucleosis and herpangina, are common offenders; diphtheria and leukemia are rare imitators. In patients with allergies, the postnasal discharge provides the basis of the sore throat. Diphtheria, rare until some parents stopped having their children immunized, is characterized by a gray pseudomembrane.

In strep throat, lymph nodes at the front of the neck are enlarged (cervical adenopathy). The beta-hemolytic streptococci that cause strep throat, the commonest bacterial exudative pharyngitis, are usually group A. When the strep produces erythrogenic toxin, susceptible individuals develop scarlet fever, exhibiting a "strawberry tongue" and a diffuse, peeling rash (desquamation), resembling a sunburn (scarlatina) except that it is most intense in the axillas and groin.

Besides fever and sore throat, patients with mononucleosis (Epstein-Barr virus) have enlarged, tender lymph nodes (posterior auricular), marked fatigue and malaise, a fine red rash, and sometimes an enlarged spleen (splenomegaly). In herpangina, caused by Coxsackie virus (serotypes A2-6, 10), petechiae or papules on the soft palate ulcerate in a few days and then heal; fever may be quite high.

Is it possible to get too much of a good thing? Nasal sprays provide some relief of rhinorrhea and nasal congestion, but they should not be used for more than a few days at a time. The rebound congestion caused by chronic use may be worse than the original symptoms and bad enough to require treatment.

If there is a moral to the story, it's that the common cold keeps us humble. From the future's perspective, ours will seem to be an age of medical ignorance. "Imagine not even being able to cure the common cold," people will chide. At least the cold is not usually fatal. We are not so lucky with other viruses. Even nonlethal ones contribute to human suffering and misery. Drinking fluids, getting plenty of rest, and taking medication for fever or sinus headaches is probably still the best approach—while we wait for the future.

BODY ART

In 1899, the British journal *Society* ran an article about the fad of nipple piercing. It was the fashion among many English women to wear thin gold rings through their nipples. They believed the rings made the breasts fuller and rounder and more stimulating to men. Jewelers performed the procedure, not doctors.

In 1996, "body art" was the sixth fastest growing retail business in the U.S. Studios are springing up near colleges and malls, the sources of eager new clients. One in ten adolescents acquires a tattoo, but as many as half are interested in getting one.

There are health risks. Tongue piercing initially causes incredible tongue swelling. Tongue studs may chip teeth and impair speech. Naval piercing can take up to 12 months to heal and is prone to infection and irritation from waistbands. Besides skin infection, other health risks of body piercing include hepatitis, nerve damage from improperly placed insertions, skin reactions from dye, and tetanus. The formation of keloids and scarring in susceptible individuals are sometimes cosmetically deforming.

Tastes in body art can be fickle. The cost of changing your mind is high: $800 to $1600 to remove tattoos by laser treatment. Sometimes multiple laser sessions are required. Black ink is usually easier to remove than green ink is. The best way of getting around the problem of removal is to avoid procedures that are meant to be permanent. Magnetic tattoo alternatives, the equivalent of "clip ons," are gaining ground.

16

The Belly of the Beast

Pain is a more terrible lord of mankind than even death himself
—ALBERT SCHWEITZER

The ultimate value of illness is that it teaches us the value of being alive
—ARTHUR W. FRANK

Everything happens to everybody sooner or later if there is enough time
—GEORGE BERNARD SHAW

Illness is the night-side of life, a more onerous citizenship. Everyone who is born holds dual citizenship, in the kingdom of the well and in the kingdom of the sick
—SUSAN SONTAG

"The Worst Part about It Is Waiting"

"I'm here for a physical. I've been putting it off and I finally got notice that my next paycheck will be held if I don't get it done." Jack Higgins sat with his arms and legs folded, looking disgruntled. He was fair, lean, and tall—well over six-feet—and, at the age of fifty-eight, in pretty good shape. His striking feature was his hair: waves and waves of silver-gray.

Okay. A work physical. Seems simple enough. H-m-m-m... Why is his body language screaming, Stay away from me!

As I went through the history I noticed he was not too cooperative, remaining silent unless asked a question and answering with almost telegraphic brevity. I gleaned he was a stockbroker who had no serious health problems. His physical examination was routine and I had no reason to suspect any difficulties.

"I plan to do a rectal exam as part of the physical examination," I said casually as I started to glove.

He motioned me away. "No, I don't think so. Not today."

I'm sure my face registered surprise. "It will take less than twenty seconds, Mr. Higgins. It's important to check for blood in your stool, feel your prostate gland, and make sure you don't have any masses in your rectum." I felt like a mother in the 1920's trying to justify cod liver oil to a child. Unlike cod liver oil, however, rectal exams could save lives.

"You're not putting your finger up inside me." He grew more resolute and brusque. "That's where this whole thing ends."

"Do you prefer to have a male health provider do the examination?"

"No one's going to do it," he growled.

"You don't want colon cancer, believe me, Mr. Higgins. Do you remember how Audrey Hepburn died? Most colon cancer can be prevented by early detection. Even Ronald Reagan had to have a polyp in his bowel removed. It was in the news. Everybody your age gets a rectal examination as part of their annual physical. That's what you came here for."

He shook his head adamantly. "Look, I'm not here by choice."

We stood for a moment like a standoff between labor and management. I sensed no amount of convincing on my part would be effective.

"How about a compromise?" I said. "Here are a few hemoccult cards. When you have a bowel movement, smear some stool on them were it tells you to. You can drop them off or mail them and I'll let you know the results. Don't say no until you think about it."

He held up a deprecating hand. "I want to get the hell out of here."

Case closed. Heavy steel doors may as well have slammed shut; Jack Higgins had heard all he was going to hear.

I filled out his employee health form while he got dressed, marking it as incomplete: patient refused rectal examination.

Taking the form, he sauntered off and disappeared—without the hemoccult cards. I fully expected never to see him again. After I completely forgot about the whole episode, some three months later, he stood at my door. "I'm surprised to see you, Mr. Higgins."

"I'm here to do that test you wanted to do."

"That's great. Why don't you have a seat." My scheduled patient was a no-show, so I took advantage of the opportunity to complete his physical.

"I also owe you an apology. I guess I was rude."

"No problem. I'm curious, though. Why'd you come back now?"

"It's a long story." He sat back in his chair and fell into easy conversation. "My wife—her name is Connie—well, she and I went to my fortieth high school reunion in Washington, DC, recently. I was really looking forward to seeing my best friend, Ray. We go way back. I was the best man at his wedding. We kept in touch as much as possible for people who don't live nearby, you know, watched each others families grow up. Time and commitments kept us from visiting often. There aren't too many people you can call friends for life, but Ray is one of them. Anyway, he and his wife had place cards at the same table as ours. I was relieved. But he showed up without his wife. I asked *Where's Joyce?*

The long pause before he answered and his pained looked—well, my mouth went dry. I couldn't have swallowed at that moment if you paid me a million dollars. Then he told me. She recently died in a head-on auto accident.

Later we went out, just the two of us, to a bar. I remember a waitress started trying to make conversation. She sensed we weren't up for small talk and left to get our drinks. Ray and I got to talking about Joyce and he wept openly. I never knew him to cry—ever. Grief made a stranger of him. That's when it really hit me: life can be taken from you at any moment. I decided I didn't want to put my wife through that kind of pain if something were to happen to me through my own stubbornness. How could I put her through that? Anyway, we ended up closing the bar. On our way out Ray said *You take good care of Connie and yourself.*

When I got back to the hotel room, my wife was already in bed. I stood looking out the window at the Washington monument for the longest time. Its two blinking red lights caught my attention: a danger signal—I knew I'd been warned twice. The first warning was from you. The second was the death of my close friend's wife. So, anyway, let's get the show on the road and get this over with."

Jack Higgins, loquacious and personable, hardly seemed to be the same man. I asked him to put on a gown and lie on his side on the examining table. Once I got him to relax, the rectal examination went well. "There, was that so bad?"

"Bad enough. It's never going to be my favorite test."

"That's fair. Why don't you clean yourself off with these tissues and I'll go test your stool sample."

When I returned, he looked like a scarred rabbit: wide-eyed, ready to jump out of the chair, so anxious I wasn't sure he was hearing. "The good news is your prostate gland feels normal, so I'm not worried about that. Your stool did test positive for blood, however, and I didn't find any hemorrhoids to explain it."

He was aghast. "So you found something wrong?"

"Yes, you're losing some blood in your stool. When the test is positive for blood, the next step is to look inside the bowel with a tube-like instrument or scope and identify where the blood is coming from. I don't do the test, but I will refer you to a specialist."

Although I questioned him again about his bowel habits, he denied any recent changes, constipation, diarrhea, bleeding, cramping, or tarry stools. I was not convinced, as worried as he was, that he would tell me the truth.

"What do I do now? Will they have to operate? I don't want a colostomy."

"Mr. Higgins, we're getting way ahead of ourselves here. It may be a polyp."

"What's that?"

"It's a fleshy lump, perhaps an inch long or so, that hangs into the bowel. Polyps may turn into cancer, but if you catch them before that happens, you can usually remove them through the scope right at the time." I answered more of his questions, but he wasn't reassured.

"I guess I should come clean with you."

"About what?"

"As a small boy I remember a great aunt who went to the hospital, and never came home. Later I found out she died of cancer. It scared the daylights out of me. I remember everyone's reaction to it, talking in hushed tones in my presence—you know how kids think—something awful had happened. For all these years I've lived with the fear that a person should avoid clinics and hospitals because once they find something in you it's too late."

How many times have I heard that view expressed in one form or another: fear of going to the health care provider. Everyone's pulse quickens in the office, worried that I'll scratch the surface a little too deeply and, boom, find something. We've all got a bit of ostrich in us, I guess.

"Let's take this one step at a time. You can do this." I sent him to a gastroenterologist.

When Jack Higgins telephoned me two weeks later, he launched into complaining. "I had to drink this horrid tasting liquid until I thought I would explode or throw up. It cleaned out my bowels all right—all evening long—not to mention the cramps. Then an enema. That wasn't too much fun either." As he went on and on, I heard the anxiety bubbling to the surface. He cleared his throat. "The doctor said I had a polyp. He removed it, but he's waiting to hear from the pathologist."

"Okay. That's all right. They want to see if it's malignant."

"The worst part about it is waiting. It's a feeling of I don't want to know, but I have to know."

"Look, try not to worry, Mr. Higgins. I'll talk to you as soon as I hear something."

Three days later, the gastroenterologist phoned me with the bottom line from the path report: the polyp was cancerous. He reassured me it was a favorable type in that it hadn't spread. Only malignant polyps with unfavorable histologic signs required surgical bowel resection.

Hurrah! It was exactly the news I hoped to hear. I asked the patient to return once more to go over the information in person. "I talked with the gastroenterologist to see how things went. It was cancerous, but he thinks he got it all and said that everything looked good. Congratulations!"

Jack Higgins' eyebrows rose like startled birds and then he took a long, deep breath and sat back to enjoy the first flush of victory. "Whew! I'm glad that's over with."

"Me, too. Now remember, the colonoscopy does need to be repeated in three years and then every five years after that. That's standard fare for this sort of thing. I know I can count on you to return for those tests. Who knows, maybe you'll acquire a taste for that special bowel-prep drink of yours."

"That remains to be seen." He laughed and then turned serious. "I guess I should thank you."

"Why?"

"The doctor said I was lucky; he got it early. It could have spread. If so—odds are—the polyp would have killed me."

"Take a glass of wine tonight and salute your friend Ray. He got you to come in here. That's what friends are for."

COLORECTAL CANCER

Colorectal cancer, the second leading cause of death by cancer in the U.S., takes hold in 6% of all Americans. Every year there are 160,000 new cases and 60,000 deaths. About 90% of those affected are over the age of 50. Most colorectal cancers are adenocarcinomas, a slowly growing tumor present for years before symptoms occur. How do they start? Usually by malignant transformation of an adenomatous polyp.

Polyps protrude into the intestinal lumen. Over 70% of polyps removed at colonoscopy are adenomatous, the only one of the three polyp types to have significant clinical implications. Large adenomas, 1 to 3 cm in size, carry a higher risk of harboring malignancy. It takes about 5 years for such a polyp to develop and another 10 years to become cancerous. Therein lies the solution.

Colon cancer can be prevented by early detection. Half of the cancers are located in the rectosigmoid region and another fourth are in the cecum and ascending colon. That means most of the cancers can be detected by visual inspection of the colon.

The flexible sigmoidoscope, a modern fiber-optic tube, snakes 60 cm into the bowel and can be used on an awake patient in the office as part of cancer screening. Sigmoidoscopy reaches about one-third to one-half of colonic adenomas and reveals polyps in 10 to 20% of all patients. Colonoscopy, which visualizes the entire colon but requires heavy sedation, detects 90 to 98% or polyps and allows biopsy or excision for pathologic confirmation. Barium enema is most useful when a tumor otherwise obstructs the colon from view.

The risk of colorectal cancer mounts with a history of adenomatous colon polyps, gynecological cancers, inflammatory bowel disease, several genetic polyposis and nonpolyposis syndromes, and a positive family history of colon cancer. The signs and symptoms of colorectal cancer depend on the location of the tumor. Cancers of the distal colon change bowel habits and leak bright red rectal blood (hematochezia). In the proximal colon they induce fecal occult blood and anemia.

The earlier the detection the better. Most patients with adenomatous polyps are completely asymptomatic. Fecal occult blood screening detects about 40% of large polyps. A complete blood count reveals anemia. Carcinoembryonic antigen (CEA) levels are high in 70% of patients with colorectal cancer and normalize after surgical resection. Endorectal ultrasound and abdominal CT scan are useful for cancer staging (stages 0 to 4). The prognosis for stages 0 (carcinoma *in situ*) and 1 (localized and not invading the subserosa) is excellent, but patients with higher stages fair less well, emphasizing the importance of early detection. Elevated liver function tests suggest metastases.

Fear or dislike of a rectal exam should *never* cost a person his or her life.

*   *   *

"No One Told Me That"

Ruth Harwood was the female version of Ichabod Crane. Long and lanky, she had a pencil neck, Adam's apple, and wispy, shoulder-length, gray hair.

"I'm sorry, I don't have an appointment, but I have this pain in my belly. It woke me up in the middle of the night."

I couldn't miss one glaring incongruity. For a woman in acute abdominal pain, she was too made up, perfumed, and decked out for a night on the town. "Can you describe the pain?"

"Have you ever had gas pains? Well, this is ten times worse. It's all over my belly and I feel kind of queasy. I'm not sick to my stomach, but I don't feel like eating either. When I try to eat, it stirs up everything. I feel like I have to move my bowels, but I can't do it."

I could tell she was used to answering medical questions because she didn't need prompting to explain the problem. "Are you passing any gas?"

"Oh, now *that* I don't have any trouble with."

"When's the last time you had a bowel movement?"

"That's my problem. I haven't gone for seven days."

"Have you tried anything?"

"I tried everything. All the over-the-counter stuff. I've even tried enemas. I'm afraid I have something bad."

"Has this ever happened to you before?"

"Over the past few months I've been having more trouble moving my bowels. Lately it's gotten worse."

Sounds like constipation. Now the question is why. Poor bowel habits? Does she have hypothyroidism? Chronically abuse laxatives or antacids? Does she eat a high fat, low fiber diet, and drink too little fluids? Is she taking medications? The possibility of a tumor seems distant.

"Mrs. Harwood, I notice in your chart that you have chronic back pain. Do you take any medication for it?"

"Why, yes, my doctor gave me a pain pill."

"What kind of pill?"

"I don't know exactly, but he said it had codeine in it. It really works."

Bingo. "Did you know that taking narcotics can cause constipation?"

She looked surprised. "No one told me that."

"Do you see what I'm getting at?"

"That would probably explain it because I've been taking those pills for about three months. Should I stop taking them?"

"I would. I can give you a prescription for something for your back pain that's not a narcotic. But let me examine you first and make sure nothing else is going on in your belly."

She laid down on the examining table without difficulty. Everything on her physical examination was normal until I reached the abdomen. Bowel sounds were present, but she was tender all over. Her abdomen was very firm. She guarded when I attempted to palpate even superficially. I could not press deeply.

I gloved for a rectal examination. The results were immediate. My finger confronted concrete-like stool. Classic fecal impaction. She was too uncomfortable for me to try to disimpact her. Her stool was negative when I tested it for occult blood.

After discussing her situation with my attending physician, we ordered an upright abdominal x-ray to be sure there was no mass or free air in the abdomen. The x-ray merely confirmed her severe constipation.

"Mrs. Harwood, to put it simply, you are full of stool."

"I always knew I was full of something, but it's embarrassing it has to be *that*." She smiled good-naturedly.

I prescribed the cathartic laxative cascara and told her to buy an oil retention enema available over-the-counter. If she still didn't have a bowel movement by the next day, I asked her to call me. I later learned that everything came out all right.

ABDOMINAL PAIN

St. Erasmus of Elmo was granted patronage of the abdomen for his martyrdom in 303 A.D. He was killed by having his intestines drawn out with a crank-driven device—some sort of windlass. The pain must have been excruciating.

It's gripped us all at one time or another: sharp, cramping, colicky, or diffuse pain in the belly. Trivial or serious, mild or severe, transient or chronic, it's an attention grabber. The memories are not fond. No one says: "Gee, I wish that pain lasted longer." Even driving to the safety of the clinic or hospital ER is not a sure bet. Hitting a bump in the road can be agonizing if the peritoneum, the abdomen's membranous lining, is inflamed (peritonitis).

A symptom of normal physiology as well as medical and surgical emergencies, abdominal pain can herald a "stomach virus" or an intestinal parasite, painful ovulation (Mittelschmerz) or a tearing abdominal aneurysm, peritonitis from a ruptured appendix or a black widow bite. Which is it? An astute clinician finds out, sometimes only with expensive tests and the passage of time. The first priority is to stabilize the patient.

The stakes are high. The health care provider must be systematic and consider the possibilities. Ask about any black or tarry stools (melena), bloating, change in bowel habits, diarrhea, dietary habits, gas (flatus), hemorrhage, vomiting, and injury. Look for abdominal bruising, insect bites, varicosities, or signs of trauma. Listen for bowel sounds. Feel for abdominal masses or fluid (ascites), abdominal bruits or rigidity. Arthritis and mouth ulcers can be clues to inflammatory bowel disease.

Borborygmi isn't an African tribe. It's the high-pitched, animalistic sound of a partial bowel obstruction heard through a stethoscope placed on the abdomen. The abdomen speaks to health care providers even when it is silent, too. Lack of peristalsis (ileus) spells trouble from drugs or disease, sometimes quite serious. Big trouble is also brewing when the abdomen swells or bruising appears over the flanks.

Home to a dozen or so major organs, the abdomen gives rise to many dozens of diseases: appendicitis, Crohn's disease, gallbladder inflammation (cholecystitis) and stones (choledocholithiasis and cholangitis), gastritis and gastric ulcers, hepatitis, inflamed colonic diverticuli (diverticulitis), irritable bowel, pancreatitis and pancreatic cancer, polycystic kidneys and kidney infections (pyelonephritis), ruptured spleen, twisted (volvulus) or telescoped (intussusception) bowel, and ulcerative colitis. If you include the adjoining pelvis, there's pelvic inflammatory disease, ruptured ovarian cyst, and urinary bladder infections (cystitis).

The nature of the pain provides clues. Pain is explosive and excruciating in patients with biliary or renal colic, ruptured aneurysm, or a ruptured viscus. A more constant but severe pain beginning rapidly characterizes acute pancreatitis, mesenteric thrombosis, or strangulated bowel. When pain starts gradually and remains steady, acute appendicitis, cholecystitis, or diverticulitis are likely. Colicky (waxing and waning) and intermittent pain are common in small bowel obstruction. The pain often localizes to the offending organ.

Some pain radiates. Gallbladder disease and pancreatitis radiate to the shoulders or back. Pain radiating from the flank to the groin may be the harbinger of ureteral colic or dissecting abdominal aortic aneurysm. Sometimes cardiac pain radiates into the upper abdomen masquerading as abdominal pain.

Peritoneal signs usually warn of the need for an operation. Involuntary guarding or rigidity of the abdominal muscles, worsening pain on coughing (cough rebound) or on straight-leg raising (psoas sign), and other signs indicate peritoneal inflammation. There are a few exceptions: bacterial peritonitis, mild diverticular disease, pelvic inflammatory disease, and ruptured ovarian (corpus luteal) cyst. Fortunately these emergencies usually can be handled medically.

Blood tests (complete blood count, serum electrolytes, tests of kidney, liver, and pancreatic function), ultrasound, urinalysis, and radiological studies cinch the diagnosis in patients with abdominal pain. Warning: always obtain a pregnancy test in a woman of reproductive age who may be pregnant. Be on the look-out for masqueraders: diabetes (ketoacidosis), heart disease (angina), strep throat (mesenteric adenitis), neurological disorders (disk disease), and psychological problems (depression).

People with severe acute abdominal pain need analgesics. Once avoided because they were thought to mask clinical signs and symptoms, appropriate pain management actually appears to increase diagnostic accuracy. Narcotics and nonsteroidal anti-inflammatory drugs are the top choices. Among the most effective of all analgesics, narcotics can be given intravenously or intramuscularly. Besides being very sedating, morphine cannot be used with biliary colic, and meperidine can agitate the elderly and unleash seizures. NSAID's cause less nausea and sedation, but ketorolac is the only NSAID available in the U.S. for parenteral use. Indomethacin and diclofenac are useful for renal and biliary colic.

CONSTIPATION

Have we overlooked the obvious? As intriguing as the possibilities are, we often forget a pedestrian one: constipation. How infrequent is infrequent? Normal individuals have from 3 to 12 bowel movements a week, so the range is broad, but excessive difficulty and straining at defecation describes constipation. It usually takes 1 day for food to traverse along the tortuous, 30-foot alimentary tract from intake to outlet.

Low-fiber diet (less than 10 to 12 grams per day) and poor bowel habits (disregard of the normal urge) are the most common causes of constipation in adults. Older people may be more prone to constipation from poor eating habits, medications that reduce motility of the colon, and medical conditions that prevent exercise or cause them to be bed-bound. Highlights of other causes would include systemic diseases (diabetes, hypothyroidism, low potassium), structural abnormalities (colonic strictures or masses, rectal prolapse), thrombosed hemorrhoids), neurological (spinal cord disorders), and psychogenic causes (cathartic abuse). The possible offending drugs are worth remembering: antacids, antibiotics, anticholinergics, calcium channel blockers, diuretics, narcotics, and psychotropic agents.

Take natural measures to keep things moving. Eat a high-fiber diet—20 to 35 grams a day. Drink enough water: as many as 8 glasses daily. Drinking a glass or two of cold water stimulates the colonic reflex to initiate a bowel movement. Exercise, follow a daily bowel routine, take vitamins, avoid laxatives, and relax your mind. Alternative medicine suggests aloe vera, flaxseed, triphala, and yoga. See what works.

*   *   *

"My One Vice Is Coffee"

Alice Padgett sat in my office, the stereotype of the successful business woman. Attractive and well-groomed, she wore a brown business suit with a light blue blouse open at the collar, revealing a thin, gold chain with a Christian cross. Hair sprayed in place, small cameo earrings dangling from her earlobes, make-up immaculately applied, she was reviewing her daily appointment book as I entered the room.

I can feel the tension level of a patient when I first walk in. It's not a conscious act, I just sense it. Alice was pensive. She started talking the minute I arrived. I barely said hello.

"So, this is what's going on. I've got this appointment with you. Then I have to run some errands and get back to the office. The problem is I've been having stomach pain and I want to make sure I don't have an ulcer."

My mind continued her train of thought: *Fix me up quickly so I can continue my lifestyle. I don't have time for this, so do it now.*

"Can you describe the pain?"

"It's like incredible hunger. Of course, it's not really hunger. I feel like my stomach is digesting itself. I have the sensation of something percolating in there all the time to the point of feeling nauseous."

"When did you first start having the pain?"

"I was at work early in the morning. I went to the coffeemaker and poured my usual brimming cup. Afterward, I got a burning feeling in my stomach; my whole stomach ignited. I blamed it on ice coffee because I was doing a lot of those over the summer."

"How much coffee do you drink?"

"I reached the point of drinking six to eight cups of coffee a day. I ended up needing more to feel alert. You have to realize, my one vice is coffee. I love the taste of fresh ground coffee. Living in NYC is torture—it has so many cafés and coffee houses. Just walk down the streets and let your nose guide you. They're calling to me, *Alice, time for another cup of coffee.*" She chuckled. "I know I can't."

She kept checking her watch. It was beginning to make me nervous.

"I've done the coffee thing on a grand scale. When I started out I took it with cream. Then I got into the habit of adding sugar. Someone at work said once you start that, you won't want it any other way. But I'm weight conscious, so I kicked that habit; I took it black. Then I got into expresso. But since my stomach's acted up, I need the milk." As she spoke, she surveyed her hands, sliding her arm bracelet toward her hand and making sure the catch was on the underside of her wrist, out of sight.

"Have you tried to cut back?"

"My fiancé pleaded with me, *Why don't you drink decaf—it tastes the same.* He's not a coffee drinker, what does he know?" She laughed. Her spring was still tightly coiled. "I was stubborn. When I finally agreed to cut back, I found that I couldn't cut back far enough. Now decaf is all I can drink, and that's only once in a while. I use lots of milk. Something's irritating about the coffee itself I think, even without the caffeine.

I'm an addict, though. The aroma. Smelling coffee gives me a warm secure feeling, like being with a good friend. Even a waft of it can put me in a terrific mood. The aroma is sometimes better than the taste."

"Do you have symptoms at night?"

"After I dose off, all of a sudden I have to sit up because something rushes up into my throat. I swallow hard because it tastes so bad. I thought I was going to vomit if I didn't sit up fast enough. It really feels like it's going to erupt." She made a face of remembering the bad taste.

"Have you ever vomited coffee-grounds colored material or blood?"

"Heavens no." She seemed concerned to hear that might happen.

Her fingers were busy touching her earrings, checking to be sure her necklace was centered, and straightening her rings.

"Have you ever had a black, tarry stool?"

She shook her head no.

"What have you done for the pain?"

"I drank gallons of milk. That only took the edge off for about a half-hour. Then I ate frozen yogurt and ice cream. They helped put out the fire—only vanilla—definitely *no* chocolate."

"Do you drink?"

"Not alcohol—no way. I was out with friends and had a gin and tonic. What a fireball; it doubled me over. I had to order milk."

"Have you tried antacids?"

"My life is an antacid commercial." She adjusted her sleeves so they were even with her suit. "I have jars of antacids at home, in my car, my purse, and at work. I've tried all the different flavors and brands because I fatigue on the taste from popping them so often. Some of the flavors have gotten repulsive. I sort through the tablets and pitch the flavors I don't like. Now I buy the jumbo size for home. I used to take the liquid antacids, but didn't like the telltale traces on the lips."

We reviewed her lifestyle and past medical history carefully. Nothing else seemed to be going on, but stress surfaced at every turn—uptight, tailored, everything cut, i's dotted, t's crossed.

"What do you do to relax?"

"I don't have much time. I'm getting the groceries, picking up my dry-cleaning, shopping for clothes or gifts, making plans."

"That sounds like a list of things to be done, but what do you do to *relax* when you go home? Do you indulge in bubble baths, read, gallivant with friends, catch movies, do crossword puzzles, surf the Internet?"

She drew a blank. "Well, no. I guess I'm a person who's always making lists and then starts working on them."

I requested she gown and lie on the examining table. Her abdomen was tender in the left upper quadrant overlying the stomach and just below the sternum. During the physical examination, her cellphone rang.

"Excuse me, I have to take this call."

"Please tell them you'll call back in about ten or fifteen minutes."

She nodded. I could hear her getting stressed over the brief phone conversation. The time bomb was ticking, growing louder as it approached the inevitable. Here was an intelligent woman, harassed, surrounded by an air of hurry, unaware that she was destroying herself.

When I got back to her examination, everything else, including checking her stool for blood, seemed normal, so I told her to get dressed while I wrote my note. When she finished she sat in the chair next to my desk.

"You have *GERD*, Alice. That's an acronym for gastroesophageal reflux disease. Your stomach acid is increased and the sphincter between your stomach and your esophagus is allowing the acid to reflux up the esophagus. It causes pain."

"What do you do for that?"

"I'm going to give you cards to smear with a stool sample to make sure you are not having any bleeding from this. I didn't find any today, but it needs to be checked a couple of times."

"I'm not seeing blood when I have a bowel movement."

"No, this test looks for blood you can't see."

"Okay."

"Then I'll schedule you for an upper GI series with small bowel follow through to make sure you don't have an ulcer. I'll start you on a medication to block stomach acid"—

"The bottom line?"

"Okay, you need to stop drinking any caffeinated or carbonated beverages, at least for now."

"Well, I knew that was coming."

"Let's see if we can't get things to quiet down."

"All right."

When Alice returned to clinic two weeks later, she was feeling worse. The x-rays were negative and so were her stool hemoccult cards. I referred her to a gastroenterologist who performed endoscopy and biopsied her stomach lining to look for *H. pylori*, a bacterial infection found in ulcers. He treated her with triple antibiotics prophylactically. When I saw her again, Alice had been taking a medication for six weeks to block acid production.

"How's it going," I inquired.

"Not so good. I'm not drinking coffee, tea, alcohol, carbonated drinks, or spicy foods. My stomach still burns."

"What's your stress level like these days?"

"It's up there." She raised her hands to her eyebrows. "The company is preparing for a federal audit, and I'm in charge of that. My performance on this project tells my supervisors how good I am."

"So when this project is over, your stress level will fall?"

"No, it's only one of my responsibilities at work. Outside of the job, I got engaged and we're preparing to buy a house. My closest aunt is in the hospital with heart problems and I recently had to have my ten-year-old pet dog put to sleep."

Alice gave me the impression she wasn't one to cry easily, but she had become more of a hapless person just over the couple of months I'd been taking care of her.

"You know the song that Frasier Crane sings—*I've got you pegged*—the second chorus at the end of the show?"

"Oh, so you know what's wrong with me? What do I have to do to get rid of this?"

"Well, let me turn the tables. Suppose I just told you what you said to me. What would you tell me?"

She looked thoughtful. "I guess I'd say you were working too hard, you're stressed-out, and you're a basket case."

"And what would you advise me to do?"

"I'd tell you to change your job and don't worry so much over the details. Things will work out." She paused. "Yeah, I would say that you worry too much."

I shrugged my shoulders as if to say, "Well."

"Oh. I guess I should take my own advice."

"It's difficult to get perspective when you're caught up in a situation. Only *you* hold the key to your medical problem. You must either change your way of coping with stress or try to eliminate the main source of stress. You're hurting yourself."

Alice Padgett looked startled at my choice of words. She gazed across the room as if through the walls into the billowing mists of aspiration and remembrance. "This is the highest paying job I've ever held." Then she looked back at me.

I raised my eyebrows. "And you're stomach is repaying you in dividends."

"Yeah, I get the point."

THE ACID PIT

In ancient Sparta, a young soldier hiding a fox under his tunic allowed the fox to chew through his stomach rather than reveal to his commander that he had broken the rules by having a pet. Stories of this kind helped make Spartan stoicism and discipline legendary. Such intense pain is not foreign to people with severe gastritis.

No wonder: inside our stomachs is an acid so corrosive it could eat through cloth and certain metals. Some people would find that alarming. Why doesn't this hydrochloric acid destroy us? Would you believe, sticky mucus? The normal stomach is coated with it. Such a thin lining is usually enough to protect us—most of us, most of the time. When it doesn't, gastritis develops, and perhaps an ulcer.

Dyspepsia refers to a group of epigastric or upper abdominal symptoms, such as bloating, burping, early satiety, "heartburn," "indigestion," nausea, or regurgitation. Although one-fourth of adults have dyspepsia, most never seek medical attention. Disorders of the gallbladder, pancreas, stomach, and thyroid, pregnancy and psychological factors all can produce dyspepsia, making the term imprecise.

Gastritis is an irritation of the stomach's mucosal surface. It refers to erosive and hemorrhagic disease, non-erosive and nonspecific disease, or other disorders. Patients with erosive gastritis may vomit "coffee grounds"-color emesis or blood. The most common causes of erosive gastritis are drugs like nonsteroidal anti-inflammatory drugs, including aspirin, the world's best selling over-the-counter drug, alcohol, caffeine, and steroids. Coffee, tea, chocolate, and most carbonated drinks contain some form of gastric acid-increasing methylxanthine, such as caffeine, theophylline, or theobromine. Stress, especially stress during medical and surgical illnesses, is another major factor in gastritis.

Then came a breakthrough: researchers discovered that certain bacteria cause gastritis and ulcers. *Helicobacter pylori* is a gram-negative rod associated with nonerosive, nonspecific gastritis. In the U.S., 50% of whites over age 60 and 10% under 30 have the infection. It is more prevalent in non-Caucasians and immigrants from developing countries, possibly acquired from childhood. About 15% of individuals with *H. pylori* infection develop a peptic ulcer, and chronic infection carries a four- to sixfold increased risk of stomach cancer (gastric adenocarcinoma and B cell gastric lymphoma).

The diagnosis of *H. pylori* infection is usually made by endoscopic biopsy. Besides endoscopy, *H. pylori* can be detected by a serologic blood test for antibodies, but quantitative titers are needed to assess response. Vitamin B_{12} malabsorption (pernicious anemia) is an unrelated cause of nonerosive gastritis.

Eight million persons in the U.S. each year develop stomach ulcers, but the lifetime prevalence of ulcers is about 10% of the population. About 80% are duodenal; 20% are gastric. Duodenal ulcers are more common in men under the age of 55, whereas gastric ulcers predominate in older individuals of either gender. Nearly 100% of patients with uncomplicated duodenal ulcers and 90% of those with non-drug-related gastric ulcers have *H. pylori* infection.

Endoscopy is the procedure of choice for confirming complete ulcer healing 12 weeks after the start of treatment. A barium upper GI series is an acceptable alternative in uncomplicated cases. Ulcers are potentially serious. Gastrointestinal hemorrhage, ulcer perforation and penetration, and gastric outlet obstruction are the cost of failure to treat or respond to treatment.

Patients with *H. Pylori* should be treated with antibiotics, which eradicate infection in about 85% of the cases. The best way to gain the upper hand is through combination therapies. Proton pump inhibitors and histamine2 (H2) receptor antagonists turn down the secretion of stomach acid. Antacids, sucralfate, prostaglandin analogues, and bismuth compounds enhance mucosal defenses. The use of antibiotics with proton pump inhibitors or bismuth compounds eradicates *H. pylori*, whereas single agents are ineffective. The FDA recently approved quadruple therapy with bismuth, metronidazole, tetracycline, and a H2 blocker.

17

Skin Deep

There is no cosmetic for beauty like happiness
—LADY BLESSINGTON

God has given you one face,
and you make yourselves another
—WILLIAM SHAKESPEARE

The worst of faces is still human
—LAVETER

Nothing in life is to be feared. It is only to be understood
—MARIE CURIE

"I Can't Even Wear My Bra"

With a frown, Mildred Hanes tented her blouse away from her chest. She was a bland-faced, obese woman. "I've got this rash. It hurts really bad. I can't stand to have my clothes touch my skin. It keeps me up at night 'cause I can't find the right position to avoid irritating it. I can't even wear my bra it hurts so bad. I swear to God, I don't tolerate anything even brushing against it."

"How did it start?"

"Before the rash I had this burning pain. It was uncomfortable. Now it's worse since the rash came. Some of it has spread under my breast. It's only on one side of me. Can you look at it and tell me what it is and give me something for pain?"

Gingerly lifting up her blouse, she exposed her chest. When she lifted her large, pendulous, right breast away from the rash, I saw clusters of vesicular lesions in a pink streak along her right mid-thorax, wrapping around the back and stopping near her spine. Some were open and weeping; others were crusting. I knew exactly what they were.

"You have shingles."

She was taken aback. "I'm not old enough to have shinglers. Isn't that an old person's disease?"

"It's pronounced *shingles*."

"Like shingles on a house?"

"Right."

Mrs. Hanes chuckled.

"Usually people get it when they're older, but shingles occurs at any age."

"How did I get it?"

"Do you remember having chickenpox?"

"I was a kid then."

"The chickenpox virus went dormant all these years and reappeared now."

"Can you make it go away and not come back?"

"I can give you antiviral medication to help heal the rash. I can't make the virus go away forever, but most people don't have a second attack."

"When will the pain stop?"

"It should subside when the rash heals. I'll give you anti-inflammatory medication to ease the pain. Sometimes the pain persists after the rash disappears." I handed her an information sheet about shingles and wrote her a prescription.

"I'm a modest woman," she said, "but I tell you. If I didn't have children at home, I'd close the blinds and walk around the house without a top until the rash is gone. I wouldn't wish this on my worst enemy." She left the room shaking her head.

SHINGLES

Twenty percent of adults get shingles (herpes zoster), an acute eruption of vesicles caused by reactivation of the chickenpox (varicella-zoster) virus. The virus, dormant in nerves near the brain and spinal cord since childhood, traverses the nerves to the skin when it is reactivated by age, illness, medications, or stress.

A blistering rash erupts in a band or streak on one side of the body, usually the back or chest, face, mouth, or extremity. Because burning, itching, or tingling may occur before the blisters appear, the wrong diagnosis is sometimes made, such as migraines if the pain is over the face or other acute illnesses depending on the location of pain. The affliction can be excruciating, but usually heals within a month.

Putting out the fire. If medical attention is sought early, within the first three days of symptoms, shingles can be treated. Anti-inflammatory drugs dampen the inflammation, anti-viral drugs (acyclovir) reduce the intensity of infection, and analgesics assuage the pain. The varicella-zoster vaccine licensed in 1995 may reduce the risk and severity of zoster.

Sometimes the pain persists due to nerve fiber damage long after the rash heals (postherpetic neuralgia), especially when the face is involved (trigeminal nerve) or patients are either immunocompromised or over the age of 60. For postherpetic neuralgia, anticonvulsants (carbamazepine, phenytoin, valproate) or antidepressants (tricyclic antidepressants), taken orally, may lessen the pain. Topical treatment with capsaicin cream, which depletes nerve terminals of the pain messenger (substance P), lidocaine and aspirin cream, or desensitization by rubbing or applying temperature changes to the skin are also recommended. Transcutaneous electrical nerve stimulation (TENS) or dorsal root surgery are last resorts for extreme treatment failures.

Skin Lesions

Don't let it's mere 0.5 to 4 mm thickness fool you. Human skin, all 6 to 10 pounds of it, provides a remarkably tough, though not impervious, 18 square foot barrier to the outside world. Many conditions predispose it to attack by infectious organisms such as bacteria, fungi, and viruses. Certain individuals are more susceptible than others. The skin is also a telltale sign of allergens and toxins we're exposed to, medications we take, and many systemic diseases.

Skin lesions come in all shapes and sizes. The primary types are macules (flat and flush), papules (small and raised), plaques (large, raised, but flat), nodules (large, raised and solid), pustules (small, pus-filled), vesicles (small fluid-filled) or bulla (large fluid-filled), and wheals (raised and edematous). They may secondarily crust (scab) and develop a fissure, erode, become erythematous or thickened (hyperkeratotic), scale, scar, or ulcerate. Telangiectasia are dilated superficial blood vessels. Skin pigment may increase, decrease, or disappear altogether. Scratching excoriates the skin and causes thickening and induration (lichenification). Combined effects and varied locations can make diagnosis challenging.

Failure to use simple office procedures to confirm the diagnosis is the most common pitfall. A Wood's black light makes ringworm (tinea) fluoresce in a darkened room. Mites (scabies), head lice (pediculosis), and ticks (Lyme disease) can be seen under the microscope. A potassium hydroxide prep reveals fungus or yeast in skin scrapings.

The distribution of skin lesions is classic. In joint flexures of the arm (antecubital fossa), axilla, groin, and wrists, one finds atopic dermatitis and scabies. On the extensor surfaces of the body, psoriasis and xanthomas are more likely. Look for seborrhea on the scalp, ears, and central face. Eczema can reside on the palms and soles.

Acne (acne vulgaris) is the most common skin condition treated by health care providers. Sunburn is the most frequent environmental exposure. Many agents cause occupational skin conditions. The principal infectious rashes are impetigo and viral exanthema.

Drug reactions range from itching without skin lesions to life-threatening skin sloughing. Common drug-induced skin lesions are erythema multiforme or nodosum, morbilliform eruptions, purpura, and urticaria (hives). Nearly half of all drug rashes are blanching, erythematous macules and papules (morbilliform).

The time-honored adage for treatment is if a skin lesion is wet, make it dry; if it is dry, wet it. The itching, silvery plaques of psoriasis need to be moisturized; weeping contact dermatitis needs to be dried. For best absorption, topical drugs should be applied after bathing or using wet soaks. The standard preparations are liquids, ointments, and powders. Topical corticosteroids are one of the main drugs prescribed for non-infectious rashes.

*   *   *

"I Would Have Stitched It Myself"

Jack Dorsey's face was a landscape. Winding furrows traversed the entire length of his weathered forehead below the thick forest of his hair. In the clinic's overhead lighting, ponderous, rugged brows cast shadows over his sunken eyes. The groves alongside his nose ran deep, coursing nearly from his eyes to his chin. His pockmarked cheeks were the piedmont to the steep slopes of his nose, which twisted capriciously at the bridge, before culminating in a bulbous summit overlooking a jutting chin. Loose skin on his neck seemed to drain his face like ravines.

"I got bitten by my dog while I was giving it a bath." The robust man extended his right hand for me to inspect. "My hand is swollen and sore now. I thought I should get it checked out. Do you think I need stitches?"

"When did the dog bite you?" I asked.

"Yesterday afternoon." Mr. Dorsey had a raspy smoker's voice.

I did the mental calculations. More than twenty-four hours had elapsed. "Let me take a look at it. We'll need to put it under the light."

His hand had four puncture wounds, two on top and two on the bottom. The palm near the thumb was swollen and reddish-purple. A jagged laceration connected the wounds. When I separated the edges of the laceration, fat globules glistened beneath the skin layer. For some reason I thought of the adage, *The hand is the servant of the mind.* Now look at it.

"This is tricky. You'd get stitches had you come by sooner."

"Oh, hell, had I known, I would have stitched it myself!"

"What do you mean?"

"I have experience with that." He must have seen my bewilderment. "I put stitches in horses, cows and pigs—it's just like human skin."

"Are you saying my skin looks like a pig's skin," I bantered.

"We've all got a touch of pig in us," he quipped.

"Speak for yourself."

He chuckled.

"Are you a veterinarian."

"Hell, no. I used to be a farmer."

"Well, I think this is a bit different. The wounds are on your hand and over tendons. That requires special care so you don't get a tendon infection and scarring."

"You sure?" he asked good-naturedly. "I think I still have some thread at home."

"Thanks for the offer, Mr. Dorsey, but not today. You need to go on antibiotics. You already have some skin infection. You might even get intravenous antibiotics."

"Intravenous? I can swallow pills."

"It's not that. A wound more than twenty-four hours old that involves tendons might require IV antibiotics. You don't want to lose any hand function."

"No, you're right about that. I need this hand for fishin'."

I discussed the details with the attending physician and arranged for Jack Dorsey's treatment. He was the fourth person in as many months to receive medical treatment for being bitten by his or her own dog.

BIG BITES

Which is more likely to become infected, a bite wound from a cat or a dog? The cats have it, paws down. Between 30 and 50% of their bites get infected, usually with *Pasteurella*, causing cellulitis, chills, fever, and swelling of local lymph nodes.

About 1% of ER visits in cities are for treatment of domestic animal and human bites. Most biting incidents are provoked, and the biting animal usually is known to its victim. Not startling. Dogs and cats are by far the two most common pets in the U.S., accounting for more than 125 million animals.

An unprovoked attack raises the possibility of rabies, a dreadful and usually fatal condition described in Mesopotamian texts as early as 2300 B.C., which was innovatively treated by Louis Pasteur. Wild animals like bats, coyotes, foxes, raccoons, and skunks are widely infected with rabies virus, but rodents and rabbits usually are not. For deep wounds it's also worth checking to be sure the bitten person is current on tetanus vaccination.

Human bites in adults often occur during drunken fights. Did the person who did the biting remember to first gargle with mouthwash? Don't take it personally, but human bites, which introduce innumerable organisms, are far more infective than dog bites are. Anaerobic mouth flora can produce an early necrotizing infection and staphylococci and streptococci cause late infections. Bites from children, which are typically superficial, usually do not get infected.

What to do: vigorous wound cleansing, irrigation, and debridement of necrotic material decrease the incidence of infection. Lacerations of the tendons or entry into joint spaces must be identified. In severe bites, x-rays should be used to find bone fractures and foreign bodies. Broad-spectrum antibiotics are recommended for cat bites in any location and for human bites. Wounds of the hand, like infected wounds, should not be sutured because they may lead to abscess formation and loss of hand function.

LITTLE BITES

Did you know that a mosquito has 47 teeth? Its bite feels like it. Or that ticks can drink 400 times their body weight in blood at one time? Disgusting.

While bites of large animals are more likely to attract attention, the bites of small creatures may be just as dramatic. Consider that there are more different kinds of insects in existence today than all other kinds of animals put together and many of them bite humans. Some insect bites are readily detected, but others are not. Bedbugs, bird mites, chiggers, fleas, ticks, and white mites are the main biting arthropods, and centipedes, fly maggots, and sand fleas also bite. Sometimes the bite is little more than an annoyance.

Instead, the bite of the brown recluse spider and the black widow may induce fatal shock (intravascular hemolysis). Ants, bees, hornets, scorpions, wasps, and yellow jackets have venomous bites, causing 50 to 100 deaths from allergic reactions (anaphylaxis) each year in the U.S. alone.

Dangerous infections like viral encephalitis and Rocky mountain spotted fever are spread by arthropods. Some tiny ticks carry Lyme disease, now the most commonly reported, vector-borne disease in the U.S.

The arthropod should be removed with a tweezer after exposure to alcohol. Calamine lotion, antibiotic and corticosteroid creams and lotions, or a cool wet dressing may be applied. A little meat tenderizer (papain) alleviates the pain. For people at risk for anaphylactic shock, injectable-drug emergency kits for the home save lives.

*   *   *

"Never This Bad"

"My foot's swollen." Thirty year-old Dave Miller gingerly pulled off his right boot. His face and the back of his neck were deeply and prematurely lined from chronic exposure to the sun.

"Why do you wear so many pairs of socks?" I asked.

"I'm trying to absorb the fluid draining from my foot." Carefully he pealed back the last athletic sock, exposing the foot.

It was a sight not even a mother could love. The lower foot was grossly swollen, like it had been injected with water, and was leaking like a sieve. The normally white skin of his ankle was taut over the top of his foot and looked angry red. His toes were so edematous he couldn't pull them apart to show me between them. The odor was foul—much worse than a locker room smell. I placed some toweling down on the floor to catch the constant drips.

"I've had problems with fungal infections before, but never this bad," he commented.

"Why did you wait so long to come here?"

He scratched his unruly beard with thick, calloused fingers. "I work nights. I sleep during the day. It's hard for me to keep a doctor's appointment."

"What do you do for a living?"

"I'm in production. I'm on my feet all day."

"Production?"

"I make culverts." His perpetually open mouth revealed his large, gaped teeth and gave him an undeservedly dull appearance.

While we talked, I cleaned Mr. Miller's foot, applied antifungal cream, and wrapped it with gauze. Surprisingly, the foot was not too painful to him. We discussed wound care and foot hygiene. "You have to leave your foot out of your shoe until this heals."

"How am I gonna do that?" He waited on my response.

"Wear a sandal or open-toed shoe. You'll also need to take two types of pills: one for the fungal infection and another to fight the bacterial infection you also have. Come back every few days so I can check your progress. We don't want the infection to spread up your leg."

"It could get worse?"

"Yes, but let's hope not."

When I summarized the findings for Dr. Carlos Santini, my clinic attending, he became animated. "You think that's bad. A resident friend of mine saw this guy from the back-woods country. He limped into the ER smelling ripe and complaining about his foot. He couldn't get his boot off, so he laid down on the examining table and the resident gave it a tug. It wouldn't budge so he yanked. To his horror, the boot came off—with the foot inside."

The thought sickened me. "You're making this up."

"No. The guy slept in his boots and hadn't bathed for who knows how long. The foot was rotted with infection."

"Is this some kind of Paul Bunyan story?"

"Not at all. It really happened. Scout's honor."

I scrutinized him carefully for signs of mirth in the corners of the eye, or mischievous turn of the mouth. I couldn't crack him.

Apparently, a boot can hide many evils.

FUNGAL SKIN INFECTIONS

Fungal infections of the skin may be superficial or deep. The common ones are superficial and are named for their location: tinea capitis (head), tinea corporis (body, "ringworm"), tinea cruris (groin, "jock itch"), tinea pedis ("athlete's foot"), tinea unguium (nailbed, onychomycosis), and tinea versicolor (trunk).

"Athlete's foot" most often presents as scaling. It may progress to burning, itching, and stinging, with fissuring and maceration of toe web-spaces. The appearance is usually typical, but fungal hyphae can also be demonstrated microscopically in skin scales treated with potassium hydroxide. Application of drying powders, avoidance of re-infection at community bathing places, careful drying of the toes after showering, and personal hygiene are essential to prevention.

Topical treatment is adequate for simple infections, but oral therapy with itraconazole or ketoconazole is recommended for recalcitrant infection. In severe cases, if the foot becomes secondarily infected with bacteria, as in cellulitis, lymphangitis, and lymphadenitis, oral antibiotics are necessary.

*   *   *

"How Did I Get This?"

The young college student lay gowned on the examining table with her legs apart in the stirrups. Her long brown hair fell at her sides as she wiped tears from her eyes. "It hurts real bad. What is it?"

I readjusted the examination lamp. She had trimmed the pubic hair over her vulva, as half of my young patients do, which made the affliction all the more glaring. In the incandescent spotlight, the whole area looked angry. A blistering rash covered her labia and had spread around her urethra and into her vagina. The sores were at different stages, some open and draining, others dried.

"You've got genital herpes, Georgette," I said, shutting off the examination lamp. "You can sit up now."

"How did I get this?"

"It's a sexually transmitted disease."

"But I only had sex once!"

I raised my eyebrows. "It takes only once."

"I can't believe this. It's so unfair."

I guessed it probably was. "Did you practice safe sex?"

She shook her head. Her skin was quite fair and her cheeks were as ruddy as a doll's. In the overhead lighting, her shiny hair assumed a red tint. "We didn't use a condom. I was on birth control pills and I thought I would be okay."

"That protects you from pregnancy, not sexually transmitted diseases."

She made no sign of understanding. "But if I got it from him, how come he didn't have pain like I do now? I had burning and tingling down there even before the rash appeared."

"The infection can be passed on when the lesions are not painful but still shedding."

Georgette cried harder. "I'm so angry at him. I'm going to call him. I'm going to tell him what he did to me."

"That's a good idea. What we need to do now is treat this."

Tears were caught in her long lashes. She dabbed her eyes and collected her thoughts. "What causes it?"

"It's a virus."

"Can it be cured?"

"No, not really. It *can* be controlled. I'm prescribing an anti-viral medication for you to take by mouth. This rash will completely go away over a couple weeks but it may reappear on its own at another time."

"You mean I'm going to have to live with this for the rest of my life?"

I hated to be the purveyor of bad news. "Without treatment most people have recurring episodes. On the optimistic side, now that you realize what this is, you can feel it coming on before the rash and call for a refill of this medication. That will shorten the episode and cut down on the pain. The rash may return in a different area, such as over your buttocks."

"And will I give this to anyone I have sex with from now on?"

"Well, we're rushing ahead of ourselves here, but the idea is that you don't have sex when you have any of these sores or lesions."

She sobbed openly. "I've ruined my whole life."

"Now, now, it's not as bad as all that," I said, trying to console her. "The more you learn about genital herpes, the better able you will be to protect yourself and others."

I counseled Georgette Thomas about AIDS and other sexually transmitted diseases. The situation was far too common. Here was another one of nature's paradoxes: something as beautiful as sex could be blighted by such dreadful conditions as the sexually transmitted diseases, and innocent youths were the usual victims.

HERPES INFECTIONS

Herpes was derived from a Greek word meaning *to creep*. The term is apt, as herpes viruses travel from repositories along nerves to do their damage. Nature lends no helping hand. Exposure to sun and wind, fatigue, fever, menstruation, stress, trauma, and viral infections trigger recurrences. Another cause is being immunocompromised, as with AIDS.

Herpes simplex virus infections, which cause searing, blistering rashes, assume two forms in adults. Herpes simplex type I infections, often referred to as "cold sores" or "fever blisters" (herpes labialis), erupt around the lips and mouth. Most adults acquire herpes simplex type I asymptomatically in childhood. Herpes simplex type II, a sexually transmitted virus, instigates genital infections (herpes genitalis). Regional lymph nodes may swell and become tender.

Oral treatment with antiviral drugs inhibits viral proliferation and staves off some but not all recurrences. For initial infections, it should be taken five times a day, but for use in preventing recurrences, it may be used two or three times a day. Topical antiviral cream is effective in reducing the duration of lesion pain and speeding lesion healing caused by recurrent herpes labialis in otherwise healthy adults.

Herpes simplex viral infections have also been linked to facial paralysis (Bell's palsy), disseminated infection, encephalitis, esophagitis, and ocular disease in susceptible hosts.

*   *   *

"It Looks Gross"

Thomas Parnes, a tall, skinny sixteen-year-old with oily, brown hair and facial acne, showed up at the clinic with his mother. His black trousers hung stylishly at half-mast. An oversize, khaki T-shirt completed the outfit. "I can't sit still in school," he complained. "This itch is driving me nuts."

"Tell me about it," I said.

He glanced at his mom.

"Well, go ahead, Tommy," she urged.

He looked down. "It's between my legs. It looks gross. I can't stop scratching it." He spoke so softly I could barely understand him.

Uncertain, I looked over at his mother. She pointed to her groin. "You should know that a few days before this started, he was out in the woods with a couple of friends goofing off."

"We weren't goofing off," he retorted quietly for the record.

She ignored him. "I think it may be poison ivy. We went to the store and got him some pink lotion."

"Did it help?"

"Not very much."

"Well, let's take a look. Do you feel uncomfortable with me examining you, Tom?'

He readjusted the baseball cap he wore reversed and tightened down on his head. "Nah, but I want my mom out of here."

Mrs. Parnes left the room, motioning she'd be right outside the door. Tom dropped his shorts. A red rash covered his penis, scrotum, and thighs. From scratching so much, he'd broken the skin, and there was mild swelling. Mrs. Parnes' speculation was correct: it *did* look like poison ivy.

"Is the rash anywhere else on you?"

"No."

I had him pull up his trousers and wrote a prescription. "How did you get it *there*, Tom?"

"I was taking a whiz in the woods near some plants." He smirked. "We were having a pissing contest. My friends got it, too. I guess we didn't figure it was poison ivy."

"Did you win?"

He smiled proudly. "Yeah."

"Well, here's your prize. Put this cream over the whole area."

CONTACT DERMATITIS

The skin is touchy about its environment. Contact dermatitis is an acute or chronic inflammation of the skin from direct contact with chemicals or allergens. In about 80% of such cases, chemical irritants, like adhesive tape, cosmetics, detergents, hair dyes or sprays, jewelry, latex, nickel, preservatives, soaps, and solvents, are to blame. The red and scaly irritant lesions are distributed on exposed body parts and their location often provides a clue to the source of irritation. Occasionally the diagnosis is confused with eczema, impetigo, or scabies.

Poison ivy or poison oak are contact allergies. They appear as crusting and weeping macules, papules, or vesicles. Shortly after exposure, prolonged washing or dousing with isopropyl alcohol may be effective. Those at risk for poison ivy and poison oak dermatitis, should use barrier creams, gloves, and protective clothing. Continual scratching of the lesions starts secondary infections.

Topical treatment is sufficient for localized involvement except on the face. During the acute weeping stage, compresses or wet dressings, alternating with calamine or starch lotions, work well. High-potency topical steroid creams or gels suppress itching. Ointments worsen skin maceration and should be avoided when weeping is extreme. As the dermatitis subsides, mid-potency steroids are useful. Severe or widespread dermatitis usually requires oral corticosteroids. Even uncomplicated allergic contact dermatitis often takes several weeks to resolve.

*   *   *

"I Have a Date Tonight"

"I brought Carol in today because she's been complaining about her eyes." Turning to her daughter, the woman said, "Tell her what's been going on."

Carol Owens, a fourteen-year-old, full-bodied girl of average height, with a heart-shaped face and big, brown eyes, had difficulty explaining her problem. "It's kind of weird," she said in a breathy voice, looking at her mother as if for confirmation. "I can't sleep in my bed, because every time I do, I wake up with both my eyes puffy. So I sleep on the recliner in our den."

"What do you mean? Is it your eyelids or around your eyes?"

She pointed to the upper eyebrow arch and under her eyes. "During the day, they get swollen again, but not as bad as the morning. They tear and get red."

"Have you had any sinus congestion? Any recent head colds?"

"My nose runs a lot and it's itchy here." She touched her nostrils.

"Do your eyes itch? Do you find yourself wanting to scratch your eyes?"

"Yeah." She denied fever, headaches, or trouble with vision.

"Ever had allergies?"

"No, I never did before, but my mom does and my nose is running like hers."

"That's true," the mother said. "She's always rubbing her nose like I do."

When it came time to examine Carol, I was reassured that her eyes moved fully in all directions and her visual acuity was normal. Her eyes did not bulge and her eyelids weren't even puffy, but she did say they were better that day. Her conjunctiva were injected and the sclera were slightly red. When I looked with a light inside her nose, the normally pink ridged turbinates were blue and covered with copious, clear nasal discharge. The back of her throat was injected and coated with the same clear drainage."

"It looks like you have allergic conjunctivitis and rhinitis, Carol. Your eye swelling could be due to allergies."

Both mother and daughter seemed reassured. I wrote prescriptions for fexofenadine and eye drops and instructed Mrs. Owens to contact me if Carol was feeling worse.

A week passed. Mrs. Owens requested another visit for the same problem. Although the medication cleared up the sinus problem and Carol's eyes were less itchy, they were still puffy in the morning and again in the afternoon. I was trying to determine what else could be going on. A sinus mass? But any process going on for three months that produced no other physical signs was probably not serious. All the same, I was on the brink of considering a CT scan of the sinuses to be sure. What was the diagnosis? Serious things were all I could seem to entertain.

Carol sat patiently on the examining table. Her eyes were slightly more swollen, nothing more. As I stared at her, it finally dawned on me. The clue was there all the time, but it hadn't registered. I glanced at the mother then back to the daughter. Both made up their eyes the same way. Carol was wearing eyeliner and mascara as well as foundation and blush.

"Have you changed your make-up recently, Carol?"

Mother and daughter looked at each other at the same time.

"Well, yeah, I bought some new mascara."

"When?"

"A couple months ago."

"About the time when your eyes started bothering you?"

"Yeah, I think so."

"Do you and your mother use the same brand of make-up?"

"I used to, but I bought some new stuff."

"How often do you apply your eye make-up?"

"I put it on twice a day, first in the morning, and then I reapply it when I come home from school in the afternoon."

"Do you wash it off at night?"

"No, I sleep with it on."

"Do you think she's allergic to her new make-up?" her mother inquired.

"It's possible. We have to do a test."

The girl looked at me straight-away as if to say *I know what you're going to do*. It took her only a split-second to respond. "I'm *not* going without my make-up," she protested. "Give me a break."

"All I'm asking you to do is not to wear any eye make-up. Use your other make-up as you wish."

"Can't I use a little eyeliner?"

"You can't use eyeliner," her mother interjected. To me she said, "She puts it all along the border of her eyelids."

"Well, *you* do it, too, mom. I'm doing it like you."

"This is only for one week," I explained. "We have to see if the make-up is the problem. If your eyes don't puff up anymore, then you're allergic to it. We have to give your eyes a chance to heal from the irritation."

"Mom-m-m. I have a date tonight."

"You can go out. You just can't wear eye make-up," Mrs. Owens replied.

Carol cupped her face with both hands like the tortured figure in *The Scream*. "I'd rather break up with him than to have him see me without make-up."

"Well, if he's that superficial, you can do better," I said. "Besides, your brown eyes are pretty even without make-up."

"Yeah, that's right," her mother agreed.

Carol looked down, a little embarrassed, but pleased nonetheless.

"It's not like you'll never wear make-up again," I added. "You may need a different kind that's hypoallergenic."

"Actually, my eyes aren't really that bad," she said.

I looked over at her mother, who smiled. "Come on, Carol, your eyes have been bugging you for months."

Carol made a face.

"If this doesn't work," I said, "I'm going to have to send you to a specialist. If you help me out here, you may not need any tests." I hoped to coax an agreement.

"Well, can I wear my eyeliner just *once* more for tonight, then I'll stop tomorrow?"

First quibbling, then bargaining. I thought of Annie in the Broadway musical singing:

> *Tooo-morrow, tooo-morrow,*
> *I love ya, tooo-morrow,*
> *you're only a day away.*

Her mother shook her head no.

"So, do we have an agreement, Carol?" I asked. "I don't hear a promise coming out of your lips."

She glanced at her mom and they looked back and forth. No words were exchanged.

"Okay, I promise," she agreed reluctantly.

A week later—guess what—no puffy eyes.

COSMETICS AND HEALTH

Beauty or youth, sexual appeal and prestige in an elegant bottle. Women are eager consumers of cosmetics, doing about $35 billion dollars of business with the cosmetic industry each year. Starting to wear make-up is one rite of passage into adolescence and womanhood and the beginning of an inextricable link between cosmetics and our concepts of feminine beauty and aging.

The product array is impressive: anti-aging creams and lotions, blushes, eyebrow pencil, eyeliner, eye shadow, foundation liquids and powders, lipsticks and glosses, mascara, and moisturizers. How much will you pay? $150 an ounce? More? According to *The Beauty Bible*, the biggest cosmetic companies spend $1 billion a year on advertising alone, collectively launching 1,700 new cosmetics a year, most of which are 80% water.

Let the buyer beware: many cosmetics irritate the eyes or skin. Cosmetics with a blemish? Moisturizers can oversaturate the skin, start infections and impair the skin's ability to heal. Some cause photosensitivity. But cosmetic labels assure: for sensitive skin, hypoallergenic, or noncomedogenic. How can that be? The FDA requires no proof of such claims.

And what do all of those "natural" ingredients—algae, eucalyptus, extracts (from cows, placenta, plants, and spleen), grapefruit, lemon, menthol, minerals, oils, peppermint, SD alcohols, vitamins, and witch hazel—do to your skin? Or the list of blatant chemicals: butylene glycol, cetyl alcohol, methylparaben, PEG 60 hydrogenated castor oil, polysorbate 40, potassium hydroxide, and stearic acid? Some cosmetics labeled as sunscreens put you at risk for skin cancer because they do not block ultraviolet radiation. Women suffer eye infections from a dangerous overgrowth of bacteria in a cosmetic product due to misuse or poor preservation.

The FDA urges the following common sense procedures. Discontinue use immediately if irritation occurs. Wash your hands before using cosmetics and apply only with clean instruments. Do not use products contaminated by being too old, being shared with others, stored in a hot place, or moistened by saliva. Avoid scratching the eyeball or skin during application.

We will never give up our cosmetics, but we can learn to use them more wisely and selectively.

COMMON EYE PROBLEMS

The eyes—"windows to the soul." One of our most crucial sensory organs, they are vulnerable to abrasions, foreign bodies, infection, inflammation, lacerations, and trauma. Besides these local conditions, many systemic diseases leave their mark on the eyes.

Although redness is the most frequent symptom, eye disorders cause burning, itching, scratching or other pain, conjunctival discharge, sensitivity to light (photophobia), and watering. From the benign to the serious, other symptoms include spots before the eyes (floaters), flashing lights, double vision (diplopia), eye bulging (proptosis or exophthalmos), and visual impairment or blindness.

Conjunctivitis, the commonest acquired eye disease seen by primary care practitioners, is the most frequent cause of red eye. Typically, bacteria or viruses inflame the conjunctiva. Extended-wear contact lenses, which are worn for seven days at a time, multiply the risk of corneal infection up to 30-fold. Good eyelid hygiene and the application of topical antibiotics may suffice. No single broad-spectrum antibiotic covers all bacterial etiologies of conjunctivitis.

Can a sexually transmitted disease such as chlamydial infection or gonorrhea cause conjunctivitis? Sure. Transmissible by eye-hand contact, STD's are becoming prevalent enough to consider routinely because they demand aggressive antibiotic therapy. Conjunctivitis due to other bacteria is usually self-limited.

"Pink-eye" is a highly contagious viral conjunctivitis. Patients should avoid contact with others for at least a week. Adenovirus is the most common agent, occurring in epidemics. Contaminated fingers, health care clinics, schools, swimming pool water, and workplaces allow the virus to spread.

Other causes of chronic conjunctivitis are also common. Allergies head the list, causing severe itching to allergen exposure. They respond to treatment with anti-inflammatory drugs, mast-cell stabilizers, or topical antihistamines. Blepharitis, an inflammation of the eyelid margin, leads to painful styes (chalazions, hordoliums). Prolonged use of contact lenses and ophthalmic medications or solutions are common non-infectious causes of chronic conjunctival irritation. A small amount of detective work will often do the trick.

18

A Plague Bridging Two Centuries

We must face what we fear;
that is the case at the core of the restoration of health
—MAX LERNER

What AIDS shows us is the limits of tolerance
—TONY KUSHNER

AIDS has taught us humility. That one little virus has reminded us
how much we still have to learn
—DONALD HENDERSON

This is a landmark in the history of medical ethics ... saying for the
first time that ... the physician may be required to violate patient
confidentiality
—JAMES E. DAVIS

The biggest disease today is not leprosy or tuberculosis, but rather
the feeling of being unwanted
—MOTHER TERESA

"I Never Noticed Them Before"

I had misgivings about Felix Pescadaro from the moment I saw him. Although I was unaccustomed to making instant value judgments, I learned to take strong first impressions seriously, especially when they were negative, even if I could not pinpoint the reason. He was dressed in black—T-shirt, jeans, boots, and a leather jacket. His hair was jet black, greased back, and wet-looking. The stubble of a beard lent him a sinister appearance. He had acne around his mouth and large black heads on his nose and forehead. His face was greasy. It wasn't his appearance though; something else about him was troublesome.

Give people a chance to show their good side before you judge them bad, a little voice in my head said. I introduced myself and settled in to take Mr. Pescadaro's history. Still wary, I had the urge to gather all the items on top of my desk and tuck them in a drawer for safe-keeping. I noted that his chief complaints were vague and hard to get a handle on.

"My back's been bothering me and I can't get no relief." He kept wiping his nose with his hand every few minutes.

I offered him a tissue and asked the obvious question: "Head cold or allergy?"

He denied both.

"What have you tried for your back?"

"The stuff at drug stores." He offered no explanation as to how or when the pain started. He was unclear where exactly it was located and what made it worse. That was distinctly unusual for a person with legitimate back pain.

"Does anything make the pain go away?"

"Demerol." That was the question he was waiting for. It had taken him less than ten minutes to reveal his agenda. He said he tried codeine and other narcotics in pill form. Now the runny nose and sniffing made sense too. He was an addict; it was that simple. Whether he ever had back pain or not was uncertain. This much was clear: he was itching to secure more narcotic.

I decided what to do. "You will need a full physical examination. Please get totally undressed behind the curtain and put on the gown facing backwards. Leave your clothes on the chair outside the curtain. If you'll have a seat on the examining table, I'll be right with you."

I waited for him to put his clothes on the chair. When he laid down the jeans, a vial fell to the floor. It looked like it could be a vial of crack. I noticed during the interview that he kept slipping his hands inside the right front pocket of his jeans as if to be reassured. I hesitated for a moment as I wondered about calling security.

Perhaps I was jaded. Patients told me about drug deals on the street corners in the neighborhood all the time. I did witness the surreptitious looks between surly people exchanging money near the hospital.

Pescadaro popped his head out from behind the curtain. His eyes were riveted on the vial. Immediately, he reached down, snatched it, and put it back in his jeans.

"Is that what I think it is?" I asked sternly.

"It depends what you think it is," he sneered.

"It's crack, isn't it."

"Don't let your imagination run wild, lady. It's my allergy medicine." He gave me an oleaginous smile.

I knew from his chart that he didn't have allergies. "Let's get on with the examination, Mr. Pescadaro." I opened the curtain and started his physical. Now I was struck with the dark circles beneath his eyes. His face looked prematurely old. Taking his blood pressure in both arms afforded the opportunity to survey his inner arms for needle punctures sites. I asked if he was right- or left-handed. He said he was right-handed, so I scrutinized his left forearm. An addict who uses oral narcotics will sooner or later move on to intravenous drugs to get that desired high. My perseverance was rewarded. I pointed to four recent needle punctures. "What are these from?"

Mr. Pescadaro wiped his nose and laughed malevolently. "They were made by hungry mosquitoes."

I tried to ignore his attitude. I was determined to give him a thorough examination. When I examined his back I noticed a crescent shaped, purple, mottled pigmented area on his right upper back flank. About the size of half a quarter, it was flush with the skin and not tender to touch. I found two others like it on his lower legs. I pointed them out. "How long have you had these purple markings on your skin?"

"I don't know, I never noticed them before. What is it with you and my skin? Read my lips: it's my *back*, my back," he said sarcastically.

I had him lie flat on his back, which he did without any apparent discomfort. I put on gloves and palpated his inguinal nodes. They were painless but swollen in both groins. *Hmmm, better check his armpits, too.* There were two, nontender, enlarged nodes in the right armpit as well. I finished the physical with a rectal examination, which was normal. Making sure that he had good anal muscle tone was important because chronic back pain could be due to a spinal cord problem. I told him I had to go over my findings with the physician so not to get dressed yet.

Dr. Mike Conley listened to the history and followed me into my office. I knew he would not be put off by the patient's recrimination. After he examined the skin lesions, felt the patient's nodes, and glanced at the needle tracks, he stepped back and folded his arms over his chest. "You're injecting yourself with drugs, aren't you."

"You're crazy!"

The air was heavy with portent. The physician looked him in the eyes and said without blinking, "Those look like needle tracks to me. Don't bullshit me, Mr. Pescadaro! Talk straight."

"It's none of your fucking business! It's my back that's killing me, remember?"

"Mr. Pescadaro, if you're doing IV drugs, you are at high risk for acquiring AIDS. The nurse practitioner and I have found suspicious skin lesions on your back and lower legs that look like Karposi's sarcoma, a type of skin cancer found in patients with AIDS. That cancer can kill you. It's not something to be ignored. Enlarged lymph nodes in your groin and armpit also point to HIV infection. You need to get those lesions biopsied as soon as possible, get tested for HIV, and stop using street drugs. You also need to detoxify, perhaps at a community program we can recommend."

"What about my back?"

"I will give you a non-steroidal anti-inflammatory medicine for your back and suggest that you try some heat on it. Your back isn't your main problem."

Mr. Pescadaro looked contemptuously at me and then at Dr. Conley. He jumped off the exam table and quickly put on his clothes. "You're all fucking *crazy* here," he shouted. "I came in for my back and you're telling me I may have AIDS. This is too fucking much! I'm out of here, man." He grabbed his leather jacket and hightailed it.

Dr. Conley looked at me and shrugged. "Document your physical exam and what we recommended in your note."

Yes, I thought, how true are the words:

What a piece of work is man...
the paragon of animals.

So no one would make a mistake in the future, I printed in Mr. Pescadaro's chart:

WARNING
!!! THIS PATIENT IS A DRUG ABUSER—NO NARCOTICS
OR OTHER ADDICTIVE DRUGS!!!
POSSIBLE KARPOSI'S SARCOMA
PATIENT REFUSES TEST FOR HIV

I learned about the outcome of some of my patients in unusual ways. Several months later, I transported an asthmatic down to the ER for treatment and passed by the x-ray view-board on my way out. Two residents huddled around a chest x-ray. I heard the name Pescadaro. When I stopped to look at it, I saw hazy infiltrates in the lungs. The residents discontinued their conversation and checked at my name tag.

"Ah, so you're the nurse practitioner who saw this guy," one said. "Your name's all over his chart."

"Why, what's the matter?" I asked.

"No, nothing. You were right."

"About what?"

"He has AIDS."

"Is this pneumocystosis?" I questioned.

"Yes."

Exactly—everything fits. I happened to look over toward the patient area and saw Pescadaro sitting in room four, coughing his head off. He looked wretched. "You know about the drug addiction?"

"Yes. I saw your note. I don't think that will be a problem much longer."

"Why?"

"He still denies he has AIDS. I doubt that he'll let us admit him for treatment."

Was it really denial or fear of being in the clutches of that merciless beast? At that moment my attitude toward Felix Pescadaro's drug addiction vanished. I felt genuinely sad for him. "That's too bad," I said with a tone of resignation. "That's how he was with us, too."

I now fully realized that nothing could be done for those who refused help. Maybe I *had* learned that one most difficult lesson after all. I could see that the resident was still bothered by Mr. Pescadaro's obstinacy. He would have to go through his own process of dealing with such patients.

BEYOND THE MYTHS ABOUT HIV AND AIDS

The conflagration of Black Death from 1347 to 1351, which was ignited by the pneumonic form of bacterial plague, killed nearly all who contracted it or about 75 million persons as it spread worldwide. Now curable with antibiotics, that plague pales next to a new, viral "plague" spanning two centuries.

First described in 1981, Acquired Immune Deficiency Syndrome (AIDS), is the devastating repercussion of infection with the Human Immunodeficiency Virus (HIV). The epidemic of HIV infection, which affects 100 million persons worldwide, will blaze into the 21st century, leaving a trail of human destruction. Its 400,000 victims in the U.S. alone, caught unaware, must suddenly face a grim diagnosis.

By 1992, AIDS already had become the leading cause of death among American men 25 to 44 years of age, the second leading cause of death among American women of the same age, and the eighth leading cause of death overall nationwide. It is the principal reason for death in half of American cities with populations above 100,000. AIDS, with its many presentations and complications, changed the face of clinical medicine. Dealing with AIDS must now be routine for health care providers.

Public figures with HIV or AIDS, such as Arthur Ashe, Greg Louganis, and Magic Johnson, as well as children like Ryan White, a young hemophiliac who lead a courageous fight, revitalized efforts aimed at public awareness, prevention, and diagnosis. Although their example has been extremely helpful, many further efforts are needed.

HIV, a retrovirus, has fewer than 10 genes compared to the 5,000 to 10,000 of bacteria and the 80,000 to 100,000 of human cells. Yet it infects and kills the very cells of the immune system that ordinarily protect against infection. More than one strain of HIV has been identified. Detection of antibodies in a blood sample confirms the presence of HIV infection.

AIDS progresses through several stages. Within a few weeks after infection with HIV, most people have the flu-like symptoms of fever, headache, malaise, skin rash, and tender lymph nodes. This "acute retroviral syndrome" lasts a couple of weeks while the virus replicates and disseminates throughout the body. Infected individuals are particularly contagious during this period. The asymptomatic phase lingers for a variable period of time, even as long as 12 years. The immune system, with T-cell counts in the low normal range, is able to limit the infection temporarily.

Then the number of helper T lymphocytes or T-cells in the peripheral blood plunges below a critical number (500 cells per cubic mm of blood) and patients enter the early symptomatic phase of AIDS. They become vulnerable to opportunistic infections and cancers. Karposi's sarcoma, a cancer of blood vessels, appears as purple skin lesions. Patients may develop evidence of neurological involvement such as dementia and a wasting syndrome with progressive weight loss and fatigue. In the advanced AIDS phase, CD4+ (helper) T-cell numbers sink below 50 per cubic mm of blood.

There is no cure for AIDS. One aim of treatment is to eradicate opportunistic cancers and infections through the use of antimicrobial drugs and chemotherapy. Another approach is to bolster the immune system. Still other drugs are directed against assailable spots in viral replication. The antiviral drugs AZT, ddl, and ddC inhibit reverse transcription, the formation of viral DNA. A new class of antiviral drugs inhibits protease, an enzyme the virus uses to cut proteins. Gene therapy and immunization for HIV are being tested. Unfortunately, HIV is becoming drug resistant.

The hard work is just beginning. The most important treatment for AIDS is prevention through education. HIV is transmitted sexually (vaginally or anally), from infected mother to fetus or infant, and by blood-to-blood contact (hypodermic needles in drug abusers). The virus does not survive when exposed to the environment. HIV-infected people are protected by the Americans with Disabilities Act, making discrimination for housing, jobs, and social benefits illegal. Research on AIDS is one of the best funded of all NIH programs and a cure should be possible in the near future.

SUBSTANCE ABUSE

By the end of the Civil War, 100,000 soldiers (of a U.S. population of 40 million) were addicted to the opium used by army doctors as a painkiller. In the war's aftermath, opium, marijuana, and cocaine could be purchased legally over-the-counter from any druggist in Virginia, Tennessee, and Kentucky. Both George Washington and Thomas Jefferson had grown *Cannabis sativa* (marijuana) on their plantations.

Even at the beginning of the 20th century, addiction, caused by inclusion of narcotics in virtually any prescription drug, was so prevalent that the U.S. government had to intercede. Cocaine was an ingredient in a popular soft drink as well as a common treatment for migraine headaches. The Food and Drug Act was the first instance of taking such a federal regulatory step.

In the U.S. today, according to the National Institute of Mental Health (NIMH), substance abuse affects nearly 10 million Americans. Half of American high school seniors polled admitted to experimenting with drugs. Now more than 90% of illegal drug use in the U.S. is marijuana (cannabis). It is no longer a drug culture, but part of mainstream America. Because growing marijuana is highly profitable, it is produced in every state. One ounce sells for about the price of an ounce of gold.

Mind-altering drugs in the form of naturally occurring hallucinogens were introduced into ancient societies as a part of rituals. In Mexico, the Aztecs exploited the hallucinogenic properties of mushrooms containing the fungus psilocybin (*Psilocybe mexicana*) and mescaline extracted from flowers of the peyote cactus. In Europe, the Vikings tapped the fungus *Amanita muscaria*. Opium poppyseeds, rich with several alkaloid narcotics besides opium, such as morphine and codeine, were native to Asia Minor, where an opium subculture developed.

In our century, LSD gained ascendancy as a prototype hallucinogen associated with a drug culture. Since then, euphemistically designated "designer drugs," such as "ecstasy" (the amphetamine derivative MDMA) or "angel dust" (phencyclidine, PCP), have emerged as the common substances of abuse from the streets to the campuses.

Drug abuse affects people of all ages in all cultural and socioeconomic groups, not just minorities, the poor, and the undereducated. Almost everyone has a friend or relative who has attempted to stop an addiction. The popular notion that addicts bring it on themselves does not deal with the biological basis of addiction.

Drug-dependency, the abuse and misuse of medications and mind-altering substances, now falls within the definition of disease. It is rooted in complex cultural, demographic, economic, medical, and political issues. Drug abuse takes an enormous toll on society, choking earnings, sabotaging physical and psychological health, and productivity, and fueling crime, social destruction, and the medical epidemic AIDS.

Why does the brain get hooked? One theory is that addiction results from drug stimulation of the brain's "reward pathways." The pharmacological and psychological effects of drugs of abuse reinforce addictive behaviors. Neuroscientists have shown that disturbances of brain neurotransmitters are involved in addiction. Drugs of abuse act on the same chemical pathways and receptors that naturally occurring compounds in the brain use. In the case of cocaine, its biological effects (on the hypothalamic-pituitary-adrenal axis) allow the design of unique interventions: a cocaine "vaccine."

Detoxification does not end addiction, but is a necessary first step in cleansing a person of drugs and withdrawal symptoms. Then the underlying disorder can be addressed. Psychosocial interventions to prevent relapse include cognitive therapy, individual drug counseling, group drug counseling, and supportive expressive therapy. The intervention success rate is about 50 to 60% for cocaine or opioid dependence. Drug-dependent patients need to understand their condition as a chronic, lifelong illness that must be treated every day.

PHYSICAL SIGNS OF DRUG ADDICTION

C, H, or 13—simple letters and numbers. But as tattoos, they may indicate an addict's choice of drug: "C" for cocaine, "H" for heroin, "13"—M being the 13th letter of the alphabet—for morphine. A heroin addict may have a monkey tattooed on the back. Some cannabis abusers prefer the tattoo of a bearded man smoking marijuana.

Drug addicts seek help under a variety of guises. Because they may deny, distort, or rationalize their problem, the health care provider must recognize the signs of drug abuse. Abnormal vital signs reflect drug intoxication or withdrawal. Substance abuse makes a person look older. The skin also reveals burns, scars, track marks, and tattoos. Superficial veins may be absent, reddened, or sclerosed from intravenous injections. Because of effects on lymphatic and venous drainage, the extremities become mushy, soft, and swollen. Antisocial emblems, such as healed scars from suicide attempts and tattoos with menacing motifs, may support other evidence of an antisocial personality.

Intoxication with stimulants, such as amphetamines or cocaine, dramatically lowers or raises the blood pressure and heart rate. Cocaine causes anginal chest pain and palpitations; a bronchitic cough and burnt fingers and lips (from smoking cocaine or "rock"); rhinitis, sinusitis, nosebleeds, and nasal septal perforation (from snorting). Pupils dilate (mydriasis), body temperature rises, and heart attack and stroke may occur. Paranoia is a common behavioral sign, and psychosis, with restlessness and stereotyped mannerisms, resembles paranoid schizophrenia.

Hallucinogens, like stimulants and anticholinergic drugs, cause perceptual changes besides the autonomic symptoms. In addition to surrealistic hallucinations, distortions and illogical cognitive leaps prevent patients from being able to ask questions.

Inhalant or solvent abusers tend to be lethargic and physically weak, unsteady in their gait, and unable to speak clearly. Their eyes may appear injected and watery.

Chronic use of cannabis (marijuana) produces an amotivational syndrome, with glazed eyes, bagginess under the eyes, and reduced lung function (vital capacity). The mental state may be dreamy or anxious and paranoid.

*   *   *

"I Thought It Was Only a Sore Throat"

I felt like I was peering into the throat of a giant cottonmouth water moccasin. Jesse Collins held his mouth wide open as I probed with my wooden tongue depressor. Thick patches of white covered the back of his throat as far down as I could see. When I scraped, some white flecks came off.

"My throat hurts when I swallow," the boyish, twenty-six-year-old complained after I finished examining him. In the office light, his skin was pale and smooth. He had delicate facial features.

"How long have you had that?'

"Maybe a week or two." He seemed to be guessing. "I thought it was only a sore throat, like a cold or something. Then it didn't go away."

"You've got thrush, Jesse."

"What's that?" His expression was quizzical. He ran his fingers through his short, wavy, brown hair. I noticed the attractive gold bracelet on his wrist.

"It's a fungal infection."

"Can you give me something for it?"

"Yes, I can. The question is why you should have thrush in the first place."

"What do you mean?"

"It's an infection that doesn't occur in otherwise healthy people unless you've been on antibiotics recently. It takes hold in someone whose immune system is compromised."

His eyes opened wide. "Why, do you think this has something to do with AIDS?" His voice was now apprehensive.

The question was a very reasonable one for someone at risk. I had a feeling he might be gay, but he hadn't told me so. "Yes, it could. Are you at risk for AIDS?"

He hesitated. "I'm gay. But I get myself HIV tested every year."

"When were you last checked?"

"I'm due." I could see his anxiety escalate. "Do you think I have it?"

"Have you had any other infections lately: pneumonia, chest colds that don't go away, diarrhea, sores on your body?"

"No."

"Do you have one steady sexual partner or multiple partners?"

He made no eye contact. It was an awkward moment. "Multiple partners."

"Do any of them have HIV infection?"

"Not that I know of. I used to have a relationship in San Francisco, but that ended. Then I moved here. I'm not in touch with anyone there anymore so I don't know what's happened to them since." His face saddened. "I didn't really care for Frisco. I felt that it was too much of'— he paused—"a meat market. I want to develop a relationship and have interests with the other person. I want it to last."

The momentary glimpse was one of earnestness.

"Are you practicing safe sex?"

"Yes, since I moved here."

"Okay, let me do a complete physical in light of our discussion." I examined him for other evidence of AIDS. He had several enlarged, non-tender lymph nodes. That was consistent. I found nothing else. "We need to get you tested and started on medication."

"Once I'm HIV positive, doesn't that become common knowledge to insurance companies and employers? I'm worried about losing my job. I'm a waiter."

"No, your medical information is confidential."

"Can I still have sex with my partners?" He looked at me keenly.

I sat back to choose my words carefully. "Exchange of body fluids can transmit HIV. If you warn the other partners, use a condom, and are *super* careful—and everyone freely consents, knowing the risks—then that's up to you."

He pursed his lips in thought. "If I do have AIDS, how long do I have to live?"

"I don't know. The new drugs can prolong life quite a while. The most important thing is to prevent opportunistic infections. The immune system is already stressed by HIV infection and can be overwhelmed by other infections. You will be vulnerable to infections you've never had before, so try to protect yourself from becoming ill."

While he sat reflecting on my words, I wondered about his psychosocial situation. "Are you quote 'out of the closet' or are you hiding this?"

"My parents know. My friends do, too."

"So you have support?"

"No, things broke off with my parents. I'm an only child and have few close friends here in NYC; I'm pretty much on my own." His smile was pained. My comment inadvertently peeled away a few protective layers, revealing a softhearted vulnerability.

I offered him some information about support groups for AIDS and gay men and sent him for blood tests to assess the status of his immune system. The thought he could have lymphoma from AIDS crossed my mind because of his diffusely enlarged nodes, but his general health seemed too good. He promised to go to the public health department for his free HIV test.

Jesse Collins phoned me a few weeks later to say he was HIV

positive. Surprisingly upbeat, he claimed his throat was feeling better since we put him on medication for thrush. However, the report on his blood work came back. His numbers were serious enough. There was no doubt now. Jesse's immune system had lowered the defense shields to bacteria, viruses, and any other microbe; he was now a sitting duck.

I made a referral to our AIDS clinic where he received antiviral drug treatment for HIV infection. I co-followed Jesse with the AIDS specialists. He did well for about six months until he developed weight loss and fatigue. When I saw him again in the clinic, he was wasting away. The rate of his deterioration was astounding. But that was the least of it.

"Jesse, can you tell me what day it is?"

"Sure." His face was blank. No answer.

"What day of the week is it, Jesse?"

He stared. I could tell he was trying to think, but he had the look of someone who has forgotten how. He didn't have the foggiest idea.

"Jesse?"

"I don't know."

"Do you know what month it is?"

Another pause without a gleam of comprehension. "Tuesday?"

"No, what month?'

Finally he shook his head. Not knowing seemed to bother him only a little; it troubled me greatly.

I stepped out to determine if anyone had accompanied him to the clinic. Thelma recollected that an older man dropped Jesse off in the waiting room and said he'd return in about an hour.

Although I had never seen it before, I wondered if this was AIDS encephalopathy, a degenerative and progressive effect of HIV infection on the brain. Because a spinal tap would be necessary to rule out the possibility of meningitis, I sent the patient to the ER. The neurology resident agreed on the phone to see him there. Unfortunately, he concurred with AIDS dementia. Here was the final tail-spin. No one could pull Jesse out of it. His disease had set a new pace for events. Who would be there for him?

From his medical chart, I got the telephone number of his parents. I dialed once and hung up before I got the nerve to stay on the line. "Mrs. Collins?'

"Yes."

"I'm calling from NYC. I'm a nurse practitioner who has been taking care of your son. This is a difficult call for me to make because I don't know you and I don't want to meddle in your business." I hesitated, trying not to be dramatic. I was now heading into the totally unknown. "I took the liberty of calling you because your son Jesse—he has AIDS. Things are not going well. I'm afraid he has lost his mental faculties and cannot contact you. He told me you were estranged and—ay-uh—I thought—well—I thought you needed to know."

"He has AIDS?" There was no sign of hostility in the voice.

"Yes."

"Is he dying?"

"Yes. I'm sorry to have to tell you that."

"Does he need money? I can wire him some money." I wondered why she was whispering. What had money to do with it?

"He needs your emotional support, Mrs. Collins. He needs to go into a hospice."

The woman was quiet. Then she began to cry.

Perhaps this was not a good idea. As I waited for something to happen to rectify the situation, I fell into a void. I took a deep breath to bolster my waning courage.

"What are you slobbering about on the phone," a gruff male voice in the background hollered. "Here, give it to me." Then he accosted me. "Who is this and why is my wife crying?"

I had the sudden inkling to hang up. Instead, after making the introductions, I repeated what I told his wife.

"I don't have a son. As far as I am concerned, he died a long time ago when he decided he liked boys. That good-for-nothing wimp's no offspring of mine."

I braced myself, involuntarily gripping the receiver harder as I ventured into a wind-tunnel of animosity. "I understand how you might feel—"

He interrupted. "Do *you* have a gay son?"

"No."

"Then you have *no* idea what it's like. You're talking off the top of your head. You *think* you know all about this. *Well, you don't know anything.*" His voice momentarily softened. "I had such hopes for him. He could have done so many things with his life... but he threw it all away. That stupid boy gave up everything. He ruined our lives, too."

"I only meant that no matter what happened previously, things are different now. He's dying from AIDS. He's losing his mind. If you want to see him again and talk to him, now is the time. Arrangements will need to be made for his care and—all too soon—his funeral."

"Well let his queer friends take care of that."

I heard his wife crying in the background.

"*Sh-h-h-h-h,*" he hissed. "As for you," he growled, "you've got a helluva lot of nerve. You've managed to stir all this up again and make my wife cry. That boy's caused her enough pain already—and me, too, for that matter. I don't want to hear anymore. Don't *ever* call here again." He slammed down the receiver.

I paused, still envenomed, as the words sank in. Now I realized why the son never went home. After I calmed down, I contacted the social workers to make arrangements for placement. They got Jesse out of his apartment lease, had his belongings boxed, and placed him in a nearby hospice. Several weeks later, on a bright but cold February day, I learned that Jesse Collins had just died.

Three days afterward I received a call. A woman with a familiar voice spoke calmly, with little emotion. She identified herself as Mrs. Collins.

"Are you in NYC?"

"Yes. I'm getting ready to go back home now."

"Are you alone?"

"Yes"—she paused—"more than ever." A sigh. "I went to the funeral, you know. I met some of Jesse's friends for the first time. They were very nice to me."

"This must be terribly difficult for you. I'm sorry."

"I knew this was going to happen a long time ago; I just didn't know when. First thing I did when I heard the news of his death was to pack a few sundries and catch a bus. My husband's upset with me, but he'll get over it."

I was waiting for the right words to cross my lips and spark the gap between us, two perfect strangers, standing over the virtual body of her only child. The pause lengthened as I wondered if any words could convey the mixture of sympathy and sorrow I felt, without cheapening, lessening, or trivializing the moment. The silence became uncomfortably long as I could only think of my own feelings and reactions or empty clichés.

"Well, I wanted to thank you for calling us a few months ago. I apologize for my husband. You must think he's a terrible man. Really, he's not. He tries, but he doesn't understand. Men don't know what it's like to be a mother. Jesse... he was still my flesh and blood... he was still my little boy. Nothing can take that away."

"I wish I could have done more, Mrs. Collins."

"You know, I got a special gift today that not many mothers get."

"Oh, what's that?"

"His male friend gave me letters that Jesse wrote to me over the years, but never sent. He said they were letters Jesse wrote when he was in therapy. They tell about the pain he felt from the way things worked out. I haven't read them all, but I can *feel* his loneliness. He was struggling to find himself...I wish things had been different. You don't know how many times I wished I could have been there for him."

In the manner of grieving people who share more of their personal lives than they otherwise might, she told me about some of his letters. "He says he drove down to see us and sat outside in his car all night long. He couldn't bring himself to come inside because he didn't want to ruin it by having a fight with my husband. Imagine that. He was so close. Then he says another time he called just to hear my voice and hung up. But this one letter is my favorite." I heard her rustling papers. "He wrote, 'I realize I can never come home, but I just want you to know how much I love you'—her voice cracked— 'mom.' I can't talk anymore. I have to go." She hung up.

For a long moment, I listened to the dial tone under the sheer weight of what she said before I slowly returned the receiver to its cradle. As her words evaporated into the silence of the day's end, I imagined all the parents who have lost their children for whatever reason and wonder how it could have happened. Those with runaways who would give anything to see them again, or hear their voices one more time, or know if they were all right. Parents who lost a child to a terrible fire, a sudden, inexplicable, senseless accident, or the cold, random, ravage of disease, who would undo time if they could. Or those parents, caught in the insidious current of work-a-day life, career-building, and living only for the future, as they drifted steadily away from their children, unaware of the widening, soon-to-be unbridgeable distance, oblivious to missed opportunities to regain contact, to forgive and to forget.

Here a father had banished his own son. I don't know if he would ever come to realize what he had done, but suddenly I felt the weight of his burden.

OPPORTUNISTIC INFECTIONS

A bad omen, the onset of opportunistic infections declares that the patient is no longer merely HIV positive, but now has AIDS. In the late symptomatic phase, opportunistic infections like fungal infections, meningitis, pneumocystosis, tuberculosis, and viruses become life threatening. Herpes viruses (cytomegalovirus and Epstein-Barr virus) presage retinal blindness and lymphomatous cancer.

Recurrent oropharyngeal and esophageal thrush (candidiasis) plague patients with HIV infection. Once-a-week fluconazole seems to be an effective strategy for prophylaxis in selected, high risk patients.

The Advisory Committee on Immunization Practices of the U.S. Public Health Services recommends that homosexual men and individuals who use injectable illegal drugs should be vaccinated both for hepatitis A and B.

NATIONALLY NOTIFIABLE INFECTIOUS DISEASES

The diagnosis of AIDS should always raise the specter of tuberculosis (TB), a burgeoning disease. More people died of TB worldwide in 1995 than in any other year in history! It ranks in the top 10 most frequently reported, nationally notifiable infectious diseases (in descending order): *Chlamydia*, gonorrhea, AIDS, salmonellosis, hepatitis A, shigellosis, TB, syphilis, Lyme disease, and hepatitis B. For people older than 65 years, TB was the most frequent disease; gonorrhea was more common in people aged 15 to 24 years, and, together with AIDS, in persons aged 25 to 44 years.

TB continues to rage globally despite the availability of effective drug therapy. Its alarming resurgence is due to HIV infection, homelessness, immigrants from developing countries, long-term care facilities, and migrant farm workers. In the U.S., more than two-thirds of the cases occur in non-white racial and ethnic groups, one-third in middle- and upper-income groups, and one-fourth in foreign-born individuals. Experts estimate that 70% of those with TB in the future will be the elderly.

Pulmonary TB, with anorexia, cough, fever, and weight loss, is the most common form of the disease, making chest radiographs useful in the diagnosis. A negative purified protein derivative (PPD) skin test does not exclude the diagnosis, but is very helpful when positive. Therapy with isoniazid (INH) and rifampin for 9 months carries a 97% cure rate. Drug-resistant TB requires the addition of pyrazinamide and either ethambutol or streptomycin.

Lightning *does* strike twice. Old TB may be reactivated by diabetes, gastrectomy, immunosuppressive therapy, and silicosis. Even with an intact immune system, a person may be re-exposed and reinfected.

Most people outside the U.S. receive the tuberculosis Bacille Calmette-Guerin (BCG) vaccine. We are not vaccinated with BCG because TB is thought to be under better control in this nation and antituberculous drugs are more readily available. BCG vaccination invalidates PPD testing for TB because the test will always be positive. Given the emergence of TB resistant to multiple drugs, our perspective may change in the future.

NEUROLOGICAL MANIFESTATIONS OF AIDS

The vascular barrier between the blood and the brain initially protects the brain from the onslaught of infection. But AIDS eventually ravages the nervous system in 90% of patients with HIV infection, according to autopsy findings. Brain, spinal cord, or nerves are targets. Neurological conditions are the presenting sign of AIDS in 5 to 10% of patients.

Coined the *AIDS dementia complex*, the combination of cognitive dysfunction, impaired motor performance, and behavioral changes has been classified on a severity scale from 1 (mild) to 4 (end stage). In stage 2, patients can no longer work, but are able to do self-care and walk. In stage 4, they are bedridden, mute, paraplegic, lack control of bowels and bladder, and lapse into coma. About 10% of those affected have seizures.

The mechanism of AIDS dementia complex is unclear, but may result from the production of neurotoxins rather than direct viral infection, although HIV has been found in the brain. Cerebrospinal fluid findings are non-specific. CT and MRI head scans exclude other potentially treatable causes of dementia and may reveal cerebral atrophy.

Infectious processes must be excluded especially when CD4+ helper cell counts are less than 100 cells per microliter. Confusion, fever, focal neurological signs, headaches, seizures, and stiff neck (nuchal rigidity), suggest meningitis due to microorganisms like cryptococcus, cytomegalovirus, syphilis, TB, and toxoplasmosis. Reactivation of latent virus results in progressive multifocal leuko-encephalopathy, a lethal brain degeneration with white matter lesions on MRI scans and positive polymerase chain reaction (PCR) on CSF testing.

AIDS also devastates the spinal cord and nerves, causing auto-nomic neuropathy, distal or demyelinating polyneuropathy, mono-neuritis, and myelopathy. About 5% of patients with AIDS develop brain lymphomas, a tumor with a poor prognosis despite treatment. Even the antiviral drugs used to treat HIV infection can provoke neurological problems.

19

Proud and Poor

The greatest of our evils and the worst of our crimes is poverty
—GEORGE BERNARD SHAW

It is not easy for men to rise whose qualities are thwarted by poverty
—JUVENAL

But I, being poor, have only my dreams
—WILLIAM BUTLER YEATS

*The other America, the America of poverty, is hidden today in a way
that it never was before. Its millions are socially invisible to the rest
of us*
—MICHAEL HARRINGTON

*If a free society cannot help the many who are poor,
it cannot help the few who are rich*
—JOHN FITZGERALD KENNEDY

"Maybe Just for Me?"

I closed the door behind me. Still wearing my white coat with the hospital logo, I told Thelma I was going to the cafeteria for lunch and asked her to take any phone messages.

As I strolled down the hallway toward the elevator, I recognized one of my patients getting off, a woman who was in the habit of arriving early for her appointments. In a desperate effort to avoid being noticed, I headed for the stairwell, but Blanche Lablanc had the eyes of a hawk.

"Doctor! Doctor!" she called out, raising her right hand. "I have an appointment to see you today at one o'clock. Can you see me now? Can you see me a little earlier?"

I explained to Mrs. Lablanc many times before that I wasn't a doctor, but it made no difference. The white clinic coat labeled me as a physician to some patients despite my name tag. I replied cordially. "Unfortunately, Mrs. Lablanc, I'm off to lunch, but I'll see you at your appointment time."

With a hint of pleading in her voice, she asked, "Maybe just for *me*?" Age had left her face with a perpetually surprised look. Her baby-fine, ashen hair was thin and long. Strands of it fell across her face as she leaned on her brown cane. Mrs. Lablanc looked vulnerable. I tried not to respond to her tug on my heartstrings. The same thing happened almost on every clinic visit, except, today, I noticed she seemed different—a little disheveled, hair slightly dirty, a look of… want.

"All right, Mrs. Lablanc," I said at the last minute in a voice of resignation.

"Oh, thank you, dear. It'll just be a quick visit."

I took Mrs. Lablanc into my office. The chart had not yet been requested. She had several new complaints. When I explored them with her, they didn't seem very definite. Something about her was bothering me…

"I like to be examined often," Mrs. Lablanc admitted. "I'm getting older now. Things can go wrong. That way, if you check me over and say I'm okay, I feel better. I sleep easier."

"Well, you can sleep soundly tonight, Mrs. Lablanc. Keep taking your medication for arthritis."

"Can you give me any free samples of that medicine?"

"You mean in addition to your prescription?"

"Yes, dear. That way I don't have to fill it right away."

I went to the drug cabinet, unlocked it, and brought back a small bag of samples. She was tickled. I smiled to myself, but couldn't stop thinking something is wrong with this picture. "Nice to see you again, Mrs. Lablanc. Take care until next time."

"Okay, Doctor."

Although Mrs. Lablanc's complaints turned out to be minor aches and pains, by the time I evaluated them and renewed her prescription, the lunch hour was gone. The busy afternoon clinic schedule could not be pushed back.

The next day, I got free to step out to a diner—this time without my white coat. Lunch à la New York City. It was a small, clean, Greek-run diner. The waiters all knew me. As I waited to be seated, I gazed longingly at the glass-encased, revolving pies and cheesecakes. I wanted a piece there and then, but was conscious of keeping my waistline. Now at the age that avaricious longing for fattening food was enough to make me gain weight, I turned my head away, avoiding further temptation.

A man with Mediterranean charm greeted me. We recognized each other. "Hello. Good to see you again."

"Hi, a window seat please."

"Yes, of course."

Once I was seated, he handed me a menu and left, returning shortly with a glass of ice water. He knew I would request it if he didn't bring it.

"Will it be the usual?"

"No. I want something different today." I continued to peruse the menu.

"Some soup perhaps?"

"No." My eyes stopped searching and I planted my finger on the menu. "How about some of your cheese blintzes with warm blueberry compote?"

"Very good. Will that be all?"

"I'd like to have a stiff drink, but I have to go back to work." I smiled.

"Too bad. I'd have one with you." He winked.

I looked at the back of the neon sign that spelled the name of the café as it hung in the window making a slight hum. Other people sat reading newspapers or books, conversing, or taking a quiet, midday reprieve from work. A waiter was wiping white-topped tables with red wooden legs. The black and white wall tiles glistened.

After the waiter returned with my order, I ate unceremoniously. Before departing I applied some lipstick and inspected my teeth for blueberry stains. When I checked my watch, I realized I had twenty-five minutes left. Now that I was fed, I could appreciate the long walk back to the hospital.

I passed a hot dog stand on the street corner just as a hot pretzel vendor was hauling his cart like a ricksha to join him. Yellow cabs pulled to the curb to drop off passengers and take on new ones, at times so rapidly, it was a mere body exchange. Steam carrying the smell of solvents rose from the sidewalk grids. I walked around them. My slow, post-meal train of thoughts was derailed only by the occasional screech of tires and battle of horns, or momentary dalliance at a store front.

A man came up to me and spoke with a Caribbean accent. "Sorry to disturb you, but I'll only take a moment of your time. I just got out of the hospital and my doctors said I need a new heart valve. I don't have any money for the surgery. If I don't get the operation right away, the doctors say I'll die. I'm asking you to give me anything you can spare, even the change in your pockets. I don't like to beg, but this is the only way I have to raise the money I need for the operation. I hope you'll think about what it would be like to be in my position. Thank you for your time." Meanwhile, he paraded around looking as healthy as a horse.

You're using the wrong pitch on me. If I had my stethoscope, I might offer you a free second opinion.

I gave him some change from my pocket, but felt like maybe I shouldn't have. Then again no one should have to beg.

Farther down the street, I saw a local merchant handing bread scraps to a woman who looked like she might be homeless. The woman accepted the bread eagerly and smiled as she tore off a piece to eat, tucking the rest into a bag. I felt like buying her a cup of coffee to go with the bread. I reached in my purse, pulled out a dollar bill and walked over to her.

As I got closer, I thought the woman looked very familiar. Then I realized who it was. Mrs. Lablanc? Yes, my own Mrs. Lablanc. I had no idea that she was homeless, or for how long. It all made sense now.

She looked embarrassed that I'd seen her, but was too close to turn away.

"Mrs. Lablanc?" I called across the distance between us.

"Hello, Doctor." She looked down at her shoes.

We stood together awkwardly for a moment. She wouldn't look up. "Would you like to go with me for a quick bite, my treat?" I asked. "I have a little time left before my afternoon patients."

"I don't wish to bother you."

"It's no bother."

Back at my usual diner, she had a slice of cherry pie à la mode and a large glass of milk. Her smile after the first bite prompted me to order pie, too, with my cup of coffee.

I made a mental note to discuss Mrs. Lablanc's situation with social services. I wasn't a social worker, but knew they would review her finances and determine her eligibility for government assistance and low-income housing. I hoped they could make temporary living arrangements for her soon.

When the waiter presented the check, all I saw was a smiley face and the words, "On the house." As he quietly retreated he turned and waved.

After that day, I never minded when Blanche Lablanc came to clinic early.

INDIGENT CARE AND HOMELESSNESS

The simple lack of access to adequate housing affects 700,000 to 7 million people in the U.S., depending on how homelessness is defined. A problem even in the Colonial Era in America, homelessness was recognized as a serious social malady in the early 1980's. In America, 37 million people live in abject poverty and 20 million are housed marginally. Despite media attention, as much as 75% of the help for the homeless comes from the private sector, especially churches, rather than from city, state, or federal sources.

The homeless are a heterogeneous population. Most are non-white men in their middle 30's, who are extremely poor and estranged from their families. About 40% are women and children. Of the adults, one-half are alcoholic, one-third are chronically mentally ill, and another third are veterans.

Homeless people are especially susceptible. Some of the factors that predispose them to illness are frequent lacerations and contusions; overcrowded shelters; poor sanitary conditions; prolonged walking or standing; shared bedding, clothes, and hairbrushes; sleeping on hard surfaces, while seated, or outside. Those who use intravenous street drugs are also at risk for abscesses of the brain and lung, AIDS, aspiration pneumonia, endocarditis (group A strep, tricuspid valve), hepatitis (A,B,C,D), pulmonary septic emboli, STD's, and TB.

With their diverse dental, medical, mental, and social problems, the homeless are an important segment of primary care, whether they are treated in clinics, emergency rooms, hospitals, or private offices. Those who provide health care to the homeless must recognize their special problems. Many homeless men and women abuse alcohol or other drugs, do not return for follow-up visits, have cultural or language barriers, are illiterate, lose their medications or have them stolen, and suffer from mental health problems. Skin disorders are perhaps the most common disorders among the homeless, affecting about one-quarter of homeless adults. The principal conditions are eczema, foot problems, infections (abscesses, cellulitis), infestations (body lice, pediculosis), lacerations, and venous stasis ulcers.

Accordingly, providers should avoid prescribing medications with an alcohol base or writing refills of potentially toxic drugs. Even for patients who are literate, instructions should be simple and direct. All medications belong in waterproof containers. Giving free medication samples encourages better compliance. For wound treatment, antibiotics should be used prophylactically. Prompt recognition and appropriate treatment can greatly improve quality of life.

You sure don't have to be homeless to lack health insurance today. About 15% of the total U.S. population is uninsured, according to Census Bureau statistics. Many in this group are indigent. They can't afford health insurance or their employers don't offer it. Serious gaps currently exist in accessibility, affordability, availability, and quality of health care for Americans.

*   *   *

"For You"

One of the clinic physicians entered my room. "I'll be taking over the care of Nilsa Lapina," he announced.

Nilsa Lapina was an elderly Hispanic woman who had an Old-World Spanish appearance. Because she spoke little English and my Spanish wasn't up to capturing the nuances I needed to take care of her medical problems, I usually had to get a translator.

"Why are you taking over?"

"She's been hospitalized."

"For what? Did I miss something?"

"No, no. You did a good job, but her medical problems are now too complex. She's developed heart failure in addition to her high blood pressure and heart arrhythmias. I was on-call the night she came in so I'll follow her."

I regretted not seeing her anymore. She'd been my patient for some time. But I realized that transferring her care under the circumstances was appropriate.

A few weeks later, someone knocked on my door. It was Mrs. Lapina. Even though the skin on her face was wrinkled, she had pretty, pierced ears. Her earrings were tiny crucifixes. "For you," she said in broken English. Without saying more she presented me with sandals, gesturing that I should take them. They were gold-colored flats with brilliant yellow netting. She came to the clinic to see the physician, but stopped by to give me the gift. Then she gave one of her *Mona Lisa* smiles.

I knew she was frail and must have gone out of her way to get them for me. I understood her to say that she planned to have me take care of her daughter. Now she had paid me the ultimate compliment.

*   *   *

"Dons't You Worry About Me"

"Can you see a patient for Dr. Conley?" Thelma asked as she stood in my doorway with a double arm load of clinic charts. "He's overbooked."

"Is it someone I've seen before?"

"No, but she's here just for a checkup. It should be a quick visit." Thelma gave me an exaggerated pleading look.

Not taken in by her innocent gestures, I asked to see the patient's chart. Dr. Mike Conley had some seriously ill patients and I felt wary.

She returned with a chart that looked as heavy as her previous load. "Now don't go giving me that look you give whenever I hand you a chart that's over two inches thick." Thelma added, "Let me know." She left abruptly.

The problem list in the front of the chart was two pages long. My lower jaw unhinged. Gladys Bordin had coronary artery disease, degenerative joint disease, early dementia, hypertension, low back pain, and supraventricular tachycardia. I gasped again when I read over the seven medications she was taking on page three. My instincts told me this wasn't going to be a quick visit, but I agreed to see her.

The patient ambled down the hall with me, using her cane to steady herself. As I turned toward my room, she tipped into the weight scales as if she never saw them. I dashed out and caught the eighty-six-year-old, black woman in the nick of time. We proceeded to the examining room arm-in-arm. She seemed relieved to sit down.

"What's the umbrella for, Mrs. Bordin? It's a beautiful, clear day."

"*Miss* Bordin!" she quickly retorted. Her forehead was lined like a musical staff and her chin was small. She wore her white hair rolled in a bun.

I repeated her name correctly.

"It keeps the sun off my head, that's why. It's too darn hot out there."

"Are you having any new problems?"

"It's my back. It's aching me so much that I's cans't stands it no more." Miss Bordin placed her right hand on the small of her back.

"How long has this been a problem?"

"Months, years, who knows anymore—a long time."

Getting the history from this patient was like pulling teeth. She was a poor historian. Eventually, through an extensive history and review of the chart, I was able to determine that her medical condition was stable. Then I noticed dried blood on her blue head wrap. "What about this blood here? What happened?"

"Well, I tends to fall a lot at home cause I dons't see so good no more."

"Do you fall because you black out?"

"No, I just trip over the 'lectricity wires, rugs, furniture, you know."

"Do you live alone?"

"My son—he's sixty-five years old—lives with me and gets my groceries, but he's never around except at night."

"How did you get here today?"

"I walks up here, 'bout ten blocks. I always try to keep my appointments, you know."

How could this woman function at home by herself? It was only a matter of time before she had an accident and seriously injured herself. That was the problem. She was very proud and independent. "I see you have Medicaid," I said. "Why don't you have a home health attendant to help you out at home?"

"Cause I dons't like them kind, always pryin' around, stealin' money or food," she replied disdainfully. "I dons't want them in my place."

"Any objection to a visiting nurse to check on you weekly?"

She reflected for a moment. "No, that would be just fine, just fine. Them ladies are professional."

When it came time to leave the clinic, Miss Bordin had no money for a cab and hadn't brought her Medicaid card with her. That meant the clinic wouldn't be reimbursed if I wrote her a cab voucher.

"I'll get home just fine, just fine. Dons't you worry about me."

As I watched her leave, cane in one hand and her dark green umbrella in the other, I thought, God, I hope so. I felt so helpless seeing the woman struggle down the main hallway, barely negotiating around all the people.

"Wait! Miss Bordin! *Miss Bordin!*" I hollered. Finally she heard me. I filled out a cab voucher and ran over to her. "Here, take this." She was appreciative.

Many of my patients have no one to look after them. They have lost their strength and yet must care for themselves. When they can no longer do that, what will happen to them? I knew that I would hear about the voucher from administration, but I couldn't let the old woman struggle home. I put it out of my mind.

*   *   *

"I Will Fight It"

Johnny Washington sported a bushy mustache and bow tie. Age

didn't leave him with wrinkles, but had tightened the skin over his face. He was smart—no flies on him at the age of ninety-two—and very proud of serving his country. His clothes were clean but old and full of patches; the cuffs were frayed and his pants were shiny and worn. He always had a two-day beard. Most the time we ended up discussing politics, although sometimes the route was circuitous.

"You're looking pretty spiffy today, Mr. Washington."

"You're looking pretty spiffy yourself."

"So, tell me, how are you doing?" I asked.

"Not so good. My brother recently died. He was a veteran, you know."

"I'm sorry to hear that."

"Yeah, I had to go to Washington, DC." He sighed.

"Is that where he lived?"

"No. There was some kind of tie-up with the government regarding who was going to pay for the burial. We couldn't bury him until they got it settled."

"Did they settle it?"

"Yes. It turned out the government eventually paid and my brother was buried in a veterans' cemetery. But for a while I thought we weren't going to be able to bury him. I don't have that kind of money. It was awful." The patient shook his head side to side in disbelief.

Mr. Washington had many somatic complaints that turned out to be manifestations of anxiety over his brother's death. When we talked more, the fear surfaced that he, too, wouldn't get properly buried when the time came.

"My sister is senile," he lamented, "my brother is in a nursing home, and I have to take care of myself and look after them. I have to make sure they're okay. I can barely get around the subways. I've outlived my wife and all my children, so I'm alone."

"I give you credit for trying so hard."

"You know, *someone* showed up at a senior citizens center and claimed he would do a free screening for old people's disease." His look was disapproving. The conversation had taken a sudden turn. I didn't know where it was headed.

"You mean Alzheimer's?"

"That's it. They put some type of gadget on my head. Later, I got a letter in the mail." He pulled the letter out of his shirt pocket and gave it to me to read. It was from a private group practice.

```
Dear Sir:

You do not have Alzheimer's disease.
Thank you for allowing us to test you.
If you have any questions please call
us.
```

Johnny Washington then displayed a bill submitted to Medicare for approximately nine-hundred dollars. He flew into a rage. "It's unfair to bill the American people for a stupid test that preys on the old people." He drew himself up proudly. "I will fight it."

I calmed him down and concluded the visit. It had been a sojourn solely for reassurance. How many people his age, I wondered, were willing to fight the fight and take on exploiters. With all the tragedy in his life, he was worried about the government's losses. While the city destroys some of its dwellers through poverty, others seem to be tempered by it and develop a powerful sense of dignity. High-spirited people like Johnny Washington were inspirational.

*   *   *

"You Don't Live Where I Do"

Marlena Lesner, just out of class, joined me for the rest of the afternoon. I enjoyed her company. She was an infusion of fresh, red blood for the day's spiritual anemia.

"Hi, Marlena. Jump in. I'm about to examine Mr. Reger."

"Great. I'm ready."

I introduced Marlena to Mr. Reger and said I would be doing some teaching. He was eager to participate. I listened carefully to Willy Reger's lungs with my stethoscope. What I heard came as no surprise. I also paused to notice he was taking much longer to exhale than to inhale. "You take a listen, too, Marlena."

She followed suit, spending more time to analyze what she was listening to.

"What do you hear?"

"Wheezes?"

"That's right," I said, proud of my protégée.

Marlena looked like a contestant on a game show who had guessed and won a Mercedes.

"Now, what else?"

Marlena had nothing else to add.

"He has asthma. His air exchange is reasonably good. Without a fever, he probably doesn't have an infection either."

"Does that mean I'm gonna live, doc?" Willy jested. He was a short, thick-chested, affable, black man in his fifties. His hairline looked razor-trimmed.

"I'm not a doctor, Willy, and yes, you *are* going to make it. But you'll need a medicated nebulizer treatment or two." Willy was one of the few people I called by first name. We'd known each other a long time.

"Here or the ER?"

"Here." Turning to Marlena, I asked, "Would you mind getting the nebulizer from the clinic nurse?"

"No problem, I'll do it," Lesner answered eagerly and departed.

"Willy, are you taking your medication regularly?"

"Yes, doc." I gave up correcting him, having failed for several years to get him to realize I was a nurse practitioner. I knew Willy meant it as a compliment. "Have you been ill with colds or flu?"

"No. Except for this, I've been healthy." He scratched his ear.

The student returned and initiated the nebulizer treatment. Willy's airways sounded less tight after the first nebulizer, but he started breathing much easier after the second. We got to talking. Marlene listened to the conversation.

"Do you have pets in the house?"

"No. The only pets we have in the house are cockroaches, loads of them."

"I read that some asthmatics are allergic to cockroaches," Malena said.

I looked at her. "Is that true?"

"Yes, a recent study says so."

"These students will teach their teachers a thing or two," I confessed to Willy. "Marlena, bring in that article. I'd like to read it."

"Okay," Marlena replied.

Willy spoke up. "The house smells of roaches."

"You can actually smell them?" the student asked innocently, but with too much enthusiasm.

"I can tell *you* don't live where *I* do," he responded with uncharacteristic sarcasm. "If you did, you'd know how the rooms smell. It'll turn your stomach. They're in the walls, under everything, even in the beds. In my kitchen, they run over anything left out, around cereal boxes, under the 'frigerator. They're all over the floor. I tries to sweep them up, but there's always plenty more the next day. If you get up at night, you crunch 'em under your bare feet in the bathroom. I don't even go down to the basement. When my daughter was little, I saw one crawl into her butt hole when she was sleepin'."

Marlena Lesner's fair skin turned a shade whiter. I cringed. You should not be so amazed, I told myself. "Can't you have something done about the roaches?" I asked.

"No. The landlord don't care. Spraying doesn't help for long and it cost too much. The whole neighborhood's that way. The guy tells me that you can't never get rid of them."

The city... alive with roaches... the stuff of nightmares.

"Why don't you see me next week, Willy, so I can see how you are coming along?" I said.

"Okay, doc." He winked.

When Willy Reger left, I told Marlena, "You can't help being sick when you live under the conditions people like Willy have to accept. Decrepit housing, overcrowding, and now major roaches."

"No one should have to live like that."

LISTENING TO ASTHMA

He fought zealously in the Spanish-American war, leading the "rough riders" to victory. He willed the Panama Canal into existence against the ravages of Yellow Fever and taunts of political opposition. With unparalleled foresight, he preserved the pristinely beautiful Grand Canyon and other wilderness areas for future generations. But Teddy Roosevelt's most endearing and inspiring campaign by far was his childhood struggle with asthma.

Once a stigma in his day, asthma is now recognized as a commonplace medical disorder to be overcome. Asthmatic former Olympic athletes, such as Amy Van Dyken, Greg Louganis, and the late Jackie Joyner-Kersee, have demonstrated what can be gained by perseverance and proper medical therapy. Asthma now afflicts about 15 million Americans, two-thirds of whom are adults. The increase in prevalence over the last decade is dramatic. Despite advances in treatment, the death toll hovers at 5,000 annually. The total estimated cost of asthma is one percent of the health care cost in the U.S., or more than 6 billion dollars. People living in urban areas, especially non-whites and the poor, are disproportionately affected.

The most common symptoms of asthma are cough, difficulty breathing (dyspnea), and chest tightness (wheezing). Asthma is a chronic lung disease that occurs when the immune system, sensitized to an allergen, starts treating it like a threat and churns out IgE antibody molecules. The antibodies attach to mast cells, which respond by releasing inflammatory substances like histamine. When the reaction extends into the bronchioles, the lung's small airways, the linings swell and produce mucus, and air passages narrow, causing difficulty breathing. Air pollution, allergens, chemicals, infections, smoking, and weather changes precipitate asthmatic attacks. Often misdiagnosed as bronchitis or pneumonia, asthma can be correctly diagnosed by patient history, physical examination, and pulmonary function tests.

Asthma is usually a problem of modern life in industrialized societies. Hospital admissions for asthma increase during times of severe air pollution, but the indoor environment has also changed. Most Americans spend at least 90% of their time indoors, corresponding to a rise in indoor entertainment. Cigarette smoke is an irritant. In humid environments, molds and pollens can trigger asthma. Dust mites, which thrive in bedding, carpets, and upholstery, have highly allergenic droppings. So do cockroaches. In one NYC study, cockroach allergies were the leading cause of asthmatic attacks.

The medical treatment of asthma is to dilate bronchi and suppress inflammation. An acute asthmatic attack with respiratory distress should be treated with oxygen, a β-2 adrenergic agonist, or an inhaled corticosteroid that is not absorbed systemically. The patient needs to be maintained on inhaled corticosteroids or a slow-release bronchodilator. Mast cell stabilizers, which are anti-inflammatory by reducing histamine release, work when used prophylactically (before exposure to allergens, cold, exercise).

When asthma is well controlled there should be no adverse medication effects, excessive use of inhaled beta-adrenergic agonists, interference with exercise or sleep, need for hospitalization, prolonged use of oral corticosteroids, or unscheduled medical care. The best way to forestall attacks is to avoid and control asthma triggers, devise a management plan for flare-ups, and schedule regular follow-up visits.

ALLERGIES

If you suffer from allergies, you can blame the dinosaurs. In the Mesozoic period they ate the gymnosperms and allowed angiosperms, or flowering plants, to dominate the earth for the next 250 million years into the present day. The male organs of plants and trees have been shedding pollen ever since. We don't know if the dinosaurs developed allergies, but the sneezes of T. Rex would have been daunting.

Man is a newcomer to the world of allergens. The appearance of humans dates back only to the more recent Quaternary period. We've had less than 2 million years to adapt. Perhaps, over time, our immune systems will evolve away from allergies—probably wishful thinking.

Today, about one-third of North America is forested, some 770 million acres with about 245 billion trees. Between sunrise and 9 A.M., pollens abound in the air. But plants don't deserve all the blame. Remember insect stings, pet dander, shellfish, and many other foods. Modern industrialized society has added a few insults to the eyes, nose, and lungs of its own: chemicals, drugs, smoke, and many more allergens.

Breathing can be hazardous if you have allergies. Invisible airborne allergens less than one-thousandth of an inch in size invade our living space, ensconce in "reservoirs" like the carpet or sofa and air ducts or the air-conditioner, and turn our own body's immune system against us.

The principal allergic diseases—asthma, rhinitis, and sinusitis—are the sixth leading cause of chronic disease. About 15% of the population has sinusitis. Hay fever (allergic rhinitis), the most common allergy, affects 35 million individuals in the U.S. Ragweed is the most troublesome pollen in North America, peaking between August and September. Six percent of Americans are allergic to cats. Sorry felines.

REMEMBERING

The music in my heart I bore
Long after it was heard no more
　　　　　　　　　—WILLIAM WORDSWORTH

[He] was like a man who stands upon a hill above the town he has
left, yet does not say "the town is near," but turns his eyes
upon the distant soaring ranges
　　　　　　　　　—THOMAS WOLFE

People are like stained glass windows. They sparkle and shine when
the sun is out; but when the darkness sets in their true beauty is
revealed only if there is a light within
　　　　　　　　　—ELISABETH KUBLER-ROSS

Tomorrow lurks in us, the latency to be all that was not achieved
before
　　　　　　　　　—LOREN EISELY

"Keep Up Your Numbers"

One morning I perused my appointment book and sighed. The schedule was booked so tightly that if anyone had a problem the least bit complicated, the whole schedule would collapse.

Thelma read my mind. "They made me book you with more patients for the morning and afternoon sessions. I told them that's not how you like to see your patients—so squeezed for time."

"What did they say?"

"Dr. Blakely said *Sorry, that's how it has to be.* What could I do?" She looked at me apprehensively.

As I thought about my time in the clinic with Thelma, I realized that nothing she could say would make me mad. Secretaries could be your best friend or your worst enemies. They could screen your calls or throw everything into your lap. Some were so good, they befriended and went to bat for the patient. Thelma was one of the good ones.

"God, I hope the patients aren't complicated or very talkative today," I said with a voice of measured equanimity. "It's not your fault, Thelma. Anyway, I have a plan. I'll save time by taking only part of the history and examining only part of the body. I'll do from the waist down today, and next week I'll do the rest."

Thelma looked horrified.

I winked at her and grabbed the chart for the first new patient. "Just kidding."

It took her a moment, but she finally laughed good-naturedly.

Later, I stopped by Dr. Patricia Blakely's office. As our clinic director, she oversaw all financial matters. We were both between patients. "Patty, you're booking my schedule too tightly," I complained. "I need more time with my patients."

"Why do you spend so much time with your patients?" she asked with a thick, Long Island accent. "These visits are supposed to be brief, fifteen-minute time slots." Her eyes were very green in the light of her office window. The girlish impression given by her short, black, wavy, hair and freckled face made be forget for a moment that she liked to take people off guard.

"It's not just me. Nurse practitioners spend time with patients to teach them about their disease, medications, what to do in emergencies, and what signs and symptoms to watch for. It's not a matter of taking a history and doing a physical exam in fifteen minutes. Many of the patients I work with are referred by physicians so I can teach them how to do a finger-stick and monitor their blood sugar level, or tell them what kind of diet they need to be on and why they need to stay on it. Pap tests and gynecological examinations on older women also take time. You need to allow time to listen to patients and answer their questions."

"Why don't you ask the social workers to handle some of the personal problems your patients tell you about?" She doodled on a piece of paper on her desk.

"Oh, but they do. They handle financial problems, check patients' eligibility for Medicare or Medicaid, and help mothers and the elderly apply for food stamps. They also deal with elder abuse. They're booked solid, overloaded. With the kind of clinic we run, we have the case loads to utilize two more social workers easily. As a result, we must handle what they can't."

"Could other personnel deal with some of these issues? Can't you refer people to psychiatry?"

"No. A person has to be floridly crazy, psychotic, schizophrenic—way out there. That's the truth. They don't have enough psychotherapists to deal with the stress of aging, chronic disease, or dying. If you want to have a patient seen acutely, they ask if it's a dire emergency. Even if you are lucky enough to get an appointment, it won't be for another four or five months."

"Surely there's a walk-in service for social work or psychiatry like our walk-in medical clinic."

"Some of the cases are viewed as too 'minor.' A lot of the patients just need to talk to someone. They don't want to admit they're depressed and usually they aren't psychotic. Some tend to place more trust in a medical person. They like talking to me. I listen to them."

Patricia Blakely looked directly at me. "Well, the financial reality is you need to increase your numbers somehow. You can't deny the business side of medicine; it pays your salary. Besides, the worst is yet to come." Her words were hardly calculated to soothe, and her tone was anything but encouraging. Then she sat back to watch my reaction.

"And how can I still give people quality care?" I stammered.

"I don't know."

I shook my head in disgust. Try as I might to bite my tongue, the words pushed their way out. "I hate to say it, but the health care system no longer puts caring first. It's too busy reaching into the wallets of our patients rather than into their hearts. No one seems worried about how all of the unfortunate people I've had the privilege to care for are shuttled through the system without concern for their inconvenience, their aches and pains, their loneliness and desperation."

"That's all well and good, but it's not my fault. It's simple. Increase your patient numbers, but don't jeopardize patient care. Now you'll have to excuse me. I have to get back to work."

How's that for a catch-twenty-two I thought as I left. Although I pondered her statement for several weeks, I found no solution. Then I knew what I had to do.

*   *   *

"You're One of the Lucky Ones"

The decision was momentous for me. I made up my mind to leave the internal medicine clinic to use my family nurse practitioner background in some other setting. Perhaps the grass across the Hudson River was greener. Maybe it was the restless itch. I gave a couple of months notice so the clinic would have time to replace me without a gap.

Each of my colleagues reacted differently to news of my impending departure. Dr. Carlos Santini was explicit. "You're one of the lucky ones who got away," he said wistfully. Dr. Mike Conley joked and teased his way out of it, but I sensed that he, in his own way, was sorry to see me go. Serai Alterman said she would miss me, gave me a hug, and seemed to mean it. Then she drifted off on a litany of her own recent adventures, not noticing that she'd lost her audience. Dr. Eva Romerez, who was not used to working with nurse practitioners and was a little wary of us anyway, seemed indifferent.

Susan Crawley's reaction to the news of my departure surprised me. Her face atypically registered some jealousy. From that moment, I sensed that Susan began to distance herself from me. Her greetings came to lack warmth. We weren't best friends, but we certainly had a good working relationship. I was a little hurt and disappointed yet understood how I might have felt if the situation were reversed. I didn't want to leave things that way.

One day I summoned enough courage to walk over to Susan's office. The door was ajar. I knocked. Susan, who was sitting at her desk finishing a chart note, looked up. "Do you have a minute?" I asked.

She motioned me to come in and sit down.

"Susan, I don't want to leave with things this way between us."

She looked relieved that the ice had been broken. Still reserved, she said, "Well, yeah, I agree with you."

"I wanted you to know how much I've appreciated your friendship and support. I feel like you're mad at me or something."

"I guess I didn't count on you leaving," Susan replied with downcast eyes. "It came as a total surprise. I always thought *I'd* be the first one to leave. I feel sort of abandoned."

"I would feel the same way, I suppose. But I didn't plan on this either. It's best for me to move on."

"Why didn't you tell me you were intending to leave? You obviously had to be thinking about this for some time."

"I wasn't sure if I would be able to do it. I've been getting more and more frustrated with the way the clinic runs—pressure to see high numbers, not enough time for complex problems, and lack of social services support. So I decided to consider my options. I made a choice to leave inner-city practice."

"What will you do?"

"I'm thinking about going to the suburbs to do more family practice and less internal medicine."

"Do you believe things will really be much different somewhere else?"

"They might be. It's worth a look. Besides, I miss taking care of kids once in a while."

"Oh, I know. It's okay. I'm not really mad. I guess I need somebody to talk to when things get crazy around here."

"You'll still have Serai to work with."

Susan rolled her eyes. "It's not the same."

"Why not?"

She paused as if on the verge of divulging an intimate secret. "Because I can't share my Martian stories with her."

We looked at each other momentarily and then broke out laughing. It felt like old times.

"Well, I guess I'd better be going," I said.

We both stood. I gave her a hug.

"Let me know what you're going to be doing."

"All right."

"Let's get together sometime, okay?"

"Sure, Susan. Take care of yourself."

*   *   *

"Who's Going to Be Taking Care of Me Next?"

I had come to know hundreds of patients; my emotions about leaving them were mixed. One of the frustrations was not knowing what happened to many of the people I'd spent a part of my life caring for. How long could patients with unraveling minds such as Nelly Fritz and Delilah Anthus hold onto a thread of reality? Would Agnes Bullock with the anal germ phobia ever lead a normal life? I didn't get follow-up. Several cases would remain loose ends.

I told everyone who came to see me I was leaving. Letters were sent to the others. I couldn't tell all of my patients because many were not scheduled to see me during my final weeks and would not have been walk-ins during that time.

The ones I did have the opportunity to tell had differing reactions. Gertrude Steuben wanted to know: *Who's going to be taking care of me next and when will I meet the new person?* Marie Acevedez wished to follow me to my new job. Blanche Lablanc asked what I was planning to do: *Are you moving to another state? Will you take some time between jobs?* Angela Guitterez and Wilma Washew said I'd been nice to them and they were going to miss me; then they got teary-eyed. Nelly Fritz broke down and cried, but she had Alzheimer's disease and cried often anyway. Willy Reger took it personally: *Don't you like taking care of me anymore?* The drug reps wanted my new address so they could tell me the name of their company's representative for that area.

*   *   *

"I Don't Like the Sound of That"

My last encounter with Dr. Janet Ressor was surreal. I'm still trying to fathom it's meaning.

I opened my desk drawer and took out a bottle of vitamins—I was into megavitamins—like I had done many other times before. That day was different: I had nothing to drink, but I attempted to swallow the caplet anyway. The caplet stuck in my throat. I inhaled and was horrified at the raspy sound I made. The caplet felt like it wedged a little more. Finally I realized the danger.

I jumped up from my desk, but my lab-coat pocket caught on the drawer. As I tore desperately at my lab-coat to free myself, I knocked things over in the room. Unable to breathe, I crouched on the floor, trying to hit myself on the back and use gravity to dislodge the pill. Salivating and drooling, I made gagging sounds as I attempted to dislodge the pill from my trachea. I couldn't think straight.

Dr. Janet Ressor, whose office was next to mine, rushed into my room. "I don't like the sound of that." She must have found me red in the face and panicking. With unexpected force, she whacked me across the back. The pill flew out of my mouth. Tears streamed down my cheeks, not from crying, but from my struggle to breathe.

"Thank you," I gasped.

"What were you trying to do?"

I explained about the vitamins in a comically hoarse voice; humor was far from my mind.

"Next time take all pills with water," Dr. Ressor said matter-of-factly and left the room.

I was quite sure she had saved my life. To her, I'll bet, it was nothing more than a reflex—a mere eye blink. I had flashbacks to a patient I saw in the ER who swallowed a pill without water in his car on the way to work and it wedged in his throat. Everyone was amazed he was able to drive himself to the ER under the circumstances. An ENT doctor had to go in and remove it. I counted myself lucky. You know, maybe I don't need vitamins after all. I tossed the bottle into the trash can.

That's the way it was in that clinic. I had a lot of respect for Dr. Ressor. She was one of the doctors I'd miss.

*   *   *

A Teacher's Farewell

Marlena Lesner handed me a folder. "Well, it's my last week working with you. I finished that patient write-up you asked me to do."

I looked it over carefully—all ten pages. "Marlena, this is good... very thorough... very conscientiously done." I hesitated.

"But what?"

"W-e-l-l, you aren't going to be able to write so much when you are out working because you won't have the time. You need to cut back on the length and focus on the critical positives. Instead of ten pages, shoot for two."

"How do you know what to exclude? It *all* seems necessary."

"You'll learn that by experience if you try to focus more. It'll take time. Nursing school teaches you how to be thorough; working in the clinic teaches you how to be succinct. I'll go over it with you later and see where it can be shortened. Why don't you give it a try first."

"Okay." Marlena looked down in the dumps.

Seeing her reaction, I added, "Everyone goes through this. I remember my first job. The attending came by and told me a transcriptionist from Medical Records complained about my dictations. They were excessive in length. I didn't know what to cut, because everything seemed important. But if *you* don't pare it, someone else will make you do it."

"No, it's not that. Not the report."

"Is something else bothering you?"

She tilted her head pensively. "Doesn't this ever get you down?"

"What?"

"These patients."

"Come on, have a seat and tell me about it." I pulled out a chair as an invitation.

Marlena plunked down. "I ache for these people," she confided. "They've become a part of my life. I feel their elation when we beat the disease. I feel their despair when we lose. When I see the elderly, I think of my own parents. When I see middle-aged patients, I realize I might have the same misfortunes. Young adults remind me of my twenties—how they would have been so altered by these diseases. Don't get me wrong. I've learned a great deal about medicine from the patients. But they are a very vulnerable group of people. I feel their vulnerability."

"Sure it bothers me, too. We all look at things referentially. That is a luxury you can no longer afford."

"What do you do about it?"

"As health care providers, we must develop our own system for preserving our optimism, our hopes, our love of life, even when we see our patients go down around us. We need to nurture ourselves. We have to realize that we are experiencing an abnormally concentrated strata of disease and bad luck. People come in with the most terrible things. We must care for them lovingly but not let it destroy us.

You also can't let the ethos of the city bring you down. Human suffering has a history and a future that exceed our own. You're trying to handle it all. We can't assume responsibility where we have none. Accept the time and resource limitations and do what you can under the circumstances."

I reflected on my own recent conversation with our financial manager Dr. Blakely on the same point. Was I being hypocritical?

"That's easier said than done," the student said with a broken smile. "We aren't taught how to do that."

"You're right. It's not in the textbooks."

"So how?" Marlena asked, raising her arms.

"I think of medical care providers as mop-up teams. Spills are happening all over, and at all hours. There are many provider teams. Each can only hope to cope with a part of the spills. We must develop the mindset that the problem is unending. When your work is done, you go home and assume a different role. It is a necessity, not an option."

"How come some other students I know aren't going through this?"

"This problem is very common among health care providers. Not everyone has as much self-insight as you do, but almost everyone comes to deal with it at one time or another. Some people are not aware of the ways...maybe automatic or instinctual...they've learned to cope. But to survive in this profession, they must have adapted to it in some way. Once aware of the process of their own pain, they usually will be able to implement the solution. Does that make any sense?"

"Yeah, in a way. I'm going to have to think it over."

"Marlena, I have enjoyed working with you. You remind me of

myself as a nurse practitioner student. If I were to sum up all of this in one sentence, I'd say that being a nurse means making a difference; delivering health care in a human way, not as a cog in some corporate machine; filling in for the system when it fails; being a patient advocate, whatever it takes to get the job done—a little bit of social worker, secretary, physician, when none is available or willing to help. That's what being a nurse means to me. I didn't go into nursing and become a nurse practitioner to do anything less."

She looked at me curiously. I know I sounded preachy, maybe even a little cynical. I wanted to tell her something about my personal experiences in that clinic and to prepare her for challenges in her own practice. At the same time, I knew she'd have to find out for herself.

It was now up to students like her to give the big city clinic a try. They would feel the burden of the city's ill's—the problems it deems insoluble or denies altogether: the abandoned, the abused, the poor, those weak in spirit or in physical strength. The challenge would be greatest for the most caring, optimistic, and motivated professionals. They would have to be strong.

Marlena thanked me, but I knew that she would not realize my contribution, if any, to her education until years later when she faced similar challenges in her own career. Then, like so many of us who wish they could find and talk to their former teachers, she would think long and hard about her experiences here. I marveled at Marlena's innocence and confidence.

At long last, I said good-bye.

*   *   *

"I'm Sorry to Bother You"

On my last day in the clinic, Thelma called to tell me I had a visitor. I went out to the front desk and brought back Nina Lopez, a wonderful, petite, middle-aged, Ecuadorian woman.

"I'm sorry to bother you." Her voice was soft, delicate, and slightly accented. "I heard you were leaving."

"Yes, today is my last day."

"My son visited me and brought me some rings—he's in the jewelry business. I wanted you to have one for all the times you have taken care of me over the years." With pride she handed me a small box. "I am going to miss you," she said.

I opened the box and found a ring inside. It had two small, lovely, emerald stones clasped in the leaves of a delicate gold setting. "I love it," I said. "Thank you so much."

The woman gave me a dignified nod. There was a simplicity and honesty about her eyes. At the last moment, I gave her a hug. Then she quickly departed.

A few hours later another patient brought me a large box all the way from home on the subway. She was Carmina Lapina, Nilsa's daughter. She reminded me so much of her mother.

When I opened it, there were silk flowers in a peach vase. I was very touched. Not knowing how to respond, I said, "You didn't have to do that. I know how hard it can be to bring things on the crowded trains."

"That's right. You obviously mean something to me."

I understood her through her accent. "Thank you. I appreciate it very much."

As my responsibilities to the clinic ebbed away, I realized that these patients had given me a heartfelt going away. I put the ring on the third finger of my right hand and looked at it again. It would be a memento of the humble, kind, and generous people like Nina Lopez and Carmina Lapina I had come to know.

*   *   *

"An Old Man's Fantasy"

The last patient I was to see in that clinic was Jose Garcia. Having taken care of him every few months for hypertension and obesity over several years, I came to appreciate his unique character and enjoyed his visits. I called to him in the waiting room. As usual, I could easily spot him. He stood over six feet tall and had a certain style of dress that reflected his native homeland of Cuba circa 1950's—the long, white pants, the white shirt and jacket with a wide tie. Even his white fedora reminded me of a tropical island's Panama Jack, which was my secret nickname for him.

Although he was in his seventies, Mr. Garcia made it known he thought of himself as a lady's man. His face, which was not deeply lined, made him look ten years younger, but his wavy salt-and-pepper hair was thinning; hence, the ever present fedora. He kept his mustache very manicured.

Mr. Garcia made his customary gesture of removing his hat with one graceful swoop of the hand while bowing before me. "Madam, I am at your service." He made me feel like a maiden in the medieval days as he, the aging knight, humbled himself before me. Always a little embarrassed, as this show was put on in front of a waiting room full of people, I usually said something like, "Oh, come along, Mr. Garcia."

Today, Mr. Garcia brought something in a brown bag. He put it aside in my office and settled in to answer the standard questions about how he was doing. After I took his blood pressure and weight and refilled his prescriptions, I noticed that he seemed preoccupied as he was rebuttoning his shirt.

"You seem deep in thought, Mr. Garcia, is anything wrong?"

"I just heard that today is your last day here. Why did you not tell me sooner you were leaving?"

"I tendered my resignation between your visits. Your last visit was two months ago. I knew I would see you before I left."

"Well, I guess this is an old man's fantasy, but I have some post-card pictures of the Virgin Islands and St. Bartholomew's Island to show you. I've been there before and was planning a little trip. Maybe you could accompany me as my private nurse since you'll have some free time for awhile. I guess you know by now I've enjoyed my visits with you." His dark eyes were vibrant.

I smiled at Mr. Garcia and graciously declined his offer to the islands, saying I didn't do private duty nursing. I did look over his postcards and said I would like to visit there someday.

Jose Garcia reached carefully into the brown bag and handed me a single, long stemmed red rose. His eyes were wet. With a cracked voice, which he strained to control, he said, "I'll miss you and so will your other patients."

Touched by his warm and sensitive gesture, I took the rose and gave Mr. Garcia a hug. I told him that I spoke with his doctor and assigned his follow up care to another nurse practitioner.

Mr. Garcia, who had regained his composure, raised his eyebrows. "And she is young, yes?"

"Yes, very young—and very married!"

He reached for his fedora and adjusted it just so on his head.

"That never stopped Don Juan." Then he smiled broadly. "Well, I must be on my way. Thank you. It has been my privilege to know you, and I count myself fortunate to have been your patient. Wherever your road takes you, I sincerely hope you find happiness and you won't be alone in that happiness."

I thanked him again for the rose and wished him well. I extended my right arm to shake hands with him as I opened the office door. Instead, Mr. Garcia gallantly took my hand and kissed the back of it. A little surprised and taken aback, I realized that Jose Garcia really could be the reincarnation of Don Juan.

Dr. Carlos Santini walked by in the hallway at that moment and saw what had just transpired and the red rose in my hand. After Mr. Garcia was well out of earshot, he teased, "Just what service *do* you provide in there for your patients?"

"I can tell you in one word," I answered.

"What?"

"Listening."

*　　*　　*

"I Hate Good-byes"

"So you finally wised up and decided to leave." Thelma attempted to sneer, but didn't quite pull it off. She entered my office as I was packing items from my desk into one of many cardboard boxes.

Stay composed and in control.

"Yeah, I'm blowing this pop-stand, as the saying goes." My throat clamped a wee bit and I felt a lump starting to form. There goes composure I said to myself as I placed my nameplate into the box.

"Well, I hate good-byes, but I stopped by to wish you luck and success in your next adventure. All these years of working with you—disagreeing, laughing, and sharing some *bizarre* moments— have left a soft spot in my heart for you. I'll miss you. She presented me a small jewelry-size box with a pink bow. She'd hidden it behind her back.

The lump was growing, my throat tightened, and now my eyes were swimming.

Blink, blink, take a deep breath and exhale slowly.

I reached out, trying not to make eye contact, but when I touched her hand, she clasped it with her other hand. I looked up to see a woman no longer able to restrain what she was feeling. Thelma's rising pool of tears, just on the verge of spilling, finally closed my throat, making it impossible to swallow. The stinging in my eyes before the hot tears was almost painful. We both dived for the tissue box at the same time and collided into each other. So much for control. After laughing, crying, and eventually hugging, we agreed we needed a make-over stat.

"Well, aren't you going to open it? It's not a Christmas gift, you know."

I opened the soft, black felt box to find a pair of gold and onyx stud earrings. They were fourteen-karat gold. I knew they weren't cheap.

"I've always noticed how your earrings amazingly matched your ensemble everyday, so I hope you have an outfit for these."

"They're beautiful, Thelma." My voice wavered as I said her name. "Thank you so much. I'll think of you whenever I wear them." I resumed dabbing and wiping.

"Well, enough of this sentimentality. I think I'd better get home and fix dinner for the mister. I can't believe I'm still here after five o'clock. You know my motto: no overtime, no Thelma." She leaned toward me, gave a quick hug, and whispered, "Take care of yourself." Turning around, she deftly grabbed a tissue and walked out.

Good-bye, Thelma Louise.

*   *   *

Remembering Their Faces

As the final hours of my last day were winding down, I found myself reassessing feelings toward my patients. I came to peace with the Daniel White's of the clinic who were trying to milk the system for disability or anything else they could get. I came to terms with patients like Amy Katz who tried to cheat their diseases, sneaking sweets at every opportunity. Even the unnerving, mentally unstable patients like Cecilia Rolanda and Roxanne Delacruz, or the angry, alcoholic Lawrence Burns, or patients like Regina Boulez, the diabetic in massive denial, who were on self-destruct missions, could not erode my growing sense of equanimity.

I finished with my paperwork and sat at my desk with hands folded in my lap. At five o'clock I stood and walked to the door. As I turned to survey the room once more—its barren walls and stark furniture—I remembered conversations I had with patients and staff, and all the human events that had played out in that cramped space. Individually, no one would ascribe too much significance to any one event, but altogether they formed an undeniable pattern. I'd learned a great deal about life. Now there was an artificial peacefulness to the room. Although I had feelings of uncertainty and loss, my work here was done at last. Today I would leave on time.

I walked out of the clinic and the hospital onto the street as I had done so many times before. The sky was no longer merely the glow of day's end; it was summer now. I looked up at the stone facade of the old hospital, remembering the faces of those with whom I'd spent part of my life. I recalled the faces of those whom I had lost—the Anna Monty's, the Alta Sweeney's, the Hector Rodriguez's, the Martha Winslow's. I saw the faces of those sentenced to die—the Gary Boone's, the Albert Green's, the Felix Pescadaro's, the Hilda Roak's, the Mary Sedgewick's, and the Frank Svelton's. I remembered those who had entertained and ennobled me—Freddie Bobbit, Gertrude Steuben, Gladys Bordin, Harold Pitts, James Whitney, Johnny Washington, Lucille Foster, Sarah Donnelly, William Robinson, and many, many others. I thought of Dr. Santini whistling down the hall, and Dr. Conley, always eager to help out. I could see Susan Crawley's face clearly as she told me about the voice from Mars. With a smile, I reflected on my special Thelma, who could read me like a book. I thought back on the people like Enrico from housekeeping who did their jobs with effort and pride on the off hours without title or recognition. All of those faces were etched firmly in my mind, and around them, the unforgettable faces of many more people off the streets of New York whose names had been eroded by time. I would remember them all. I would go home now and keep them in a special place in my heart ...

This time I would never come back.

APPENDIX

Notes on Quotations and Citations
Source Notes
Resources for Patients
Internet Information Websites
National Nurse Practitioner Organizations
Index

NOTES ON QUOTATIONS AND CITATIONS

BEGINNINGS
Coleridge, Samuel Taylor (1772-1834), English poet, critic, and theologian, *Additional Table Talk*

1

Baruch, Bernard Mannes (1870-1965), American stock broker, political adviser, and public official
Cousins, Norman (b. 1915), American editor and writer, *Anatomy of an Illness*, Norton, 1979
Kubler-Ross, Elisabeth (b. 1926), Swiss-born, U.S. psychiatrist and writer, *On Death and Dying*, 1969
Rossetti, Christina Georgina (1830-1894), English poet, *Song*, 1862
Saunders, Cicly, Dame, established modern day hospice prototype, St. Christopher's, London, 1967

2

Chase, Alexander (b. 1926), American journalist, *Perspectives*, 1966
du Maurier, George Louis Palmella Busson (1834-1896), *Petter Ibbetson*, 1891
I Did It My Way, song popularized by the late Frank Sinatra
Knebel, Fletcher (b. 1911), American journalist and writer, *Reader's Digest*, December, 1961
Lamb, Charles (1775-1834), English essayist and critic, *A Farewell to Tobacco*, 1805
Thoreau, Henry David (1817-1862), American essayist and poet
Terry, Luther L., MD, first U.S. Surgeon General's report, January 11, 1964
Van Duyn, Mona, first woman to be U.S. Poet Laureate, 1992

3

Castenada, Jesse, set 24 hour walking record in Albuquerque, MN, 1976, *The Guinness Book of World Records*, New York: Bantam Books, 1998
Dickinson, Emily Elizabeth (1830-1886), American poet
Franklin, Benjamin (1706-1790), American statesman, diplomat, author, scientist, and printer, *Poor Richard's Almanack*, 1749
Graham, Billy (b. 1918), American Southern Baptist TV evangelist

Keats, John (1795-1821), English poet, *Endymion*, 1817
Maudsley, Henry, contemporary psychologist and author

4

Dix, Dorothy (1861-1951), U.S. journalist and writer, in Martha Lupton's *The Speaker's Desk Book*, 1937
Emerson, Ralph Waldo (1803-1882), American poet, essayist, philosopher, 1834
Rainsbury, Paul, Dr., 1992
Rosch, Paul, Dr., American Institute of Stress
Schuller, Robert, contemporary, American minister and author
Tolstoy, Leo (1828-1910), Russian novelist and moral philosopher, *Anna Karenina*

5

Bell, Alexander Graham (1847-1922), Scottish-born American inventor
Brody, Jane E., journalist, *New York Times*, 1987
Byron, George Gordon (1788-1824), English romantic poet
Calment, Jeanne Louise (1875-1997), record longevity, died in France, *The Guinness Book of World Records*, 1998
Nathan, George Jean (1882-1958), American drama and social critic, *Cosmetics vs. Humor, American Mercury*, 1925
Renoir, Pierre August (1841-1919), French painter
Swift, Jonathan (1667-1745), English satirist, *Thoughts on Various Subjects*, 1711
Waugh, Evelyn (1903-1966), English novelist
West, Mae (1892-1980), American actress
World Health Organization, Constitution, 1948

6

Desai, Anita, contemporary writer
Didion, Joan (b. 1934), American writer
Holmes, Sr., Oliver Wendell (1809-1894), American physician, professor, writer, *The Autocrat of the Breakfast Table*, 1858
Reagan, Ronald Wilson (b. 1911), actor and 40th U.S. President (1981-89)
Roach, Marion (b. 1956), U.S. writer, *Another Name for Madness*, 1985
Weinpur, Sally, attorney-at-law, Congressional testimony,1995

7

Bortz, Walter M., II, *Dare to be 100*, New York:Simon & Schuster, 1996

Burroughs, William (b. 1914), American writer, *Testimony Concerning a Sickness*, Deposition, 1959

Cicero, Marcus Tullius (106-43 B.C.), Roman statesman, orator, and philosopher

Faulkner, William (1897-1962), American writer, *Essays, Speeches and Public Lectures*, accepting Nobel Prize, 1949

Horace [Quintus Horatius Flaccus] (65-8 B.C.), Roman poet, *Epistles*

Morris, Desmond (b. 1928), English zoologist and writer, *The Human Zoo*

Virgil [Publius Vergilius Maro] (70-19 B.C.), Roman poet, *Aeneid*

8

Bradford, Rosalie, heaviest female recorded, *The Guinness Book of World Records*, 1998

Cheever, John (1912-1982), American writer, *The Falconer*, 1977

Minnoch, Jon Brouser, heaviest male recorded, *The Guinness Book of World Records*, 1998

Place, Jonathan, highest blood glucose level recorded, 1997, *The Guinness Book of World Records*, 1998

Rebeta-Burditt, Joyce (b. 1938), U.S. programming executive, novelist, *The Cracker Factory*, 1977

Russell, Bertrand (1872-1970), English philosopher, mathematician, social reformer, *The Conquest of Happiness*, reprinted 1996

Shakespeare, William (1546-1616), English playwright, *Macbeth*, Act II, Scene 3

Shaw, George Bernard (1856-1950), Irish-born British playwright, critic, social reformer

9

Conrad, Joseph (1857-1924), Polish-born English novelist

Gershwin, George (1988-1937) American jazz composer

Howe, Edgar Watson (1857-1937), American journalist and writer

Kennedy, John Fitzgerald (1917-1963), 35th U.S. President

Lindbergh, Charles Augustus (1902-1974), American aviator, first solo transatlantic flight

Plato (428-348 B.C.) Greek philosopher

Shakespeare, William, *Hamlet*, Act III, Scene 1

10

Beauvoir, Simone de (1908-1986), French existentialist novelist, essayist, political activist, feminist, *Les Belles Images*, 1966

Camus, Albert (1913-1960), French philosopher, novelist, playwright, journalist

Enright, D. J., *The Oxford book of death*. Oxford: Oxford University Press, 1983

Greene, Graham (1904-1991), English writer, *The Heart of the Matter*

Humphry, Derek, *Final Exit: The Practicalities of Self-Deliverance and Assisted Suicide for the Dying*, New York: Dell Publishing, 1992

In re Conroy, New Jersey Supreme Court; Claire Conroy was a demented, 84 year-old woman

In re Quinlan, New Jersey Supreme Court seminal case; Karen Quinlan was a 22 year-old woman in a persistent vegetative state, 1976

Kevorkian, Jack, American physician, credited with first assisted suicide, June 4, 1990; patient was Janet Adkins

Lawrence, David Herbert (1885-1930), English novelist and poet

Proust, Marcel (1871-1922), *The Sweet Cheat Gone*

Sexton, Anne (1928-1974), American poet

Styron, Jr., William Clark Styron (b. 1925), American writer, 1990

11

Butler, Samuel (1612-1680), English poet, satirist

Johnson, Samuel (1709-1784), English conversationalist, critic, lexicographer, writer, *Russelas*

Rand, Ayn (1905-1982), Russian-born American novelist, *The Fountainhead*, 1943, reprinted 1996

Reik, Theodor (18888-1969), Austrian-born American psychologist and writer, *The Need to be Loved*, 1963

12

Bierce, Ambrose Gwinett (1842-1914), American author

Charcot, Jean-Martin (1825-1893), French neurologist

Poe, Edgar Allen (1809-1849), American author, *The Tell-Tale Heart*

13

Emerson, Ralph Waldo, *Journals*, 1836

Hammerschmidt, Rosalie, R.N., & Meandor, Clifton K., M.D., *A Little Book of Nurse's Rules*, Rule #28, Philadelphia: Hanley & Belfus, Inc., 1993

Huxley, Aldous Leonard (1894-1963), English author

Kesey, Ken, *One Flew Over a Cuckoo's Nest*, 1984

Menninger, William, Dr.

Syrus, Publilius (1st century B.C.)

Szasz, Thomas (b. 1920), Hungarian-born, American psychiatrist, *The Second Sin*, 1974

Valery, Paul Ambroise (1871-1945), French poet, critic, writer, 1942

14

Abel, Elie, *The Missile Crisis*, 1966

Askey, Vincent, M.D., former President of American Medical Association

Charlemagne (742-814), Charles I, Charles the Great, King of the Franks, Emperor of the West

Chekhov, Anton Pavlovich (1860-1904), Russian playwright and author

Duke, James, *The Green Pharmacy*, reprinted 1998

Hammerschmidt, Rosalie, R.N., *A Little Book of Nurse's Rules*, Rule #114, 1993

Leeuwenhoek, Anton van (1632-1723), Dutch microscopy pioneer and naturalist

Sacks, Oliver (b. 1933), English neurologist and author, quoted by Walter Clemons "Listening to the Lost," *Newsweek*, 20 August, 1984

Sydenham, Thomas (1624-1689), English physician, as quoted in the *New York Academy of Sciences*, Vol. IV, p. 923, 1928

Terence [Publius Terentius Afer] (190-159 B.C.), *The Woman of Andros,* 166 B.C.

15

Auden, Wystan Hugh (1907-1973), English-born American poet and playwright

Butler, Samuel (1612-1680), English poet and satirist, *The Way of All Flesh*

Fleming, Alexander, Sir. (1881-1955), British bacteriologist, Nobel Laureate, 1945

Medawar, Peter Brian, Sir (b. 1915), Brazilian-born, British biologist, Nobel Laureate, 1960

Osler, Sir William (1849-1919), Canadian-born British physician and educator, *Aphorisms from His Bedside Teachings*

Shaw, George Bernard, *Back to Methuselah*, 1921

Sydenham, Thomas, as quoted in the *New York Academy of Sciences*, Vol. IV, p. 922, 1928

16

Frank, Arthur W., contemporary author

Frasier, an NBC television sitcom

Jones, Willy, highest recorded fever, Grady Memorial Hospital, Atlanta, GA, 1980, *The Guinness Book of World Records*, 1998

Schweitzer, Albert (1875-1965), French music scholar, philosopher, physician, theologian

Sontag, Susan (b. 1933), American author and critic, *Illness as a Metaphor*, 1978

17

Annie, Broadway musical
Begoun, Paula, *The Beauty Bible*, Seattle: Beginning Press, 1997
Blessington, Marguerite, Countess of, Irisk writer, salon host
Curie, Marie (1867-1934), French chemist, Nobel Laureate, 1903
Munch, Edvard (1863-1944), Norwegian artist, *The Scream*
Pasteur, Louis (1822-1895), French chemist
Shakespeare, William, *Hamlet,* 1600

18

Centers for Disease Control, Morbidity and Mortality Weekly
Report, Friday, June 5, 1981, the first report on the epidemic we now call
AIDS (then known as "GRID," Gay Related Immune Disease) based on 5
cases seen by Drs. Michael Gottlieb and Joel Weisman
    Davis, James E., contemporary author and editor
    Henderson, Donald, Dr.
    Kushner, Tony (b. 1956), American playwright
    Lerner, Max (b. 1902), Russian-born, American journalist and teacher
    Teresa, Mother (b. 1910), Albanian-born, Roman Catholic nun, founder
of the Missionaries of Charity, and Nobel Laureate, 1979

19

Harrington, Michael (1928-1989), American social critic and writer, *The Other America; Poverty in the United States*, 1962
    Kennedy, John Fitzgerald, *Inaugural Address*, 1961
    Juvenal [Decimus Junius Juvenalis] (55-130 A.D.)
    Yeats, William Butler (1865-1939), Irish author, producer, politician, and Nobel Laureate, 1923

REMEMBERING

Eiseley, Loren, *Man Against the Universe, The Star Thrower*, 1978
    Wolfe, Thomas (1900-1938), American novelist, *Look Homeward Angel,* 1929
    Wordsworth, William (1770-1850), English poet, *The Solitary Reaper*

SOURCE NOTES

General Sources

Asimov, I. (1992). *Isaac Asimov's Book of Facts*. Mamaroneck, NY: Hastings House Book Publishers.

Cartwright, F. F., & Biddiss, M.D. (1991). *Diseases and History*. New York: Barnes & Noble Books.

Kiple, K. F. (Ed.). (1993). *The Cambridge World History of Human Disease*. Cambridge University Press.

Louis, D. (1983). *2201 Fascinating Facts*. New York: Wing Books.

Oldstone, M.B.A..(1998). *Viruses, Plagues, and History*. New York: Oxford University Press.

Rybacki, J. J., & Long, J. W. (1998). *The Essential Guide to Prescriptive Drugs*. New York:Harper Perennial.

Tierney, L. M., McPhee, S. J., & Papadakis, M.A. (Eds.). (1997). *Current medical diagnosis & treatment*. Stamford, CT: Appleton & Lange.

Chapter 1

Cater, J. (1996). Can hospice care be provided to people who live alone? *Home Healthcare Nurse*, 14(9), 710-716.

Caudill, M. A., Holman, G. H., & Turk, D. (1996). Effective ways to manage chronic pain. *Patient Care*, June 15, 154-172.

Fisher, R. (1996). Tools of the heart. *American Journal of Nursing*, 96(7), 56-57.

Harwood, K. (1996). Straight talk about breast cancer. *Nursing96*, October, 39-44.

Hirsch, M. A. (1995). Uniquely hospice: Policies and procedures of terminal care at home. *Caring Magazine*, November, 20-26.

Lamendola, F. P. (1996). Keeping your compassion alive. *American Journal of Nursing*, 96(11), 16R-16T.

Oesterling, J. E. (1995). Benign prostatic hypertrophy. Medical and minimally invasive treatment options. *New England Journal of Medicine*, 332, 99-109.

Pasero, C. L., & McCaffery, M. (1996). Pain in the elderly. *American Journal of Nursing*, 96(10), 39-45.

Reese, C. D. (1996). Please cry with me. Six ways to grieve. *Nursing96*, August, 56.

Special article. (1996). Statement of the American Socirty of Clinical Oncology: Genetic testing for cancer susceptibility. *Journal of Clinical Oncology*, 14, 1730-1736

Vetrosky, D. T., Gerdom, L., & White, G. L. (1997). Prostate cancer. Pathology, diagnosis, and management. *Clinical Reviews*, 7(5), 79-100.

Weiss, M. C., & Weiss, E. T. F. (1997). *Living Beyond Breast Cancer. A
Survivors Guide for When Treatment Ends and the Rest of Your Life Begins*. New York:Time Books Random House.

Chapter 2

American Thoracic Society. (1995). Standards for the care of patients with
chronic obstructive pulmonary disease. *American Journal of Respiratory Critical Care Medicine*, 152, S78.

Droppleman, P. G., & Thomas, S. P. (1996). Anger in nurses. *American
Journal of Nursing*, 96(4), 26-31.

Guthery, D., & Schumann, L. (1998). Congestive heart failure. *Journal of
the American Academy of Nurse Practitioners*, 10(1), 31-38.

Hafner, J-P., & Ferro, T. J. (1998). Recent developments in the management of COPD. *Hospital Medicine*, January, 29-38.

Hamm, C.W., Goldmann, B.U., Heeschen, C., et al. (1967). Emergency
room triage of patients with acute chest pain by means of rapid testing
for cardiac troponin T or troponin I. *New England Journal of Medicine*,
337(Dec 4), 1648-1653.

Hollis, J. F., Lichtenstein, E., Vogt, T. M., et al. (1993). Nurse-assisted
counseling for smokers in primary care. *Annals of Internal Medicine*,
118(7), 521-525.

Larson, D. (1997). Smoking cessation. Counseling your patients. *Clinician
Reviews*, 7(6), 57-80.

Moreyra, E., Taheri, H., & Wasserman, A. (1995). Chest pain. Is it life-
threatening—or benign? *Consultant*, December, 1819-1826.

Morgan, W. C., & Hodge, H. L. (1998). Diagnostic evaluation of dyspnea.
American Family Physician, 57(4), 711-716.

Rose, J. E. (1996). Nicotine addiction and treatment. *Annual Review of
Medicine*, 47, 493-507.

Chapter 3

Foody, J., & Sprecher, D. (1997). Current concepts in preventative car-
diology. *Cortlandt Forum*, November, 232-244.

Fromm, R. E., Jr., Varon, J., & Gibbs, L. R. (1995). Congestive heart failure
and pulmonary edema for the emergency physician. *Journal of Emergency Medicine*, 13(1), 71-87.

Masley, S. C. (1998). Dietary therapy for preventing and treating coronary artery disease. *American Family Physician*, 57(6), 1299-1306.

Vaczek, D. (1997). The personal touch: Addressing noncompliance in the elderly. *Pharmacy Times*, August, 35-40.

Whitten, C. (1995). Vegetarian diets and ischemic heart disease. *Topics in Clinical Nutrition*, 19(2), 27-33.

Chapter 4

(1997). *Overcoming infertility. A compassionate resource for getting pregnant.* NY: WH Freeman.

American College of Obstetricians and Gynecologists. (1997). Sexual assault. *ACOG Educational Bulletin No. 242.* Washington, DC: American College of Obstetricians and Gynecologists.

Busch, P. E. (1996). Panic disorder. The overlooked problem. *Home Healthcare Nurse*, 14(2), 111-116.

Catanzarite, V., Deutchman, M., Johnson, C. A., & Scherger, J. E. (1995). Pregnancy after 35: What's the real risk? *Patient Care*, January 15, 41-51.

Freeman, E. W. (1996). Can antidepressants be used to tame psychological symptoms of PMS? *Medscape Women's Health*, 1(10).

Hanson, V., & Talarico, L., D., (1997). How to provide postcoital contraception. *Patient Care*, April 15, 81-85.

Royce, C. F. (1995). Breaking through to the adolescent patient. *American Journal of Nursing*, Decemeber, 19-23.

Chapter 5

Butler, R. N., Collins, K. S., Meier, D. E., Muller, C. F., & Pinn, V. W. (1995). Older women's health: Clinical care in the postmenopausal years. *Geriatrics*, 50(6), 33-41.

Col, N. F., Eckman, M. H., Karas, R. H., et al. (1997). Patient-specific decisions about hormone replacement therapy in postmenopausal women. *Journal of the American Medical Association*, 277, 1140-1147.

Daniel, C. R., Dolan, N. C., & Wheeland, R. G. (1996). Don't overlook skin surveillance. *Patient Care*, June 15, 90-107.

Galsworthy, T., & Wilson, P.L. (1996). Osteoporosis. It steals more than bone. *American Journal of Nursing*, 96(6), 27-33.

Jerger, J., Chmiel, R., Wilson, N., & Luchi, R. (1995). Hearing impairment in older adults: New concepts. *Journal of the American Geriatrics Society*, 43, 928-935.

Kanacki, L. S., Jones, P. S., & Galbraith, M. E. (1996). Social support and depression in widows and widowers. *Journal of Gerontological Nursing*, February, 39-45.

Leetun, M. C. (1996). Wellness spirituality in the older adult. *Nurse Practitioner*, 21(8), 60-70.

Oparil, S., & Calhoun, D. A. (1998). Managing the patient with hard-to-control hypertension. *American Family Physician*, 57(5), 1007-1014.

Chapter 6

Brandt, E. N., Hadley, S., & Holtz, H. A. (1996). Family violence: A covert health crisis. *Patient Care*, September 15, 138-165.

Consensus Statement. (1997). Diagnosis and treatment of Alzheimer's disease and other related disorders. *Journal of the American Medical Association*, October 22/29.

Cummings, J.L., & Kaufer, D.I. (1996). Neuropsychiatric aspects of Alzheimer's disease: the cholinergic hypothesis revisited. *Neurology*, 47(4), 876-883.

Hall, G. R., & Wakefield, B. (1996). Acute confusion in the elderly. *Nursing96*, 26(7), July, 32-37.

Sano, M., Ernesto, C., Thomas, R.G., et al. (1997). A controlled trial of selegiline, alpha-tocopherol, or both as treatment for Alzheimer's disease. The Alzheimer's Disease Cooperative Study. *New England Journal of Medicine*, 336(17), 1216-1222.

Shea, C. A., Mahoney, M., & Lacey, J. M. (1997). Breaking through the barriers to domestic violence intervention. *American Journal of Nursing*, 97(6), 26-33.

Stewart, W.F., Kawas, C., Corrada, M., & Metter, E.J. (1997). Risk of Alzheimer's disease and duration of NSAID use. *Neurology*, 48(3), 626-632.

Tang, P.N., Jacobs, D., Stern, Y., et al. (1996). Effect of oestrogen during menopause on risk and age at onset of Alzheimer's disease. *Lancet*, 348(9025), 429-432.

Vernarec, E. (1998). The high cost of hidden conditions. *Strategic Medicine*, 2(3), 30-35.

Chapter 7

Cantor, M. H., & Brennan, M. (1993). Volume four: New York City as a place of residence for older people: Life space, environment, and impact of crime. In J. R. Dumpson (Ed.). *Growing older in New York City in the 1990s*. New York: The New York Center for Policy on Aging of the New York Community Trust.

Young, M. A., & Stein, J. H. (1990). Elderly crime victims: The double sorrow. *Aging*, 360, 36-37.

Chapter 8

Armstrong, D. G., & Lavery, L. A. (1998). Diabetic foot ulcers: Prevention, diagnosis and classification. *American Family Physician*, 57(6), 1325-1332.

Bradley, K.A. (1992). Management of alcoholism in the primary care setting. *Western Journal of Medicine*, 156, 273.

Bussey, B. F., & Morgan, S. L. (1997). Obesity: Is there effective treatment now? *Consultant*, November, 2945-2957.

Centers for Disease Control and Prevention. (1997). *National Diabetes Fact Sheet*, November.

Centers for Disease Control and Prevention. (1997). Update. Prevalence of overweight among children, adolescents and adults—United States, 1988-1994. *Morbidity & Mortality Weekly Report*, 46(9), 199-202.

Council on Scientific Affairs, American Medical Association. (1996). Alcoholism in the elderly. *Journal of the American Medical Association*, 275, 797-810.

Daher, G.C., Cooper, D.A., Zorich, N.L., et al. (1997). Olestra ingestion and dietary fat absorption in humans. *Journal of Nutrition*, 127, 1694S-1698S.

Gibbs, W. W. (1996). Gaining on fat. *Scientific American*, August, 88-94.

Report of the Expert Committee on the Diagnosis and Classification of Diabetes Mellitus. (1997). *Diabetes Care*, 20, 1183-1197.

The World Health Organization. (1997). Conquering suffering suffering, enriching humanity. *World Health Report*. Executive summary.

Thun, M.J., Peto, R., Lopez, A.D., et al. (1997). Alcohol consumption and mortality among middle-aged and elderly U.S. adults. *New England Journal of Medicine*, 337 (December 11), 1705-1714.

Chapter 9

Baloh, R. W. (1997). When your patient complains of dizziness: An overview. *Family Recertification*, 19(11), 14-60.

Berman, G. D., Saper, J, R., & Solomon, G. D. (1996). Chronic headache: Management strategies that make sense. *Patient Care*, January 30, 54-66.

Connaughton, P. N., McKhann, G., & Walker, M. D. (1995). Decade of the brain: A midpoint status report. *Patient Care*, July 15, 94-114.

Kelley, R. E. (1998). Stroke prevention and intervention. *Postgraduate Medicine*, 103(2), 43-62.

Loeffler, J. S., Morantz, R. A., & Posner, J. B. (1995). Brain tumor care: Vigilance and teamwork. *Patient Care*, April 15, 45-69.

Maas, J.B., Wherry, M.L., Axelrod,D.J., Hogan, B.R., & Blumin, J.A. (1998). *Power sleep: The revolutionary program that prepares your mind for peak performance.* New York: Villard Books.
Nowell, P. D., Buysse, D. J., Reynolds, C. F., et al. (1997). Clinical factors contributing to the differential diagnosis of primary insomnia and insomnia related to mental disorders. *The American Journal of Psychiatry,* 154(10), 1412-1416.

Chapter 10

Antidepressants: One of many drug classes used in suicide attempts. (1997). *Drugs & Therapy Perspectives,* 10(7), 14-16.
Block, M., Gelenberg, A. J., & Malone, D. A. (1997). Rational use of the newer antidepressants. *Patient Care,* March 30, 49-77.
Centers for Disease Control. (1997). Regional variations in suicide rates—United States, 1990-1994. *Morbidity & Mortality Weekly Report,* 46(34), 789-793.
Hall, J. K. (1996). Assisted suicide: Nurse practitioners as providers? *Nurse Practitioner,* 21(10), 63-71.
Komaroff, A. L., Fagioli, L. R., Geiger, A. M., et al. (1996). An examination of the working case definition of chronic fatigue syndrome. *American Journal of Medicine,* 100(1), 56-64.
Kutner, M. (1998). Terminal care for elderly patients. *Clinical Geriatrics,* 6(2), 46-57.
Lavretsky, H. (1998). Late-life depression: Risk factors, treatment, and sex differences. *Clinical Geriatrics,* 6(3), 13-30.
Post, K., Zhang, M., Fortney, J., et al. (1998). Persistently poor outcomes of undetected major depression in primary care. *General Hospital Psychiatry,* 20(January), 12-20.
Saeed, S. A., & Bruce, T. J. (1998). Seasonal affective disorders. *American Family Physician,* 57(6), 1340-1346.

Chapter 11

Bromber, W. D. (1998). Urinary tract infections: Part I-The basics. *Cortlandt Forum,* January, 160-174.
Galindo, D., & Kaiser, F. E. (1995). Sexual health after 60. *Patient Care,* April 15, 25-38.
Junnila, J., & Lassen, P. (1998). Testicular masses. *American Family Physician,* 57(4), 685-692.
Majeroni, B. A. (1998). Bacterial vaginosis: An update. *American Family Physician,* 57(6), 1285-1289.
Plourd, D. M. (1997). Practical guide to diagnosing and treating vaginitis.

Medscape Women's Health, 2(2).

Stevens, P. E., Tatum, N. O., & White, J. C. (1996). Optimal care for lesbian patients. *Patient Care*, March 15, 121-141.

Uy, S., & McNicoll, K. (1998). Are you up-to-date on Pap smears? *Family Practice Recertification*, 20(1), 53-80.

Vincent, M. T., & Adeyele, E. (1998). Are you comfortable taking the sexual history? *Family Practice Recertification*, 20(1), 87-101.

Chapter 12

Aboaf, A.B., & Wolff, P.S. (1996). Paroxysmal atrial fibrillation: A common but neglected entity. *Archives of Internal Medicine*, 156:362-366.

Franklyn, J.A. (1994). The management of hyperthyroidism. *New England Journal of Medicine*, 330:1731-1734.

Herbert, M. (1998). Atrial fibrillation: Handling the acute emergency. *Emergency Medicine*, May, 18-42.

Kastor, J.A. (1993). *Arrhythmias*, Saunders.

Tietgen, S.T. & Leinung, M.C. (1995). Thyroid storm. *Medical Clinics of North America*, 79:169-180.

Chapter 13

Hubbard, J.R. et al. (1995). Recognizing borderline personality disorders in the family practice setting. *American Family Physician*, 52, 908-915.

O'Brien, P. G. (1996). The manipulative patient: A behavioral conceptualization. *The American Journal for Nurse Practioners*, 13-30.

Sobel, S.V. (1996). What's new in the treatment of anorexia nervosa and bulimia? *Medscape Women's Health*, 1(9).

Weiden, P., & Olfson, M. (1995). Cost of relapse in schizophrenia. *Schizophrenia Bulletin*, 21, 419-428.

Chapter 14

Anderson, L. G. (1998). Aspirating and injecting the acutely painful joint. *Emergency Medicine*, January, 16-38.

Chapron, D. J., & Tselikis, P. (1998). Reducing adverse drug effects in the elderly. *Strategic Medicine*, 2(3), 13-24.

Clinical update. (1997). Managing back pain. New clinical guidelines. *Clinician Reviews*, 7(11) 57-72.

Espino, D. V., Jules-Bradley, C. A., Johnston, C. L., & Mouton, C. P. (1998). Diagnostic approach to the confused elderly patient. *American Family Physician*, 57(6), 1358-1366.

Hughes, E. F. (1997). Alternative medicine: What works, and what do you tell patients? *Family Practice Recertification*, 19(11), 63-87.

Youngkin, E. Q., & Israel, D. S. (1996). A review and critique of common herbal alternative therapies. *Nurse Practitioner*, 21(10), 39-49.

Chapter 15

Graber, M. A. (1998). Dealing with acute abdominal pain: part 1: Clues to the diagnosis. *Emergency Medicine*, February, 74-100.

Laine, L., & Fendrick, A. M. (1998). Helicobacter pylori and peptic ulcer disease. *Postgraduate Medicine*, 103(3), 231-243.

Proceedings of a symposium. (1998). Gastrointestinal protection in NSAID therapy. *The Journal of Musculoskeletal Medicine*, March, Supplement.

Chapter 16

American Thoracic Society. (1993). Guidelines for the initial management of adults with community-acquired pneumonia: Diagnosis, assessment of severity, and initial antimicrobial therapy. *American Rev Respiratory Dis*, 148, 1418-1426.

Centers for Disease Control and Prevention. (1997). Immunization of health-care workers: recommendations of the Advisory Committee on Immunization Practices and the Hospital Infection Control Practice Advisory Committee. *Morbidity & Mortality Weekly Report*, 46(RR-18), 4-9.

Centers for Disease Control and Prevention. (1997). Prevention and control of influenza: recommendations of the Advisory Committee on Immunization Practices (ACIP). *Morbidity & Mortality Weekly Report*, 46(No. RR-9).

Centers for Disease Control and Prevention. (1997). Prevention of pneumococcal disease: recommendations of the Advisory Committee on Immunization Practices (ACIP). *Morbidity & Mortality Weekly Report*, 46(RR-8), 1-24.

Farr, B. M. (1997). Prognosis and decisions in pneumonia. *New England Journal of Medicine*, 336, 288-289.

Fune, L., Shua-Haim, J. R., Ross, J. S., & Frank, E. (1998). Infectious diseases in the elderly. *Clinical Geriatrics*, 6(3), 31-50.

Institute for Clinical systems Integration. (1998). Viral upper respiratory tract infections in adults. *Postgraduate Medicine*, 103(1), 71-80.

Mehta, J. B., & Dutt, A. K. (1995). Tuberculosis in the elderly. *Infect Med*, 12(1), 40-46.

Niederman, M. S., Skerrett, S. J., Yamauchi, T., & Pinkowish, M. D. (1998). Antibiotics or not? Managing patients with respiratory infections. *Patient Care*, January 15, 60-89.

Saab, S., & Martin, P. (1998). Hepatitis C: A practical approach to diagnosis and management. *Family Practice Recertification*, 20(1), 21-44.

Chapter 17

Goldstein, B. G., & Goldstein, A. O. (1997). *Practical Dermatology*. Second Edition. St. Louis, MO: Mosby.

Morrow, G. L., & Abbott, R. L. (1998). Conjunctivitis. *American Family Physician*, 57(4), 735-746.

Reisman, R.E. (1994). Insect stings. *New England Journal of Medicine*, 331, 523-526.

Chapter 18

Centers for Disease Control and Prevention. (1996). Ten leading nationally notifiable infectious diseases—United States, 1995. *Morbidity & Mortality Weekly Report*, 45(41), 883-884.

Centers for Disease Control and Prevention. (1997). Update: trends in AIDS incidence—United States, 1996. *Morbidity & Mortality Weekly Report*, 46(37), 861-867.

Centers for Disease Control and Prevention. (1997). 1997 USPHS/IDSA guidelines for the prevention of opportunistic infections in persons infected with human immunodeficiency virus. *Morbidity & Mortality Weekly Report*, 46(RR-12), 1-46.

Cusack, J.R., & Anderson, T.W. (1998). Physical signs of addiction. *Emergency Medicine*, May, 120-130.

Gasbarro, R. (1996). Issues in addiction. *Pharmacy Times*, December, 28-35.

Meyer, R. E. (1996). The disease called addiction: emerging evidence in a 200-year debate. *The Lancet*, 347, 162-166.

O'Brien, C. P. (1997). A range of research-based pharmacotherapies for addiction. *Science*, 278, 66-70.

Nutt, D. J. (1996). Addiction: brain mechanisms and their treatment implications. *The Lancet*, 347, 31-36.

Rachlis, A. R. (1998). Neurologic manifestations of HIV infection using imaging studies and antiviral therapy effectively. *Postgraduate Medicine*, 103(3), 147-161.

Chapter 19

Middleton, A. D. (1997). Managing asthma. It takes teamwork. *American Journal of Nursing*, 97(1), 39-43.

Richman, E. (1997). Asthma diagnosis and management. New severity classifications and therapy alternatives. *Clinician Reviews*, 7(8), 76-110.

Rosentreich, D. L., Eggleston, P., Kattan, M., et al. (1997). The role of cockroach allergy and exposure to cockroach allergen in causing morbidity among inner-city children with asthma. *New England Journal of Medicine*, 336, 1356-1363.

RESOURCES FOR PATIENTS

The following are only some of the many national organizations and available sources of information about health care and medical disorders. Omissions to this list are unintentional. Inclusion does not signify endorsement by the publisher or authors. We focused on the disorders presented in this book rather than on all possible medical diseases. Patients should explore local resources in their community as well and discuss all questions about the information they obtain with their health care provider. While we have made a reasonable effort to assure that the addresses, telephone numbers, and websites listed are current and correct, such information is subject to change beyond our control.

Aging

American Association of Retired People (AARP)
601 E Street, NW
Washington DC 20049
(202) 434-2277
(800) 424-3410
(202) 434-6561 (TDD)
http://www.aarp.org

Alcohol and Drug Abuse

Alcoholics Anonymous
475 Riverside Drive
New York NY 10015
(212) 870-3400
(888) 645-0677 (for California)
http://www.alcoholics-anonymous.org

American Council for Drug Education (Phoenix House Foundation)
164 West 74th Street
New York, NY 10023
1-800-378-4435 (DRUGHELP)
(English; Spanish Tuesday through Thursdays)
http:/www.acde.org

National Clearinghouse for Alcohol and Drug Information
Substance Abuse and Mental Health Service Administration (SAMSHA)
PO Box 2345
Rockville MD 20847-2345
(800) 729-6686
(800) 458-5231, extension 5377
(Spanish) (800) 487-4889 (TDD)
http://www.health.org/resref.htm

National Drug and Alcohol Treatment Referral Routing Service
US Department of Health and Human Services
Center for Substance Abuse Treatment
National Drug Abuse and Treatment Hotline
(800) 662-4357 (662-HELP)
(800) 662-9832 (66-AYUDA) (Spanish)

Allergic and Autoimmune Disorders

Asthma and Allergy Foundation of America
1125 15th Street NW, Suite 502
Washington DC 20005
(202) 466-7643
(800) 727-8462 (7-ASTHMA)
http://www.aafa.org

Lupus Foundation of America, Inc. Information Line
1300 Piccard Drive, Suite 200
Rockville MD 20850
(301) 670-9292
(800) 558-0121
http://www.lupus.org/lupus

Lyme Disease Foundation Information Hotline
1 Financial Plaza, 18th Floor
Hartford CT 06103-2601
(800) 886-5963
http://www.aldf.com

The Food Allergy Network
10400 Eaton Place, Suite 107
Fairfax VA 22030
(702) 691-3179
(800) 929-4040

http://www.foodallergy.org

Alternative Medicine

American Botanical Council
PO Box 201660
Austin TX 78720
(512) 331-8868
http://www.herbalgram.org

American Massage Therapy Association
National Information Office
820 Davis Street
Evanston IL 60201
(312) 761-2682
(800) 696-2682
http://www.amtamassage.org

Aromatherapy Institute and Research (AIR)
PO Box 2354
Fair Oaks CA 95628

Association for Applied Psychophysiology and Biofeedback
Biofeedback Certification Institute of America
10200 W 44th Ave, Suite 304
Wheat Ridge CO 80033
(303) 422-8436
(800) 477-8892
http://www.aapb.org

Blindness and Eye Care

National Eye Care Project Helpline
PO Box 429098
San Francisco CA 94142-9098
(880) 222-3937
http://www.eyenet.org

Prevent Blindness America
500 East Remington
Schaumburg IL 60173
(800) 331-2020
http://www.preventblindness.org

Bone and Joint Diseases

National Osteoporosis Foundation
2100 M Street, NW, Suite 602
Washington DC 20037
(202) 223-9994
http://www.nof.org

The Arthritis Foundation
National Office
1330 West Peachtree Street
Atlanta, GA 30309
(404) 872-7100
(800) 283-7800
http://www.arthritis.org

Cancer

American Cancer Society, Inc.
National Headquarters
1599 Clifton Road, NE
Atlanta GA 30329
(800) 227-2345 (ACS-2345)
htttp://www.cancer.org

Breast Cancer, Y-Me, National Organization Hotline
212 West Van Buren
Chicago IL 60607
(800) 221-2141
(800) 986-9505 (Spanish)
http://www.y-me.org

National Alliance of Breast Cancer Organizations (NABCO)
Information Services Department
9 East 37th Street, 10th Floor
New York NY 10016
(800) 719-9154
nabcoinfo@aol.com (e-mail)
http://www.nabco.org

National Cancer Institute
Cancer Information Service
(800) 422-6237 (4-CANCER)
(English, Spanish)
http://www.nci.nih.gov

Gilda Radner Familial Ovarian Cancer Registry
Roswell Park Cancer Institute
National Ovarian Cancer Coalition
Elm and Carlton Streets
Buffalo NY 14263
(800)-682-7426 (OVARIAN
http://www.ovarian.org

Chronic Pain

American Academy of Pain Management
13947 Mono Way #A
Sonora CA 95370
(209) 533-9744
www.aapainmanag.org/index.
html

Diabetes

American Diabetes Association
1660 Duke Street
Alexandria VA 22314
1-800-342-2383 (DIABETES)
www.diabetes.org

National Diabetes Foundation
(800) 726-8459

National Diabetes Information Clearinghouse
1 Information Way
Bethesda MD 20892-3560
(301) 654-3327
http://www.niddk.nih.gov

Digestive Diseases

Crohn's and Colitis Foundation
386 Park Avenue South, 17th Floor, New York NY 10016
(800) 343-3637 (brochure hotline)
(800) 932-2423
http://www.ccfa.org

National Digestive Disease Education
and Information Clearinghouse
1555 Wilson Blvd, Suite 600
Rosslyn VA 22209

Domestic Violence

The National Coalition Against Domestic Violence
PO Box 18749
Denver CO 80218
(303) 839-1852

National Workplace Resource Center on Domestic Violence
Family Violence Prevention Fund
(415) 252-8900

Family Violence Prevention Fund
There's No Excuse for Domestic

Violence
Work to End Domestic Violence Kit
(800) 363-2287 (END-ABUSE)
(English, Spanish)
http://www.igc.apc.org/fund

National Domestic Violence Hotline
(800) 799-7233 (799-SAFE)
(English, Spanish)
(800) 787-3224 (TDD)
http://www.inetport.com/~ndvh

Eating Disorders

American Anorexia Nervosa Association, Inc.
133 Cedar Lane
Teaneck NJ 07666
(201) 836-1800

Fertility

American Society for Reproductive Medicine
1209 Montgomery Highway
Birmingham AL 35216-2809
(205) 978-5000
http://www.asrm.com

Grief Counseling

The Compassionate Friends (TCF) (death of children)
PO Box 3696
Oak Brook IL 60522-3696
(708) 990-0010
http://www.jjt.com/~tcf_national

Hearing Disorders and Deafness

Hearing Aid Helpline
International Hearing Society
16880 Middlebelt Road, Suite 4
Livonia MI 48154
(800) 521-5247
http://www.hearingihs.org

Hearing, Dial-a (Screening Test)
Occupational Hearing Service
PO Box 1880
Media PA 19063
(800) 222-3277 (222-EARS)
dahst@aol.com (e-mail)

National Information Center on Deafness
Gallaudet University
800 Florida Avenue, NE
Washington DC 20002
(202) 651-5051
(202) 651-5052 (TDD)

Heart Disease

American Heart Association
National Center, 7272 Greenville Avenue
Dallas TX 75231
(214) 373-6300/6308
(800) 242-8721
http://www.americaheart.org

Home Care

National Association for Home Care
228 Seventh Street, SE
Washington, DC 20003
(202) 547-7424
http://www.nahc.org

Hospice Care

National Hospice Organization
1901 North Moore Street, Suite 901
Arlington VA 22209
(800) 658-8898
http://www.nho.org

Infectious Diseases and Vaccinations

Centers for Disease Control and Prevention
1600 Clifton Road, NE
Building 1, SSB249, MS A 34
Atlanta, GA 30333
(404) 639-3492
(888) 329-4232
http://www.cdc.gov

World Health Organization
International Travel and Health
Advice to Travelers
(518) 436-9686
http://www.who.it/gpv-dvacc/
    travel/travel

Kidney and Urologic Disease

American Foundation for Urologic Disease
1128 North Charles Street
Baltimore MD 21201
(800) 242-2383
www.access.digex.net/~afud

Geddings Osbon Foundation Impotence Resource Center
(800) 433-4215
http://www.impotence.org

National Kidney Foundation
30 East 33rd Street, 11th Floor
New York, NY 10016
(800) 622-9010
www.aerie.com/netahtml/nihdb/
    kudetail.html

*National Kidney and Urologic
Diseases Information
Clearinghouse*
Let's Talk About Bladder
Control for Women Campaign
National Institutes of Health
(800) 891-5388

Liver Disease

American Liver Foundation
Hepatitis/Liver Disease Hotline
1425 Pompton Avenue
Cedar Grove, NJ 07009
(800) 223-0179
(800) 465-4837 (GO-LIVER)
http://www.liverfoundation.org

Lung Disease

American Lung Association
1740 Broadway
New York, NY 10019-4374
(800) 586-4872 (LUNG-USA)
http://www.lungusa.org

Medicare Information

Medicare Hotline
(800) 638-6833

Mental Health

National Mental Health

Association
10221 Prince Street
Alexandria VA 22314-2971
(703) 684-7722
(800) 228-1114
http://www.nmha.org

*National Institute for Mental
Health*
Depression Awareness,
Recognition and Treatment
Program
(301) 443-3720
http://www.nimh.nih.gov

*Obsessive-Compulsive
Foundation*
(203) 878-5669
http://www.centerpt.org/search/
    m50jkpwt.htm

Minority Health Issues

*Office of Minority Health
Resource Center*
PO Box 37337
Washington DC 20013
(800) 444-6472 (English,
Spanish)
(301)589-0951 (TDD)
www.omhrc.gov

Neurological Disorders

*American Brain Tumor
Association*
2720 River Road, Suite 146
Des Plaines IL 60018
(800) 886-2282
www.abta.org

American Council for Headache Education (ACHE)
875 Kings Highway, Suite 200
West Deptford NJ 08096
(800) 255-2243 (255-ACHE)
http:/www.achenet.org

Alzheimer's Disease Education and Referral Center (ADEAR)
PO Box 8250
Silver Spring MD 20907-8250
(800) 438-4380
http:/www.alzheimers.org

Alzheimer's Disease and Related Disorders Association (ADRDA)
919 North Michigan Avenue, Suite 1000
Chicago IL 60611-1676
(800) 272-3900
(312) 335-8882 (Spanish)
http://www.alz.org

American Paralysis Association
(Associated with Christopher Reeve Foundation)
500 Morris Avenue
Springfield NJ 07081
(800) 225-0292
http://www.apacure.com

Epilepsy Foundation of America, Information Center
4351 Garden City Drive, Suite 406
Landover MD 20785
(301) 459-3700
(800) 332-1000 (English, Spanish)
(800) EFA-4050 (EFA library)
http://www.efa.org

Muscular Dystrophy Association (MDA)
3300 East Sunrise Drive

Tuczon AZ 85718
(520) 529-2000
(800) 572-1717
http://www.mdausa.org

Myasthenia Gravis Foundation
222 South Riverside Plaza
Chicago IL 60606-9524
(213) 887-0056 (Spanish)
(800) 541-5454
http://www.med.unc.edu/mgfa

National Multiple Sclerosis Society (NMSS)
205 East 42nd Street
New York NY 10017-5706
(800) 344-4867
www.nmss.org

National Stroke Association (NSA)
96 Inverness Drive East, Suite I
Englewood CO 80112-5112
(800) Strokes
http://www.stroke.org

The National Headache Foundation (NHF)
428 West St James Place
Chicago IL 60614
(800) 843-2256
http:/www.headaches.org

Parkinson's Disease Association
1250 Hyland Boulevard
Staten Island NY 10305
(800) 223-2732 (223-APDA)
http://www.pdaparkinson.com

Spinal Cord Injury Association
8300 Colesville Road, Suite 551
Silver Spring MD 20910
(800) 962-9629
http://www.erols.com/nscia

Nutrition

American Dietetic Association
Consumer Nutrition Hotline
216 West Jackson Boulevard
Chicago IL 60606-6995
(800) 366-1655 (in English and
Spanish)

Center for Food Safety and
Applied Nutrition
Food and Drug Adminsitration
(800) 332-4010 (English,
Spanish)
http://www.fda.gov

Pain

American Chronic Pain
Association (ACTA)
PO Box 850
Rocklin CA 95677
(916) 632-0922

National Chronic Pain Outreach
Association (NCPOA)
7979 Old Georgetown Road,
Suite 100
Bethesda MD 20814
(301) 652-4948

Rare Diseases

National Information Center for
Orphan Drugs and Rare
Diseases
PO Box 1133
Washington DC 20013-1133
(800) 456-3505

National Organization for Rare
Disorders (NORD)
PO Box 8923

New Fairfield CT 06812
(203) 746-6518
(800) 999-6673
http://www.pcnet.com/~orphan

Referrals

National Health Information
Center (NHIC)
Office of Disease Prevention and
Health Promotion
U.S. Department of Health and
Human Services
PO Box 1133
Washington DC 20013-1133
(800) 336-4797
http://nhic-nt.health.org

Rehabilitation

National Rehabilitation
Information Center (NARIC)
8455 Colesville Road, Suite 935
Silver Spring, MD 20910-3319
(800) 346-2742
http://www.cais.net/naric

Self-Help

National Self-Help
Clearinghouse
25 West 43rd Street, Room 620
New York NY 10036
(212) 354-8525
http://192.217.234.202/iris/omoz
oj9w.htm

National Center for Health
Statistics
Department of Health and
Human services
(301) 436-8500
http://www.cdc.gov/nchs

Sexual Function and Health

Sexual Function Health Council
American Foundation for
Urologic Disease
300 West Pratt Street, Suite 401
Baltimore MD 21201
http://www.afud.org/sfunctn.html

*Sex Information and Educational
Council of the United States
(SIECUS)*
130 West 42nd Street Suite 350
New York NY 10036-7802
(212) 819-9770
http://www.siecus.org

Sexually Transmissible Diseases

*AIDS Clinical Trials Information
Service (ACTIS)*
(800) 874-2572 (English,
Spanish)
http://www.actis.org

CDC National HIV/AIDS Hotline
(800) 342-2437
(800) 344-7432 (Spanish)
(800) 243-7889 (TDD)
http://www.thebody.com/cdc/hiv
    news/hivnews10.html

*CDC National Sexually
Transmitted Disease Hotline*
PO Box 13827
Research Triangle Park NC
(800) 227-8922
(800) 344-7432 (Spanish)
(800) 243-7889 (TDD)
http://www.thebody.com/cdc/hiv
    news/hivnews10.html

*Centers for Disease Control and
Prevention*
HIV/AIDS educational resources
(800) 458-5231
http://www.thebody.com/cdc/cdc
    page.html

Skin Diseases

Skin Cancer Foundation
(212) 725-5176
(800) 754-6490 (SKIN-490)
info@skincancer.org (e-mail)
http://www.skincancer.org

Sleep Disorders

National Sleep Foundation
(202) 347-3471
natsleep@erols.com (e-mail)
http://www.sleepfoundation.org

*The American Sleep Disorders
Association*
1610 14th Street, NW, Suite 300
Rochester MN 55901
(507) 287-6006
http://www.asda.org

Smoking Cessation

*National Center for Health
Promotion*
Smoke Stoppers Program
3920 Varsity Drive
Ann Arbor MI 48108
(313) 971-6077
http://www.welltech.com/nchp/
    welcome.htm

Support Groups

Well Spouse Foundation
PO Box 801
New York NY 10023
(212) 644-1241
(800) 838-0879
http://www.healthy.net/pan/cso/
    cio:/wsf.htm

Victim Assistance

National Organization of Victim Assistance (NOVA)
(202) 232-6682
www.access.digex.net/~nova

Visiting Nurses

Visiting Nurses Association of America
11 Beacon Street
Suite 910
Boston MA 02128
(800) 426-2547
http://www.vnaa.org

Women's Health and Related Issues

Jacobs Institute for Women's Health
409 12th Street, SW
Washington DC 20024-2188
(202) 863-4990
http://www.jiwh.org

National Women's Health Network
1325 G Street, NW
Washington DC 20005
(202) 347-1140

The PMS and Menopause Self-Help Center
101 First Street, Suite 441
Los Angeles CA 94022
(415) 964-7268

INTERNET INFORMATION WEBSITES

In deference to those who prefer to go directly to the Internet, this list includes Websites listed under the previous section as well as additional resources. There are many other valuable Internet resources not listed here. We excluded entreprenurial sites, unless the information they provided was particularly helpful, Websites of organizations that charge for information, and sites that were not very informative or patient/consumer-friendly.

Acne/Eczema
http://freenet.uchsc.edu/2000/
    adolescent/acne.html

Addictions
http://www.addictions.org

Aging
http://www.aarp.org
http://www.alz.uci.edu
http://www.arclab.org

AIDS
http://www.thebody.com

Alcoholism
http://www.alcoholics-
    anomymous.org

Alzheimer's Disease
http://med-www.bu.edu/
    Alzheimer/home
http://www.alz.org
http://www.alzheimers.org

Arthritis
http://www.arthritis.org

Asthma and Allergies
http://www.aaaai.org
http://www.aafa.org
http://www.foodallergy.org

Biofeedback
http://www.aapb.org

Birth Control
http://gynpages.com/ultimate
http://www.arhp.org

Blindness Prevention
http://www.preventblindness.org

Botanicals
http://www.herbalgram.org

BrainTumors
http://www.abta.org

Breast Cancer
http://nysernet.org/bcic

www.feminist.org/other/bc/bcho
me
http://www.nabco.org
http://www.y-me.org

Cancer
http://cancer.med.upenn.edu
http://www.cancer.org
http://www.nci.nih.gov

Crohn's Disease and Colitis
http://www.ccfa.org

Deafness
http://deafworldweb.org/dww

Depression
www.execpc.com/~corbeau

Diabetes
http://niddk.nih.gov
http://www.diabetes.com
http://www.diabetes.org

Dieting and Weight Loss
http://www.cyberdiet.com

Domestic Violence
http://www.igc.apc.org/fund
http://www.inetport.com/~ndvh

Eating Disorders
http://www.members.aol.com/
edapine/facts.html
www.ndmda.org/eating

Epilepsy
http://www.efa.org

Eye Care and Disorders
http://www.aoanet.org
http://www.eyenet.org
http://www.glaucoma.org
http://www.nei.nih.gov

Gastroenterologic Diseases
(colon, esophagus, gallbladder, liver, pancreas, stomach)
http://www.gastro.org
http://www.niddk.nih.gov/health/
digest/digest.htm

Geriatrics
americangeriatrics.org/pated

Grief Counseling
http://www.jjt.com/~tcf_national

Headaches
http://www.achenet.org
http://www.headaches.org

Health Information Resources
http://healthnet.ivi.com
http://www.healthatoz.com
http://www.ama-assn.org
http://www/cdc.gov/nchswww
http://www.ebig.com
http://www.medicinenet.com
http://nhic-nt.health.org
http://www.who.org/home/
map_ht
http://192.217.234.202/iris/omoz
oj9w.htm

Hearing
http://www.hearingihs.org

Heart Disease
http://www.americanheart.org
http://www.amhrt.org

Home Care
http://www.nahc.org

Hospice Care
http://www.nho.org

Impotence
http://www.impotence.org

Infectious Diseases and Vaccinations
http://www.cdc.gov
www.cdc.gov/travel/travel.html

Infertility
http://www.asrm.com
http://www.ihr.com/infertility

Kidney Disease
www.access.digex.net/~afud
http://www.aerie.com/netahtml/
  nihdb/kudetail.html

Liver Disease
http://www.liverfoundation.org

Lung Disease
http://www.lungusa.org

Lupus
http://www.lupus.org/lupus

Lyme Disease
http://www.aldf.com

Massage Therapy
http://www.amtamassage.org

Medical Reference and Journal Access
www.cdc.gov/epo/mmwr/mmwr
www.invivo.net/bg/medline
http://www.nejm.org
http://www.nlm.nih.gov

Mental Health
http://www.cmhc.com
http://www.nmha.org
http://nimh.nih.gov

Minority Health
http://www.omhrc.gov

Multiple Sclerosis
http://www.msfacts.org
http://www.nmss.org

Muscular Dystrophy
http://www.mdausa.org

Myasthenia Gravis
http://www.med.unc.edu/mgfa

Natural Death
http://dspace.dial.pipex.com/com
  /town/square/aco26/ndcusa

Obsessive-Compulsive Disorders
http://www.centerpt.org/search/
  m50jkpwt.htm

Osteoporosis
http://www.nof.org

Pain Management
http://www.aapainmange.org/
   index.html

Panic/Anxiety Disorders
http://www.algy.com/anxiety/
   index.html
http://www.paems.com.au/abo
   ut/info.html

Paralysis
http://www.apacure.com

Parkinson's Disease
http://www.pdaparkinson.com

Pharmaceutical Information
http://pharminfo.com
http://www.fda.gov
http://www.rxlist.com

Prostate Cancer
http://www.comed.com/prostate

Rare Disorders
http://www.pcnet.com/~orphan

Rehabilitation
http://www.cais.net/naric

Sexual Function
http://www.afud.org/sfunctn.html
http://www.siecus.org

Sexually Transmissible Diseases
http://www.actis.org
http://www.thebody.com/cdc/hiv
   news/hivnews10.html

www.thebody.com/cdc/cdcpage

Skin Diseases
http://www.pinch.com/skin
http://www.skincancer.org

Sleep Disorders
http://www.asda.org
http://www.sleepnet.com

Smoking Addiction
http://www.con.ohio-
   state.edu/tobacco
http://www.lungusa.org/tobacco/
   index.html
http://www.welltech.com/nchp/
   welcome.htm

Spouse Support
http://www.healthy.net/pan/cso/
   cio:/wsf.htm

Stress
http://www.teachhealth.com

Stroke
http://www.stroke.org

Student Health
http://www.columbia.edu/cu/heal
   thwise/alice.html

Substance Abuse
http://www.acde.org
http://www.adhl.org/callus.html
http://www.health.org/resref.htm

Suicide Prevention
http://www.afsp.org

Thyroid Diseases
http://www.thyroid.org/patient/
    patient.htm

Veterans Affairs
http://www.va.gov/medical.htm

Victim Assistance
http://www.access.digex.net/~
    nova

Visiting Nurses
http://www.vnaa.org

Widowed Persons Service
www.aarp.org/griefprograms/
    wps
http://www.aarp.org/griefandloss
    /bereavementprog.html

Women's Health
http://www.jiwh.org
http://www.yahoo.com/health/
    women_s_health
http://www.papsmear.org

NATIONAL NURSE PRACTITIONER ORGANIZATIONS

This list includes only organizations with primarily nurse practitioner membership. Nurse Practitioners also belong to many other national nursing organizations.

American Academy of Nurse Practitioners (AANP)
Capitol Station, LBJ Building
P.O. Box 12846
Austin, TX 78711
(512) 442-4262
(512) 442-6469 (Fax)
Email: admin@aanp.org
http://www.aanp.org

American College of Nurse Practitioners (ACNP)
503 Capitol Ct. NE, #300
Washington, DC 20002
(202) 546-4825
(202) 546-4797 (Fax)
Email: acnp@nurse.org
http://www.nurse.org/acnp

American Nurses Association (ANA)/ Council of Advanced Practice Nurses
600 Maryland Avenue, SW, #100 West
Washington, DC 20024
(202) 651-7000
(202) 651-7001 (Fax)
(800) 274-4ANA
Email: see address listings under "contact us"
http://www.nursingworld.org

National Association of Nurse Practitioners in Reproductive Health (NANPRH)
1090 Vermont Avenue, NW, #800
Washington, DC 20005
(202) 408-7025
(202) 408-0902 (Fax)
Email: nanprh@nurse.org
http://www.nurse.org/nanprh

National Association of Pediatric Nurse Associates and Practitioners (NAPNAP)
1101 Kings Highway North, #206
Cherry Hill, NJ 08034-1912
(609) 667-1773
(609) 667-7187 (Fax)
Email: info@napnap.org
http://www.napnap.org

National Conference of
Gerontological
Nurse Practitioners
(NCGNP)
P.O. Box 270101
Fort Collins, CO 80527-0101
(970) 493-7793
(970) 416-0910 (Fax)
Email: ncgnp@frii.com
http://www.ncgnp.org

National Organizations of
Nurse Practitioners
Faculties (NONPF)
One Dupont Circle, NW, #530
Washington, DC 20036
(202) 452-1405
 (202) 452-1406 (fax)
Email: nonnpf@aacn.nche.edu
http://www.nonpf.com/home.htm

INDEX

TO ORDER

UNFORGETTABLE FACES:
Through the Eyes of a Nurse Practitioner

Visit Our Website at

http://www.unforgettablefaces.com

➤ Place Orders On-line

➤ Major Credit Cards and Purchase
Orders Accepted

➤ Academic Volume Discounts Available

➤ Autograph by First Author

Questions about Ordering?
E-mail: info@unforgettablefaces.com